Understanding Psychiatry

Understanding Psychiatry

Edited by **Harvey Wilson**

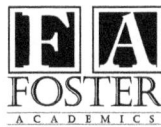

FA
FOSTER
ACADEMICS

New Jersey

Published by Foster Academics,
61 Van Reypen Street,
Jersey City, NJ 07306, USA
www.fosteracademics.com

Understanding Psychiatry
Edited by Harvey Wilson

International Standard Book Number: 978-1-63242-439-6 (Hardback)

Printed in the United States of America.

Contents

Preface

Every book is initially just a concept; it takes months of research and hard work to give it the final shape in which the readers receive it. In its early stages, this book also went through rigorous reviewing. The notable contributions made by experts from across the globe were first molded into patterned chapters and then arranged in a sensibly sequential manner to bring out the best results.

This book provides comprehensive insights into the field of Psychiatry. It elucidates new techniques and their applications in a multidisciplinary approach. Psychiatry is an extensive field of study related to the diagnosis and treatment of mental, emotional and behavioral disorders. It is an area of medical science which deals with all kinds of mental problems and works to provide mental well-being to every human. This book is an essential guide for readers who want a detailed analysis of this subject. It will serve as a valuable source of reference to graduate and post-graduate students. Case studies of various countries across the globe have also been discussed in this book, in order to provide it a global perspective.

It has been my immense pleasure to be a part of this project and to contribute my years of learning in such a meaningful form. I would like to take this opportunity to thank all the people who have been associated with the completion of this book at any step.

Editor

Broader Role for Antipsychotics in the Treatment of Obsessive Compulsive Disorder and Schizophrenia—A Malaysian Case Series

Benedict Francis[1], Stephen Thevananthan Jambunathan[1,2], Subash Kumar Pillai[1]

[1]Department of Psychiatry, University Malaya Medical Center, Kuala Lumpur, Malaysia
[2]The Mind Faculty, Solaris Mont Kiara, Kuala Lumpur, Malaysia
Email: ben.franciscan@gmail.com

Abstract

Obsessive compulsive disorder (OCD) and schizophrenia have been considered to be variants of the same disorder. At the advent of psychiatry, there was a distinction between neurotic, mood disorders and psychotic disorders. As perceptions and thoughts evolve in this dynamic field, there has been a paradigm shift in the way these disorders are being perceived. Of particular interest is that concerning OCD and schizophrenia. In a much anticipated and very welcomed move, DSM V has now included delusional beliefs as a specifier of OCD. However the much spoken about schizo-obsessive syndrome is yet to be explored and addressed. Recurrent and intrusive thoughts, impulses and images are key experiences seen in OCD. How we differentiate these vivid images from visual hallucination is a question yet to be answered. The following case series is an example of how difficult the boundaries between severe OCD and schizophrenia can be, and the promising usage of atypical antipsychotic in controlling obsessive compulsive symptoms. Whether untreated OCD is a significant prodromal symptom of schizophrenia, a subtype of schizophrenia or an initial indicator of various syndromes, remains to be seen, depending on environmental effects on the neuroplasticity of the mind and brain. The cases discussed will highlight the role of antipsychotics in patients diagnosed as having OCD, and gives strength to the idea that perhaps antipsychotics should be used more liberally in the treatment of OCD in schizophrenia. Here, we present a case series to show the use of atypical antipsychotics as monotherapy or augmenter in quelling obsessive-compulsive symptoms in patients who fulfilled the DSM V criteria for both schizophrenia and OCD. The efficacy of antipsychotics in reducing OCD symptoms in psychotic patients, as shown in this case series, contributes to the body of evidence that OCD and schizophrenia are really spectrum disorders with a common denominator. It is hoped that this exciting finding will lead to a

paradigm shift in the usage of antipsychotics in OCD and eventually change how this disease is viewed and treated.

Keywords

Antipsychotics, Obsessive Compulsive Disorder, Schizophrenia, Monotherapy

1. Introduction

It is interesting to decipher the link between OCD and schizophrenia. In earlier classifications, OCD was categorized under "anxiety disorder". However, reflecting a paradigm shift, DSM-V has reclassified OCD under "obsessive-compulsive and related disorder" [1]. It is controversial that the latest classification does not include a specifier for schizophrenia. It does, however, include a specifier for delusional belief. In these four cases, there is a link between the development of OCD and schizophrenia as all of our patients fulfilled the diagnostic criteria for both OCD and Schizophrenia.

The existence of the so called "schizo-obsessive" disorder has been postulated for the past decade or so but has never been properly classified [2] [3]. This is understandable as there is a difficulty in distinguishing OCD with poor insight and OCD with delusional belief, particularly that which may point towards a more holistic diagnosis of schizo-obsessive disorder [4]-[6]. Once the schizo-obsessive disorder is accepted as a clinical entity, this will create new vigour into definitive pharmacological treatment of this disorder and promote the possible usage of antipsychotics as a monotherapy agent and at the same time broaden the usage for antipsychotics in OCD for not only treatment resistant cases but regular cases. The early usage of antipsychotics in patients who fit into the diagnostic category of "schizo-obsessive" syndrome might lead to a decrease in OCD symptoms.

The objective of this case series is to demonstrate that earlier and broader usage of antipsychotics in patients with OCD and schizophrenia may be beneficial and this may in turn give strength to the idea that these two disorders are indeed of the same spectrum.

1.1. Case 1

A 25-year-old Chinese lady, with an underlying OCD diagnosed one year ago, required acute psychiatric treatment because of compulsive hand washing and refusal to talk for 3 days. She was referred for acute in-patient care from a psychiatrist because of suspected Serotonin Syndrome due to the high doses of serotonin enhancers. She was then on sertraline 150 mg, escitalopram 20 mg and fluvoxamine 100 mg. She was relatively well until 6 months before admission, when she had to defer her studies because of her worsening hand washing compulsion and behaviour. For the past two weeks, she had difficulty sleeping and had only been able to sleep at four in the morning. During this hospitalization, she talked very minimally and spent most of her time staring at the ceiling. There were sporadic episodes where she exhibited disorganized behaviour such as smiling inappropriately, talking to herself, grimacing and gesticulating. At times she jumped off her bed without reason. Besides that, she started ruminating before she ate. She believed that Satan was under her pillow after her father put Buddhist prayer chants under her pillow. She also heard a voice speaking to her. The voice "haunts" her, but did not give specific instructions. She was subsequently put on olanzapine 10 mg daily. All antidepressants were withheld. By the 1st week, her hand washing frequency, hallucinations and delusions improved. She had very poor insight and rationalized her behaviour and preferences as very practical practices. A week after she was discharged, she was back in medical school. However she had two isolated episodes of delusions of reference. The first episode was in a restaurant where she felt people were talking about her. The second episode was in the clinic when she began singing at the lobby and got violently upset when people smiled at her. In psychological rehabilitation, she now participates in all the activities and feels she is getting better. After one month of olanzapine 10 mg daily, her hallucinations, delusions and hand washing compulsions were gone. She continued to show improvement with only the antipsychotic. Her insight had improved significantly. Six months after first contact with us, she is now functioning in full remission with only olanzapine. Her insight is now very good and she remains highly motivated to complete her degree.

1.2. Case 2

A 36-year-old Chinese lady, diagnosed in the past as having schizophrenia was admitted in the psychiatric ward due to poor sleep for six months and excessive hand washing which started 2 years back, worsening over the past two months. In the past months, she stayed awake for thirty hours a day for most days in a week. For the past six months, she became increasingly suspicious of the people around her, particularly her parents, and had poor concentration. She felt that washing dishes is a sign of dislike towards her and sometimes walked softly so that people will not hear her coming. She also felt that everyone was talking about her or referring to her, and that everyone was able to read her mind. She was first diagnosed with schizophrenia ten years ago when she presented with negative symptoms, agitation and suicidal ideation. It started when she became depressed after she broke up with her first boyfriend. In the following years, she has been involved in a series of relationships, all of which failed. 10 years into her illness, she became obsessed with making bookmarks and made close to 4000 bookmarks, all of which are unsold. Around the same time, her excessive hand washing started. She was started on escitalopram. This compulsion to wash hands had worsened over the last six months prior to this admission. At times she spent up to five hours in the toilet washing her hands. During this current admission, she was noted to be very manipulative, guarded and suspicious. She was started on olanzapine and sertraline during this admission. She had poor insight and blamed her parents for her poor health. She attributed coarse skin of her hands to food allergy, though it was obvious that her skin problem was contact dermatitis from detergent usage. Risperidone 1 mg bd was added to her regime and it was noted that her hand washing decreased with the commencement of risperidone. She was eventually discharged reasonably well with intra-muscular paliperidone 100 mg 4 weekly and sertraline 200 mg od. Her OCD symptoms improved tremendously but her persecutory feelings towards her parents remain.

1.3. Case 3

A 15-year-old boy with an underlying OCD for 2 years was brought in by police escort because he refused to come out of his father's car for 10 days. He only left the car to use the toilet facilities at home. One week prior to admission he began to show disorganized behaviour such as demanding that his mother repeatedly turn the car engine on and off until he felt calm and insisted that his mother threw away the plastic bags that he had filled up with his urine. He was first seen by a psychiatrist at the age of 10 due to frequent washing of his hands, with each session lasting more than 30 minutes. He also spent as long as 3 hours in the bathroom bathing. Subsequently, he was diagnosed with OCD but treatment was not started then as he was young and symptoms were manageable. Currently, he does not have any delusion, hallucination or suicidal ideation. He comes from a small family of 3 siblings but has a poor relationship with his father. He described his father as being a very strict person and short tempered. During this admission, he was quiet and did not respond to questioning. He denied having any hallucinations or delusions but kept mostly to himself. The nurses however reported that he frequently appeared to be talking to somebody even when he was alone. Although he seemed to have psychosis, he never admitted to this experience. He was started on escitalopram 10 mg od and lorazepam 1 mg bd. Later on, risperidone 1 mg bd was added to his treatment regime as his symptoms were not resolving. The eventual addition of risperidone made a significant improvement in his symptoms, particularly the hand washing. The eventual diagnosis on discharge was OCD with the differential diagnosis of schizophrenia.

1.4. Case 4

A 25-year-old man, with a known case of schizophrenia for the past 4 years, was admitted to the psychiatric ward because of aggressiveness towards his parents. He had hit his mother and father on the head several times. He said that he felt a compulsion to behave in this way because he was angry towards them. His mental illness first started at the age of 20 when he was initially diagnosed as having recurrent and intrusive impulses to hit people. His reason was that he had to hit them before they harmed him. A diagnosis of schizophrenia was eventually made and he was started on intramuscular paliperidone, olanzapine and lorazepam. He began seeking opinions from numerous psychiatrists all of whom agreed that he had OCD as well. He was then prescribed clomipramine 100 mg daily, sertraline 10 mg daily, olanzapine 5 mg daily and 1mg of lorazepam for sleep. Over the last one year he developed the delusions of reference and persecution. In fact, during this admission, he had begun to have delusions of persecution as he felt his college mates were calling him extremely derogatory and rude names. He continued to feel the urge to hit anyone near him before they hit him. He is currently on olanzapine 5 mg od, sertraline 150 mg od, clonazepam 1 mg on, perphenazine 4 mg bd and asenapine 10 mg bd. His obsessive symptoms reduced when the olanzapine was increased to 10 mg daily. Currently, in a psychological rehabilitation centre, he continues to show improvement with strict behavioural modification.

2. Discussion

OCD has been reported to be a common co-morbidity in schizophrenia which adversely affects patient outcomes. Regardless of the cause-effect factor, both these conditions seem to co-exist with each other at some point or the other. In a related study, the investigators set out to determine the rate of OCD in patients with first-episode schizophrenia. They found that 14% of 50 Schizophrenic patients screened met the diagnostic criteria for OCD. They also went on to conclude that OCD is relatively frequent in patients with first-episode schizophrenia and may have a protective effect on some schizophrenic symptoms [7]. Another study involving 50 adolescent patients with either schizophrenia or schizoaffective disorder showed that 26% of them met DSM IV criteria for OCD [8]. Byerly, M., et al. assessed one hundred schizophrenic or schizoaffective patients and found that nearly one third of them exhibited clinically significant obsessive-compulsive symptoms. They also found that the obsessive-compulsive symptoms began concurrently with or after the onset of the psychotic disorder [9]. Faragian, S., et al. analysed 133 patients who met DSM-IV criteria for both schizophrenic disorder and OCD. They found that in 48% of patients, obsessive compulsive symptoms (OCS) preceded the first psychotic symptoms and only 27% had OCS post psychotic symptoms. In 24% of the patients, both OCS and psychosis occurred simultaneously [10].

Recognizing the presence of psychotic symptoms in OCD patients and vice versa alters treatment options, especially when it comes to augmenting medication. In all of the cases above, antipsychotics were used together with Selective Serotonin Reuptake Inhibitors (SSRIs), resulting in positive results in reduction of OCD symptoms. In fact, antipsychotics are one of the most common augmenters used in treatment of OCD, as illustrated by a study done in 2014. In this study, 361 participants reported taking medication; 77.6% were taking a selective serotonin reuptake inhibitor; 50% reported use of at least one augmentation strategy. Antipsychotics were most often prescribed as augmenters (30.3%), followed by benzodiazepines (24.9%) and antidepressants (21.9%) [11]. Amongst the antipsychotics, risperidone seems to be more efficacious to treatment resistant OCD, as illustrated by McDougle, C.J., et al. In their study, 36 patients who were refractory to SSRI were given a course of risperidone for 6 weeks. They found that risperidone addition was superior to placebo in reducing OCD (P < 0.001), depressive (P < 0.001), and anxiety (P = 0.003) symptoms in the subjects [12]. The patient in case 3 responded well when risperidone was added to his treatment regime. Currently, antipsychotics are used as augmenters in treatment resistant OCD. However, these case series illustrate that when antipsychotics are started earlier on in the treatment regime, patients respond in a more rapid fashion.

However, the question remains whether antipsychotics can be used effectively as monotherapy for the treatment of OCD. Several older case studies have shown improvement in OCD symptoms with antipsychotic use alone. The antipsychotics used in these studies were chlorpromazine, loxapine and haloperidol [13]. These treatment modalities are grossly outdated. A quick search in an online database revealed little recent publication to support the notion that antipsychotic can be used as a monotherapeutic agent. Of note was a study done by Bystritsky et al. They showed that olanzapine was significantly superior to placebo in treatment refractory OCD who were unresponsive to SSRIs [14]. McDougle et al., however, suggested that antipsychotic monotherapy is not useful in the management of treatment resistant OCD [15].

Perhaps the key to understanding the role of antipsychotics in OCD patients is to decipher how Clozapine, an atypical antipsychotic induces obsessive compulsive symptoms in its users. De Haan et al. noted that more Clozapine treated subjects compared to non-Clozapine treated subjects develop obsessions [16]. Some, such as Poyurovsky et al. noted that up to 70% of schizophrenics treated with atypical antipsychotics such as clozapine, olanzapine or risperidone develop secondary obsessive compulsive symptoms (OCS) [17]. There have been more than a few hypotheses to explain this phenomenon. A dysregulation of serotonergic pathways have been attributed to this. Antiserotonergic antagonism at the 5-HT1C, 5-HT2A and 5HT2C receptors induces obsessive compulsive symptoms [18]. Specific genetic properties may also dispose schizophrenic patients to develop secondary OCS during treatment with atypical antipsychotics. For example, one polymorphism has been located in a particular gene (SLC1A1) that encodes the neuronal glutamate transporter, which has been associated with a genetic risk for OCD [19]. This altered glutamate neurotransmission contributes to obsessive compulsive symptoms in patients, as suggested by Cai, J., *et al.* In their study, they concluded that polymorphisms in the genes that control glutamate transmission, SLC1A1, GRIN2B, and GRIK2, contribute towards clozapine induced OCD [20]. Since deficient serotonin function is important in the pathophysiology of OCD, the dopaminergic and serotonergic regulatory effect exhibited by atypical antipsychotics could explain why it is effective in treatment-resistant OCD.

3. Conclusion

In conclusion, there is still much work to be done in comprehensively defining the relationship between OCD and schizophrenia. If OCD and schizophrenia are indeed a variant of the same disease, it paves the way for broader usage of antipsychotics in the treatment of OCD in schizophrenia. It will also facilitate fresh pharmacological research into development of new antipsychotics that could be used as monotherapy for OCD. Finally, these case studies and the associated references of this article suggest evidence that the schizo-obsessive disorder may be a syndrome that needs to be recognized.

Acknowledgements

Thanks to the Department of Psychiatry, University Malaya Medical Center, for their support in the development of this case series.

References

[1]   American Psychiatric Association (2013) Diagnostic and Statistical Manual of Mental Disorders. 5th Edition.

[2]   Hwang, M.Y. and Hollander, E. (1993) Schizo-Obsessive Disorders. *Psychiatric Annals*, **23**, 396-401. http://dx.doi.org/10.3928/0048-5713-19930701-11

[3]   Zohar, J. (1997) Is There Room for a New Diagnostic Subtype: The Schizo-Obsessive Subtype? *CNS Spectrums*, **2**, 49-50.

[4]   Solyom, L., DiNicola, V.F., Phil, M., Sookman, D. and Luchins, D. (1985) Is There an Obsessive Psychosis? Aetiological and Prognostic Factors of an Atypical Form of Obsessive-Compulsive Neurosis. *Canadian Journal of Psychiatry*, **30**, 372-380.

[5]   Insel, R.T. and Akiskal, H.S. (1986) Obsessive-Compulsive Disorder with Psychotic Features: A Phenomenologic Analysis. *American Journal of Psychiatry*, **143**, 1527-1533.

[6]   Bottas, A., Cooke, R.G. and Richter, M.A. (2005) Comorbidity and Pathophysiology of Obsessive-Compulsive Disorder in Schizophrenia: Is There Evidence for a Schizo-Obsessive Subtype of Schizophrenia? *Journal of Psychiatry Neuroscience*, **30**, 187-193.

[7]   Poyurovsky, M., Fuchs, C. and Weizman, A. (1999) Obsessive-Compulsive Disorder in Patients with First-Episode Schizophrenia. *American Journal of Psychiatry*, **156**, 1998-2000.

[8]   Nechmad, A., Ratzoni, G., Poyurovsky, M., Meged, S., Avidan, G., Fuchs, C., *et al.* (2003) Obsessive-Compulsive Disorder in Adolescent Schizophrenia Patients. *American Journal of Psychiatry*, **160**, 1002-1004.

[9]   Byerly, M., Goodman, W., Acholonu, W., Bugno, R. and Rush, A.J. (2005) Obsessive Compulsive Symptoms in Schizophrenia: Frequency and Clinical Features. *Schizophrenia Research*, **76**, 309-316.

[10] Faragian, S., Fuchs, C., Pashinian, A., Weizman, R., Weizman, A. and Poyurovsky, M. (2012) Age-of-Onset of Schizophrenic and Obsessive-Compulsive Symptoms in Patients with Schizo-Obsessive Disorder. *Psychiatry Research*, **197**, 19-22. http://dx.doi.org/10.1016/j.psychres.2012.02.024

[11] Van Ameringen, M., Simpson, W., Patterson, B., Dell'Osso, B., Fineberg, N., Hollander, E., *et al.* (2014) Pharmacological Treatment Strategies in Obsessive Compulsive Disorder: A Cross-Sectional View in Nine International OCD Centers. *Journal of Psychopharmacology*, **28**, 596-602.

[12] McDougle, C.J., Epperson, C.N., Pelton, G.H., Wasylink, S. and Price, L.H. (2000) A Double-Blind, Placebo-Controlled Study of Risperidone Addition in Serotonin Reuptake Inhibitor-Refractory Obsessive-Compulsive Disorder. *Archives of General Psychiatry*, **57**, 794-801.

[13] Fineberg, N.A., Gale, T.M. and Sivakumaran, T. (2007) A Review of Antipsychotics in the Treatment of Obsessive Compulsive Disorder. *FOCUS*, **5**, 354-360.

[14] Bystritsky, A., Ackerman, D.L., Rosen, R., Vapnik, T., Gorbis, E., Maidment, K.M., *et al.* (2004) Augmentation of SSRI Response in Refractory Obsessive-Compulsive Disorder Using Adjunctive Olanzapine: A Placebo-Controlled

Trial. *The Journal of Clinical Psychiatry*, **65**, 565-568. http://dx.doi.org/10.4088/JCP.v65n0418

[15] McDougle, C.J., Barr, L.C., Goodman, W.K., Pelton, G.H., Aronson, S.C., Anand, A., *et al.* (1995) Lack of Efficacy of Clozapine Monotherapy in Refractory Obsessive-Compulsive Disorder. *American Journal of Psychiatry*, **152**, 1812-1814.

[16] de Haan, L., Linszen, D. and Gorsira, R. (1999) Clozapine and Obsessions in Patients with Recent-Onset Schizophrenia and Other Psychotic Disorders. *The Journal of Clinical Psychiatry*, **60**, 364-365.

[17] Poyurovsky, M., Weizman, A. and Weizman, R. (2004) Obsessive-Compulsive Disorder in Schizophrenia: Clinical Characteristics and Treatment. *CNS Drugs*, **18**, 989-1010. http://dx.doi.org/10.2165/00023210-200418140-00004

[18] Meltzer, H.Y. and Huang, M. (2008) *In Vivo* Actions of Atypical Antipsychotic Drug on Serotonergic and Dopaminergic Systems. *Progress in Brain Research*, **172**, 77-97. http://dx.doi.org/10.1016/S0079-6123(08)00909-6

[19] Dickel, D.E., Veenstra-Vander, W.J., Cox, N.J., Wu, X., Fischer, D.J., Etten-Lee, V.M., *et al.* (2006) Association Testing of the Positional and Functional Candidate Gene SLC1A1/EAAC1 in Early-Onset Obsessive-Compulsive Disorder. *Archives of General Psychiatry*, **63**, 778-785. http://dx.doi.org/10.1001/archpsyc.63.7.778

[20] Cai, J., Zhang, W., Yi, Z., Lu, W., Wu, Z., Chen, J., *et al.* (2013) Influence of Polymorphisms in Genes SLC1A1, GRIN2B and GRIK2 on Clozapine-Induced Obsessive-Compulsive Symptoms. *Psychopharmacology*, **230**, 49-55.

Health Care Students' Attitudes towards People with Schizophrenia— A Survey of Eight University Training Programs

Bengt Svensson[1], David Brunt[2], Ulrika Bejerholm[1], Mona Eklund[1],
Amanda Lundvik Gyllensten[1], Christel Leufstadius[1], Urban Markström[3],
Mikael Sandlund[4], Margareta Östman[5], Lars Hansson[1]

[1]Department of Health Sciences, Lund University, Lund, Sweden
[2]School of Health Sciences and Social Work, Linnean University, Växjö, Sweden
[3]Department of Social Work, Umeå University, Umeå, Sweden
[4]Department of Clinical Sciences/Psychiatry, Umeå University, Umeå, Sweden
[5]Faculty of Health and Society, Malmö University, Malmö, Sweden
Email: bengt.svensson@med.lu.se

Abstract

Background: Discrimination and stigmatization of people with mental illness are a global and complex phenomenon and there is evidence that negative attitudes and discrimination are also prevalent among health care staff and health care students. Methods: Attitudes towards people with schizophrenia among 1101 students in eight different university programs providing training for work in the health care and social sectors were explored, using a cross-sectional design. Results: In five of the eight training programs the majority of the students' perceived people with schizophrenia as a danger to others. In several aspects police students were found to hold more negative attitudes than students from other programs. Students with previous experiences of work in mental health services and students knowing a person with schizophrenia showed more positive attitudes. Discussion: In order to decrease negative attitudes and prejudices towards people with schizophrenia among students, it is essential that the training includes personal contact with people with experience of being mental illness.

Keywords

Attitudes, Stigma, Schizophrenia, Students

1. Introduction

Discrimination and stigmatization of people with mental illness are a global and complex phenomenon linked to problems of knowledge, attitudes and behaviour [1]. Negative attitudes, stereotypes and discrimination are still highly prevalent in the population [2]. In fact there is evidence that public attitudes have not changed during the last two decades, or even turned worse in the case of people with schizophrenia [3]. Stigma and discrimination in many ways affect people with a mental illness causing a lowered self-esteem and quality of life [4], and affecting possibilities of adequate housing, work and financial situation in a negative way [5] [6]. Stigma is also a major barrier to help seeking [7] and cause delays, dropout and non-adherence in treatment [8] [9]. Recurrent studies during the last decades in the general population have further shown that people with mental illness are perceived as strange, frightening, unpredictable, aggressive and lacking self-control. Particularly people with schizophrenia are associated with negative stereotypes [10]-[12]. In repeated studies schizophrenia has been identified as the most stigmatizing condition among all types of mental illness [13] [14], closely linked to perceptions of fear, violence and being unpredictable.

Although stigmatizing attitudes is prominent among the general population it could be expected that professionals within the health care system would have a more knowledge-based, reflected and realistic view of persons with mental health problems. However, there is evidence that people with mental illness feel patronised, humiliated and punished in contact with services and that patients point out mental health staff as one of the groups which are the most stigmatizing [1]. Studies on mental health staff's attitudes have mainly focused on the prevalence of stereotypes and desire for social distance from people with mental illness. A review of studies focusing attitudes of mental health staff revealed that a majority of these studies constituted comparisons between staff and the general population [15]. One of the main findings from this review is that a majority of the studies show that beliefs of mental health providers do not differ from the general population or are more negative. This is in contradiction with a hypothesis that professionals' knowledge of mental illness and regular contact with people with a mental illness would result in more favourable attitudes. However it seems that this does not act as a protective factor when it comes to the prevalence of stereotypes regarding people with a mental illness or a greater willingness to interact with these people [16] [17]. A Swedish study not included in this review showed that attitudes towards mental illness and people with mental illness among nursing staff in psychiatric and somatic health care were similar [18]. Related studies from somatic health care also illustrate the phenomenon of diagnostic overshadowing. Persons with mental health problems report experiences of being treated with disrespect, being ignored, and being subjected to the suspicion that their physical complaints may be related to their mental illness [19]-[21].

Students' attitudes toward schizophrenia have only been scarcely studied, although a few studies have been presented. A study in Germany with focus on teenagers in secondary and grammar school showed that only a few students actually endorsed negative views about people with schizophrenia [22]. Another study of teenager's attitudes however presented quite high percentages of students who had stigmatizing attitudes and a desire for social distance [23]. In a study comparing stigmatization of schizophrenia as perceived by nurses, medical doctors, medical students and patients it was found that medical students reported the highest level of stigmatizing attitudes including assumptions of dangerousness, unpredictability and a desire for social distance [24]. On the other hand Linden and Kavanagh [25] did not find any significant differences, when comparing attitudes toward persons with schizophrenia, between registered mental health nurses and mental health nurse students. A study of pharmacy students revealed that a large majority of the participants would be unwilling to share a flat with a person with a diagnosis of schizophrenia ask such a person to be baby sitter. In the same study a majority also believed that people with schizophrenia are unpredictable and dangerous [26]. The results of studies of student's attitudes are so far inconclusive and performed in different cultural contexts that might be of importance. In the context of the negative attitudes from different groups in society towards persons with mental illness, it is important to investigate and to understand the attitudes held by those university students, who are preparing for work in the health care and adjacent fields, and who will bring these attitudes into their chosen profession. No theories have to our knowledge been presented concerning the differences in attitudes and intentional behaviour between student groups and an explorative study might shed more light on this field.

2. Aims

The aim of the present study was to investigate attitudes towards people with schizophrenia among students in eight different university programs providing training for work in the health care and social sectors.

Further research questions were: do attitudes towards people with schizophrenia differ with regard to type of university program, the students' sex, age, living conditions, familiarity with mental illness or past experience of work in the mental health sector? Our hypothesis was that students having a familiarity with people with schizophrenia would show more positive attitudes.

3. Methods and Subjects

This study is part of a research project aiming at investigating attitudes towards mental illness among different categories of university students. A sample of students in training for a broad range of health professions, not yet in the part of their training that focused on psychiatry and mental illness was aimed for. Thus, universities with training programs for nurses, occupational therapists, physiotherapists, physicians, psychologists, public health workers and social workers were approached. The selection of student categories was based on the strategic reasoning that these form the vast majority of professional categories working with health care and support for people with mental illnesses. Furthermore, since we aimed at participation also from other professions in regular contact with people with mental illness, training programs for police officers were approached as well. Universities from all over Sweden were approached and asked for participation, and strategic sampling was used in order to obtain heterogeneity. The principles utilized in the sampling process were also those of age and size of the university and their geographical distribution in the country. Six universities were initially selected, four agreed to participate and two declined due to bad timing. A further two universities were approached and both were willing to participate, and by these measures the variations in the sample needed was reached. This study complied with stipulations in the Swedish Act Ethical Review of Research Involving Humans (SFS, 2003), and informed consent was applied.

3.1. Procedure

The procedure for selection of subjects was the same at all universities. A member of the research team made contact with a teacher working with the targeted student group. The teacher asked for the students' informed consent and explained that participation was voluntary. The teacher scheduled the data collection, which was timed to occur prior to but close to a course that focused on mental illness in each programme or a more comprehensive course where mental illness formed a part. The contact teacher distributed the instrument to the students at the beginning of an ordinary lecture. The instruments were completed immediately and the responses were placed in a box, which was subsequently collected or sent to the research team. Information about the exact number of dropouts is uncertain due to the procedure used. Comparisons of the number of students enrolled for the courses with the number of participating students showed, however, that the number of dropouts was fairly low.

3.2. Measures

Level of familiarity with people with mental illness was elicited by using a slightly modified version of the Level of Familiarity Questionnaire [27]. The questionnaire contains 11 statements about familiarity with mental illness. Answer on each statement is yes or no. If more than one statement is affirmative, the highest level of familiarity is used for ranking. The highest rank is 11 = high familiarity with a person with mental illness, 7 = medium familiarity, 1 = little familiarity.

In order to investigate opinions about persons with schizophrenia, a Swedish version of the Attitudes to Persons with Mental Illness questionnaire was used [10]. In the first part of the questionnaire questions about familiarity with specific mental illness are requested. The following part of the questionnaire elicits attitudes towards seven different mental illnesses: severe depression, panic attacks, schizophrenia, dementia, eating disorders, alcohol addiction and drug addiction. For each mental illness eight statements are included where the respondent can choose to answer on a five-point scale including extreme statements, for example "1 = not dangerous to others, 5 = dangerous to others". A high rating always indicate a more stigmatizing attitude A study of the psychometric properties of the Swedish version revealed dubious test-retest reliability for some of the disorders and attitudes items [28]. Thus, in this study, only attitudes towards schizophrenia were analyzed and the statements regarding "unpredictable" and "difficult to talk with" were excluded. If the students marked one of the two answer alternatives on the negative side of the five-point scale they were regarded as having a "negative attitude".

In addition information about sociodemographic characteristics was obtained.

3.3. Statistics

Pearson product-moment correlation was used to investigate associations between variables.

Student's t-test was used to analyze relationships of attitudes to socio-demographic variables where the variable had two categories (e.g. sex). One-way analysis of variance with Scheffe's *post-hoc* test was used to test for differences in attitudes between students in different educational programs. The statistical software package used was SPSS 20.0 for Windows. The Alpha level was set to <0.05.

4. Results

Table 1 shows the number of participants in the study, divided in type of training programs and sociodemographic characteristics. A majority of students were female (75%) and the three most common student groups were social worker, nurse and police students comprising 68% of the participants. A minority (35%) had experiences of previous work with people with mental illness and the length of work experience in mental health services varied greatly (1 month - 20 years).

Attitudes among students in different education programs showed that irrespective of program a great majority of the student's perceived people with schizophrenia as unusual (**Table 2**). In five of eight education programs a majority of the students perceived people with schizophrenia as a danger to others, and with regard to prospects of recovery more than a third of the students in seven of eight education programs were pessimistic about the possibilities to recover from schizophrenia. Differences between the educational programs were few. Police students were more negative than nurse students, social work students, occupational therapist students and physiotherapist students in three of the items and physiotherapist students had more negative attitudes than

Table 1. Sociodemographic characteristics of the sample (n = 1101).

Variable	n (%)
Sex (n = 1100)	
Male	269 (24.5)
Female	831 (75.4)
Age md (range) (n = 1096)	25 (19 - 53)
Civil status (n = 1090)	
Married/cohabiting	571 (52.4)
Alone	518 (47.6)
Student groups	
Nurse students	210 (19.1)
Police students	203 (18.4)
Social work students	342 (31.1)
Occupational therapist students	95 (8.6)
Physiotherapist students	81 (7.4)
Physician students	78 (7.1)
Psychologist students	62 (5.6)
Public health students	30 (2.7)
Familiarity md (range) (n = 961)	7 (0 - 11)
Experiences of previous work in mental health services (n = 1088)	
Yes	376 (34.6)
No	711 (65.4)
Length of work in mental health services (*months*) md (range)	8.0 (1 - 239)

nursing students and social work students concerning the aspect of "pulling themselves together" (**Table 3**).

The influence of sociodemographic factors on attitudes to persons with schizophrenia revealed that a larger percentage of male students (n = 269) stated that persons with schizophrenia have themselves to blame for their disorder (1.5 ± 0.8 vs. 1.3 ± 0.6; p = 0.001) while female students (n = 831) to a higher degree perceived persons with schizophrenia as "unusual" (4.4 ± 1.0 vs 4.1 ± 1.2; p = 0.001). Younger students had to a higher degree the perception that persons with schizophrenia have themselves to blame for their disorder r = −0.06 (p = 0.05) and that they are unpredictable r = −0.17 (p = 0.01).

A larger proportion of students living alone perceived persons with schizophrenia as more unpredictable than students who were married or cohabiting (4.3 ± 0.7 vs 4.1 ± 0.8; p = 0.005) and students with experience of work in mental health services (n = 377) perceived persons with schizophrenia as less dangerous (3.5 ± 1.1 vs 3.6 ± 0.9; p = 0.01) than students with no such experience (n = 710).

Students who claimed that they knew a person with schizophrenia (n = 131) perceived persons with the disorder as less dangerous (3.3 ± 1.1 vs 3.6 ± 0.9; p = 0.003), and were more optimistic about improvement if treated (1.8 ± 0.9 vs 2.1 ± 0.9; p = 0.003). When comparing this group with those who had work experience of mental health no significant differences were found.

5. Discussion

Negative attitudes and prejudices towards people suffering from mental illness is an important obstacle for inclusion and participation on equal conditions into the society. In the present study we asked students, whose future occupation would be in the social and health care fields about how they perceived people suffering from schizophrenia, being as they are part of one of the most exposed subgroups of people with mental illness. The rather large sample representing eight different university programs with a nation wide coverage must be considered as a fairly representative sample. That the sample also consisted of mostly female participants is also a strength since the distribution of sex reflects the labour situation with regard to the student's future professions.

Table 2. Attitudes to people with schizophrenia among students divided in different education program (n = 1101) (%)[*].

Student groups	Danger to others	Themselves to blame	Not improved if treated	Perceived as unusual	Pulling themselves together	Never recover
Nurse students	42	1	5	54	2	30
Police students	69	2	9	75	2	34
Social work students	55	1	11	76	4	40
Occupational therapist students	50	1	6	84	6	33
Physiotherapist students	54	3	1	77	6	26
Physician students	46	1	4	90	5	42
Psychologist students	44	1	10	86	1	55
Public health students	60	1	20	70	13	47

[*]If the students marked one of the two answer alternatives on the negative side of the five-point scale they were regarded as having a "negative attitude".

Table 3. Significant differences in attitudes between students in the different programs (n = 1101). The numbers in the cells indicate which item the difference concern. See text below the table.

Student group	Nurse students	Social work students	Occupational therapist students	Physiotherapist students
Police students	2[**]	2[**]	1[*]	3[*]
Physiotherapist students	5[**]	5[**]	n.s	-

1. Danger to others; 2. Themselves to blame; 3. Not improved if treated; 4. Perceived as unusual; 5. Pulling themselves together; 6. Never recover. One-way Anova, [*]p < 0.05, [**]p < 0.01, [***]p < 0.001. Programs in left column (police students and physiotherapy students) showing more negative attitudes.

In five of the eight education programs the majority of the students perceived people with schizophrenia as a danger to others, and with regard to prospects of recovery more than a third of the students in seven of the eight education programs were pessimistic about prospects of recovery from this disorder. These results present a picture of a rather negative apprehension of people suffering from schizophrenia, but at the same time they are in accordance with the findings in studies by Björkman *et al*. [18] and Crisp *et al*. [10] who found negative perceptions about persons with schizophrenia among nursing staff and the general population, respectively.

With regard to variations between the education programs, police students in several aspects seem to hold more negative attitudes than students from other training programs. A plausible interpretation may be that police students to a greater extent during their university education are trained in handling difficult situations where security has a higher priority, rather than training how to treat persons with schizophrenia. Studies among police officers about attitudes towards people suffering form mental illness partly support these findings. Watson *et al*. [29] found that a label associated with schizophrenia increased perceived dangerousness among police officers. However, studies among police officers are rare and it is not evident that police officers hold more negative attitudes towards people with mental illness than the general population [30].

Our hypothesis that greater familiarity with people with schizophrenia will contribute to less negative attitudes was confirmed. Students with experience of past work in mental health service and students knowing a person with schizophrenia showed less negative attitudes compared to those without such work experience or such personal knowledge. This finding is in line with earlier studies which found that personal contact with people suffering from mental illness contribute to less negative attitudes [27] [31]. This could be made through cooperation with consumer organizations. To invite consumers to give lectures or to participate in discussion groups could easily be included in course curriculums.

6. Conclusion

In summary, attitudes among students towards people with schizophrenia are in several instances comparable with attitudes as presented by the general population. In order to decrease negative attitudes and prejudices towards people with schizophrenia among students it is essential that the training includes personal contact with people with experiences of being mentally ill.

Acknowledgements

The study was financially supported by the Swedish Council for Working Life and Social Research.

References

[1]   Thornicroft, G., Rosem D. and Kassam, A. (2007) Discrimination in Health Care against People with Mental Illness. *International Review of Psychiatry*, **19**, 113-122. http://dx.doi.org/10.1080/09540260701278937

[2]   Angermeyer, M.C. and Dietrich, S. (2006) Public Beliefs about and Attitudes towards People with Mental Illness: A Review of Population Studies. *Acta Psychiatrica Scandinavica*, **113**, 163-179. http://dx.doi.org/10.1111/j.1600-0447.2005.00699.x

[3]   Schomerus, G., Schwahn, C., Holzinger, A., Corrigan, P.W., Grabe, H.J., Carta, M.G. and Angermeyer, M.C. (2012) Evolution of Public Attitudes about Mental Illness: A Systematic Review and Meta-Analysis. *Acta Psychiatrica Scandinavica*, **125**, 440-452. http://dx.doi.org/10.1111/j.1600-0447.2012.01826.x

[4]   Livingston, J.D. and Boyd, J.E. (2010) Correlates and Consequences of Internalized Stigma for People Living with Mental Illness: A Systematic Review and Meta-Analysis. *Social Science & Medicine*, **71**, 2150-2161. http://dx.doi.org/10.1016/j.socscimed.2010.09.030

[5]   Rüsch, N., Angermeyer, M.C. and Corrigan, P. (2005) Mental Illness Stigma. Concepts, Consequences and Initiatives to Reduce Stigma. *European Psychiatry*, **20**, 529-539. http://dx.doi.org/10.1016/j.eurpsy.2005.04.004

[6]   Sharac, J., McCrone, P., Clement, S. and Thornicroft, G. (2010) The Economic Impact of Mental Health Stigma and Discrimination: A Systematic Review. *Epidemiologia e Psichiatria Sociale*, **19**, 223-232. http://dx.doi.org/10.1017/S1121189X00001159

[7]   Gulliver, A., Griffiths, KM. and Christensen, H. (2010) Perceived Barriers and Facilitators to Mental Health Help-Seeking in Young People: A Systematic Review. *BMC Psychiatry*, **10**, 113. http://dx.doi.org/10.1186/1471-244X-10-113

[8]   Andrews, G., Henderson, S. and Hall, W. (2001) Prevalence, Co-Morbidity, Disability and Service Utilisation. Over-

view of the Australian National Mental Health Survey. *British Journal of Psychiatry*, **178**, 145-153. http://dx.doi.org/10.1192/bjp.178.2.145

[9] Sirey, J.A., Bruce, M.L., Alexopoulus, G.S., Perlick, D.A., Raue, P., Friedmann, S.J. and Meyers, B.S. (2001) Perceived Stigma as a Predictor of Treatment Discontinuation in Young and Older Outpatients with Depression. *American Journal of Psychiatry*, **158**, 479-481. http://dx.doi.org/10.1176/appi.ajp.158.3.479

[10] Crisp, A.H., Gelder, A.G., Rix, S., Meltzer, H.I. and Rowlands, O.J. (2000). Stigmatisation of People with Mental Illnesses. *British Journal of Psychiatry*, **177**, 4-7. http://dx.doi.org/10.1192/bjp.177.1.4

[11] Link, A.G., Phelan, J.C., Bresnahan, M., Stueve, A. and Pescosolido, B. (1999) Public Conceptions of Mental Illness: Labels, Causes, Dangerousness and Social Distance. *American Journal of Public Health*, **89**, 1328-1333. http://dx.doi.org/10.2105/AJPH.89.9.1328

[12] Phelan, J.C. and Link, B.G. (1998) The Growing Belief That People with Mental Illnesses Are Violent: The Role of the Dangerousness Criterion for Civil Commitment. *Social Psychiatry and Psychiatric Epidemiology*, **33**, 7-12. http://dx.doi.org/10.1007/s001270050204

[13] Dickerson, F.B., Sommerville, J., Origoni, A.E., Ringel, N.B. and Parente, F. (2002) Experiences of Stigma among Outpatients with Schizophrenia. *Schizophrenia Bulletin*, **28**, 143-155. http://dx.doi.org/10.1093/oxfordjournals.schbul.a006917

[14] Mann, C.E. and Himelien, M.J. (2004) Factors Associated with Stigmatization of Persons with Mental Illness. *Psychiatric Services*, **55**, 185-187. http://dx.doi.org/10.1176/appi.ps.55.2.185

[15] Schulze, B. (2007) Stigma and Mental Health Professionals: A Review of the Evidence on an Intricate Relationship. *International Review of Psychiatry*, **19**, 137-155. http://dx.doi.org/10.1080/09540260701278929

[16] Lauber, C., Nordt, C., Braunschweig, C. and Rössler, W. (2006) Do Mental Health Professionals Stigmatize Their Patients? *Acta Psychiatrica Scandinavica*, **113**, 51-59. http://dx.doi.org/10.1111/j.1600-0447.2005.00718.x

[17] Nordt, C., Rössler, W. and Lauber, C. (2006) Attitudes of Mental Health Professionals towards People with Schizophrenia and Major Depression. *Schizophrenia Bulletin*, **32**, 709-714. http://dx.doi.org/10.1093/schbul/sbj065

[18] Björkman, T., Angelman, T. and Jönsson, M. (2008) Attitudes towards People with Mental Illness: A Cross-Sectional Study among Nursing Staff in Psychiatric Care and Somatic Care. *Scandinavian Journal of Caring Sciences*, **22**, 170-177. http://dx.doi.org/10.1111/j.1471-6712.2007.00509.x

[19] Brinn, F. (2000) Patients with Mental Illness: General Nurses' Attitudes and Expectations. *Nursing Standard*, **14**, 32-36. http://dx.doi.org/10.7748/ns2000.03.14.27.32.c2792

[20] Liggins, J. and Hatcher, S. (2005) Stigma toward the Mentally Ill in the General Hospital: A Qualitative Study. *General Hospital Psychiatry*, **27**, 359-364. http://dx.doi.org/10.1016/j.genhosppsych.2005.05.006

[21] Schulze, B. and Angermeyer, M.C. (2003) Subjective Experiences of Stigma. A Focus Group Study of Schizophrenic Patients, Their Relatives and Mental Professionals. *Social Science & Medicine*, **56**, 299-321. http://dx.doi.org/10.1016/S0277-9536(02)00028-X

[22] Schulze, B., Richter-Werling, M., Matschinger, H. and Angermeyer, M.C. (2003) Crazy? So What! Effects of a School Project on Students' Attitudes towards People with Schizophrenia. *Acta Psychiatrica Scandinavica*, **107**, 142-150. http://dx.doi.org/10.1034/j.1600-0447.2003.02444.x

[23] Economou, M., Louki, E., Peppou, L.E., Gramandani, C., Yotis, L. and Stefanis, C.N. (2012) Fighting Psychiatric Stigma in the Classroom: The Impact of an Educational Intervention on Secondary School Students' Attitudes to Schizophrenia. *International Journal of Social Psychiatry*, **58**, 544-551. http://dx.doi.org/10.1177/0020764011413678

[24] Serafini, G., Pompili, M., Haghighat, R., Pucci, D., Pastina, M., Lester, D., Angeletti, G., Tatarelli, R. and Girardi, P. (2011) Stigmatization of Schizophrenia as Perceived by Nurses, Medical Doctors, Medical Students and Patients. *Journal of Psychiatric and Mental Health Nursing*, **18**, 576-585. http://dx.doi.org/10.1111/j.1365-2850.2011.01706.x

[25] Linden, M. and Kavanagh, R. (2012) Attitudes of Qualified vs. Student Mental Health Nurses towards an Individual Diagnosed with Schizophrenia. *Journal of Advanced Nursing*, **68**, 1359-1368. http://dx.doi.org/10.1111/j.1365-2648.2011.05848.x

[26] Volmer, D., Mäesalu, M. and Bell, J.S. (2008) Pharmacy Students' Attitudes toward and Professional Interactions with People with Mental Disorders. *International Journal of Social Psychiatry*, **54**, 402-413. http://dx.doi.org/10.1177/0020764008090427

[27] Corrigan, P.W., Green, A., Lundin, R., Kubiak, M.A. and Penn, D.L. (2001) Familiarity with and Social Distance from People Who Have Serious Mental Illness. *Psychiatric Services*, **52**, 953-958. http://dx.doi.org/10.1176/appi.ps.52.7.953

[28] Svensson, B., Markström, U., Bejerholm, U., Björkman, T., Brunt, D., Eklund, M., Hansson, L., Leufstadius, C., Gyllensten, A.L., Sandlund, M. and Östman, M. (2011) Test-Retest Reliability of the Swedish Version of Two Instruments for Measuring Public Attitudes towards Persons with Mental Illness. *BMC Psychiatry*, **11**, 11.

http://dx.doi.org/10.1186/1471-244X-11-11

[29] Watson, A.C., Corrigan, P.W. and Ottati, V. (2004) Police Officers' Attitudes toward and Decisions about Persons with Mental Illness. *Psychiatric Services*, **55**, 49-53. http://dx.doi.org/10.1176/appi.ps.55.1.49

[30] Cotton, D. (2004) The Attitudes of Canadian Police Officers toward the Mentally Ill. *International Journal of Law and Psychiatry*, **27**, 135-146. http://dx.doi.org/10.1016/j.ijlp.2004.01.004

[31] Corrigan, P.W., Edwards, A.B., Green, A., Diwan S.L. and Penn D.L. (2001) Prejudice, Social Distance and Familiarity with Mental Illness. *Schizophrenia Bulletin*, **27**, 219-225. http://dx.doi.org/10.1093/oxfordjournals.schbul.a006868

3

Attention-Deficit/Hyperactivity Disorder in Adults with High-Functioning Pervasive Developmental Disorders in Japan

Yasuko Takanashi[1], Hirobumi Mashiko[1,2], Hirohide Yokokawa[3,4], Yoko Kawasaki[5],
Shuntaro Itagaki[1], Hiromichi Ishikawa[1], Norihiro Miyashita[1,6], Yasuaki Hayashi[7],
Asako Kudo[8], Kentaro Oga[9], Rieko Matsuura[10], Shin-Ichi Niwa[1*]

[1]Department of Neuropsychiatry, Fukushima Medical University School of Medicine, Fukushima, Japan
[2]Fukushima General Health and Welfare Center, Fukushima, Japan
[3]Department of Public Health, Fukushima Medical University School of Medicine, Fukushima, Japan
[4]Department of General Medicine, Juntendo University School of Medicine, Tokyo, Japan
[5]Musasino Child Development Clinic, Tokyo, Japan
[6]Hanawakousei Hospital, Fukushima, Japan
[7]Landic Nihonbashi Clinic, Tokyo, Japan
[8]Hoshigaoka Hospital, Fukushima, Japan
[9]Surugadai Nihon University Hospital, Tokyo, Japan
[10]Shiba Clinic, Tokyo, Japan
Email: *si-niwa@fmu.ac.jp

Abstract

Aims: This study was designed to verify the proportion of Japanese adults with pervasive developmental disorder (PDD) who met the diagnostic criteria (other than E) for attention-deficit/hyperactivity disorder (ADHD) in the Diagnostic and Statistical Manual of Mental Disorders, Fourth Edition, Text Revision (DSM-IV-TR). Furthermore, we examined to what extent adults with PDD think that they exhibit ADHD symptoms. Methods: We developed an original Japanese self-report questionnaire to determine the presence or absence of 18 symptoms from the diagnostic criteria for ADHD in the DSM-IV-TR. We administered the questionnaire to 64 adults with high-functioning PDD (45 men and 19 women) and 21 adults with ADHD (10 men and 11 women), aged 18 to 59 years, with a full-scale intelligence quotient ≥75. Target patients were evaluated for ADHD by their psychiatrists. Results: Twenty-nine (45.3%) adults with PDD also had ADHD. The percentage of these adults who had over six perceived inattention symptoms from the DSM-IV-TR was 96.6%. The percentage of these adults who had over six perceived hyperactivity-impulsivity symptoms

---

*Corresponding author.

was 65.5%. Thirty-five (55.6%) adults with PDD responded that they were aware of having ADHD symptoms at the level of the relevant diagnostic criteria. **Conclusions:** The present study is the first to examine the frequency of objective and perceived ADHD symptoms in adults with PDD in Japan. Our results show that both objective and perceived ADHD symptoms frequently appear in a large number of adults with PDD. This suggests that it is necessary to attend to concomitant ADHD symptoms in the medical care of adults with PDD.

Keywords

Adults, Attention-Deficit/Hyperactivity Disorder (ADHD), High-Functioning, Pervasive Developmental Disorders (PDD), Self-Report

---

1. Introduction

The essential feature of attention-deficit/hyperactivity disorder (ADHD) is a persistent pattern of inattention and/ or hyperactivity-impulsivity that interferes with functioning or development [1]. Pervasive developmental disorders (PDD) are characterized by severe and pervasive impairment in several areas of development: reciprocal social interaction skills, communication skills, or the presence of stereotyped behavior, interests, and activities [2]. In 2013, the Diagnostic and Statistical Manual of Mental Disorders, Fourth Edition, Text Revision (DSM-IV-TR) [2] was revised to the Diagnostic and Statistical Manual of Mental Disorders, Fifth Edition (DSM-5) [1]. Due to this revision, the general terminology for autism, PDD not otherwise specified, childhood disintegrative disorder, and Asperger's disorder, all of which were included under the classification for PDD in the DSM-IV-TR [2], was changed to Autism Spectrum Disorder (ASD) in the DSM-5. Moreover, the revision recognizing the comorbidity of PDD and ADHD in the DSM-5, which was not recognized in the DSM-IV-TR, is another significant difference between the two versions of the DSM. The concurrence of PDD and ADHD has been commonly recognized in clinical settings, especially within the field of pediatrics [3]-[6]. Among the youths with PDD, 40% - 78% [3]-[6] experience ADHD symptoms to a degree that meets the DSM-IV criteria for ADHD, a markedly higher rate than the 3% - 7% [2] prevalence of ADHD among school-age children.

It is widely known that PDD is a persistent disorder that can extend beyond childhood [7]. However, only Sweden has examined adults with PDD, reporting that 37% - 43% of adults with PDD also have ADHD symptoms [7]-[10].

To date, ADHD has been recognized as a childhood disorder that improves over time. However, research in some countries shows that in 49% - 66% of individuals, some symptoms persist until adulthood [11]. Furthermore, a large epidemiologic survey of adults in 10 countries (not including Japan) conducted between 2001 and 2003 showed that the prevalence of adult ADHD was 3.4% [12]. Thus, ADHD is emerging as an important disorder in adults.

Few reports have estimated the prevalence of ADHD or PDD in adults in Japan; however, based on our clinical experiences, a relatively high prevalence of PDD with ADHD symptoms is expected. At the same time, we feel that a considerable number of adults with PDD complain about ADHD symptoms, such as those who visit a clinic with the main complaint of ADHD symptoms.

It is necessary to prepare a comprehensive and effective treatment plan for symptoms related to both PDD and ADHD [4] [13], and to treat the symptoms of inattention and hyperactivity individually, as required [14]. Since studies have reported that drugs used for ADHD have therapeutic efficacy in children with PDD with ADHD symptoms [15]-[19], it is meaningful to examine ADHD symptoms in individuals with PDD to develop an appropriate therapeutic strategy.

Now that the DSM has been revised to recognize the concurrence between ADHD and ASD (including what was previously referred to as PDD) even in the diagnostic criteria, there is a need to examine the concurrence between ADHD and ASD further in a wide range of subjects, including children and adults.

In this study, we aimed to estimate the proportion of Japanese adults with PDD who met the diagnostic criteria for ADHD except for criterion E in the DSM-IV-TR. Furthermore, we examined to what extent adults with PDD think that they exhibit ADHD symptoms. Since this study began before the DSM-IV-TR was revised to the

DSM-5, all of the diagnoses made within this study adhered to the DSM-IV-TR.

2. Methods

2.1. Subjects

We asked psychiatrists, including those in charge of an outpatient clinic specializing in developmental disorders at the Department of Neuropsychiatry, Fukushima Medical University Hospital, and those working at seven affiliated institutions that were familiar with the medical and psychiatric care of developmental disorders, to help gather data for this study. Eleven psychiatrists working in the eight institutions provided informed consent and conducted this study. Psychiatrists included in this study had a median of 16 years of experience in the clinical practice of psychiatry (range, 6 - 37 years). The study period was from June 2007 to March 2008. Study subjects were individuals attending outpatient clinics in the Department of Neuropsychiatry at Fukushima Medical University Hospital, or at the seven institutions that were affiliated with the cooperating psychiatrists.

We chose subjects who met the following inclusion criteria: 1) met the diagnostic criteria for PDD or ADHD in the DSM-IV-TR [2], 2) age of 18 to 60 years, and 3) Full Scale Intelligence Quotient (FIQ) $\geq$ 75. As mentioned previously, the subjects for this study were limited to patients whose diagnoses were affirmed by obtaining sufficient objective information (*i.e.*, maternity health record book and report cards) and subjective information concerning their childhood (*i.e.*, information provided by one or both parents).

The exclusion criteria were as follows: 1) regular medication treatment for chronic physical disease, 2) under treatment for bipolar disorder, 3) under treatment for schizophrenia, and 4) pregnant or lactating. Inclusion criteria 2 and 3 were included to raise the validity of subjects' self-evaluations. Consecutive individuals who met the inclusion criteria and who did not meet the exclusion criteria during the study period (June 2007 to March 2008) were asked to participate, and informed consent was obtained from those who agreed.

2.2. Questionnaire

We developed a self-report questionnaire to determine the presence or absence of 18 symptoms listed from (a) to (i) in criterion A (1), and from (a) to (i) in criterion A (2) of the diagnostic criteria for ADHD in the DSM-IV-TR [2]. The questionnaire was devised so that responses would be "yes" if the symptom was perceived to be present and "no" if the symptom was perceived to be absent (see **Table 1**). In addition, the questionnaire asked subjects for their sex, age, and occupation. Answers of "yes" were scored as 1 and "no" answers were scored as 0. The total score from the nine questions concerning symptoms in criterion A (1) in the DSM-IV-TR [2] served as the total score for inattention, and the total score from the nine questions related to criterion A (2) served as the total score for hyperactivity-impulsivity. In addition, an overall score was determined for all 18 questions.

2.3. Procedure

The questionnaire, explanatory documents, an envelope to return the completed questionnaire, and a ballpoint pen were distributed to subjects via their psychiatrists. We asked subjects to return their sealed envelope with the completed questionnaires to their psychiatrists. The attending psychiatrists provided basic information about the diagnosis, the results of the intelligence test, age at diagnosis of ADHD or PDD, and information regarding the medical care of the subject. We asked the attending psychiatrists to classify the subjects with ADHD based on four sub-classifications: combined type, predominantly inattentive type, predominantly hyperactive-impulsive type, and in partial remission (psychiatrists' classification). If the subject was diagnosed with PDD, we asked the attending psychiatrist whether the subject satisfied the diagnostic criteria for ADHD in the DSM-IV-TR except for criterion E, and if the subject met the criteria, we then asked the psychiatrist to classify that subject using the same four ADHD sub-classifications. Based on the intelligence test, the psychiatrists provided the subjects' verbal IQ (VIQ), performance IQ (PIQ), and FIQ.

In this study, we divided subjects into three groups as per the psychiatrists' judgments regarding the presence of ADHD symptoms: ADHD, PDD with ADHD, and PDD without ADHD. In addition, for the subsequent data analysis, we categorized the subjects with PDD, as observed by the attending psychiatrists, as "inattention PDD subjects" if they fulfilled the diagnostic criteria for inattention, and as "hyperactivity-impulsivity PDD subjects" if they fulfilled the diagnostic criteria for hyperactivity-impulsivity. Moreover, based on subjects' responses to the questionnaire in this study, we categorized subjects with a total inattention score of $\geq$6 or a total hyperac-

Table 1. Details of the 18 questions prepared based o the diagnostic criteria for ADHD in the DSM-IV-TR.

1) Nine questions about inattention:

   1   Do people often tell you that you "make many careless mistakes" in schoolwork, work, or other activities?

   2   Do you often have difficulty sustaining attention at work or in play activities?

   3   Do you often fail to hear someone speaking to you directly?

   4   Do you often fail to accomplish tasks because you missed the instructions?

   5   Do you often have difficulty organizing tasks and activities?

   6   Are you particularly weak at tasks that require sustained mental effort?

   7   Do you often lose things necessary for tasks or activities?

   8   Are you easily distracted?

   9   Do you often forget your plans or appointments?

2) Nine questions about hyperactivity-impulsivity:

   1   Do you often fidget with your hands or feet or squirm in your seat?

   2   Do you often leave your seat in situations in which you are expected to remain seated?

   3   Do you often feel very restless?

   4   Are you often unable to play or engage in leisure activities quietly?

   5   Do you often spend too much time bustling about?

   6   Do people often tell you that you "talk a lot"?

   7   Do you often blurt out answers before questions have been completed?

   8   Do you often have difficulty waiting for your turn?

   9   Do you find yourself butting into conversations or games at times?

Abbreviations: ADHD, attention-deficit/hyperactivity disorder; DSM-IV-TR, Diagnostic and Statistical Manual of Mental Disorders, Fourth Edition, Text Revision.

tivity-impulsivity score of ≥ 6 as "perceived ADHD subjects" (see **Figure 1**).

2.4. Analysis

For inter-group comparisons of the number of subjects, the chi-square test was conducted, and for inter-group comparisons of age at diagnosis, age at completing the questionnaire, the respective scores, and the respective IQs, t-tests were used for comparing the groups. Analyses were conducted using the Statistical Package for the Social Sciences (SPSS 16.0, SPSS Inc., Chicago, IL), and the level of significance was set at $P < 0.05$.

3. Results

One hundred and five subjects recruited from the eight institutions completed the questionnaire. Among the 105 respondents, 20 were excluded from analysis (one whose age was inappropriate, three with an FIQ < 75, ten whose intelligence test results were unknown, and others who lacked a diagnosis of ADHD by the attending psychiatrist). Thus, 85 subjects (81%) were included in the final analysis. Of these, 37 did not take medication, while 48 were undergoing medication treatment. Prescribed medicines, in the order of highest to lowest usage frequency, were sodium valproate, fluvoxamine maleate, and methylphenidate hydrochloride. Among the eligible subjects, 64 had PDD (45 men and 19 women), and 21 had ADHD (10 men and 11 women). Among the 64 subjects with PDD, 13 had autistic disorder (9 men and 4 women), 38 had Asperger's disorder (30 men and 8 women), and 13 had PDD not otherwise specified (6 men and 7 women). Among the 21 subjects with ADHD, 8 (4 men and 4 women) had the combined type, 9 (4 men and 5 women) had the predominantly inattentive type, and 4 (2 men and 2 women) were in partial remission. None of the subjects had the predominantly hyperactive-impulsive type ADHD. The response rate to each question was high (97.6% to 100%), indicating that all of the questions were appropriate.

3.1. Subject Characteristics

Subject characteristics are shown in **Table 2**. Overall, for men, the number of subjects with PDD was signifi-

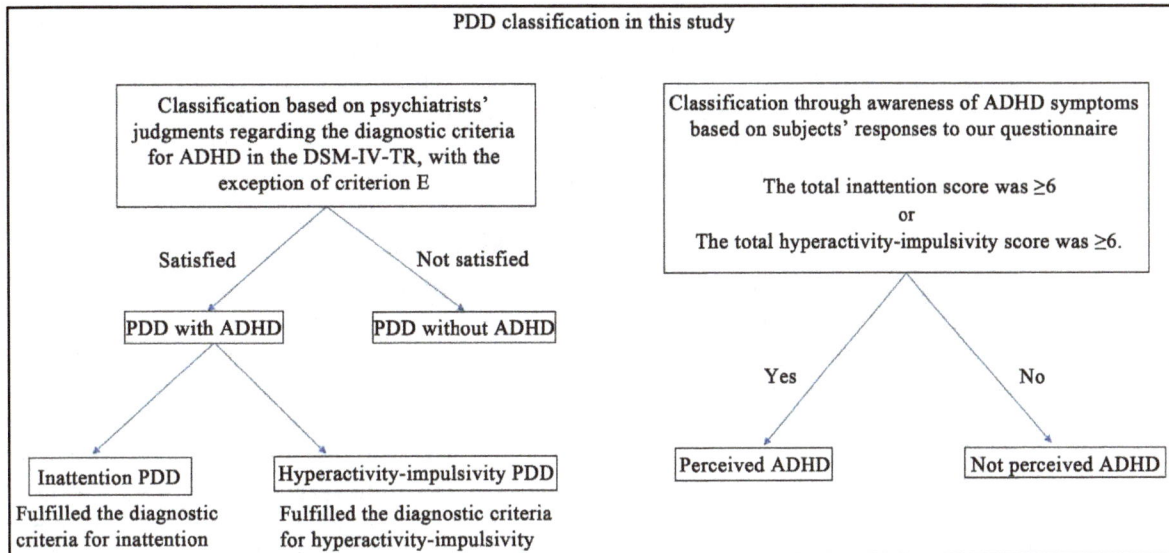

Figure 1. PDD classification in this study.

Table 2. Subject characteristics.

Variable		ADHD		PDD	P^c
	n	n (%) or M (SD)	n	n (%) or M (SD)	
Number of subjects		21 (100)		64 (100)	**
Male		10 (47.6)		45 (70.3)	**
Female		11 (52.4)		19 (29.7)	ns
Age at diagnosis[a]	21	32.76 (9.74)	64	17.91 (14.39)	**
Male	10	28.60 (10.35)	45	15.09 (13.70)	**
Female	11	36.55 (7.75)	19	24.58 (14.14)	*
Age at answering[b]	21	36.29 (9.49)	64	27.53 (8.46)	**
Male	10	31.50 (9.12)	45	26.27 (8.19)	ns
Female	11	40.64 (7.85)	19	30.53 (8.53)	**
Verbal IQ	20	99.15 (10.35)	60	102.20 (14.61)	ns
Male	10	96.90 (12.29)	42	103.33 (15.19)	ns
Female	10	101.40 (8.00)	18	99.56 (13.18)	ns
Performance IQ	20	96.70 (14.10)	60	98.38 (15.56)	ns
Male	10	90.70 (17.88)	42	98.62 (16.15)	ns
Female	10	102.70 (4.45)	18	97.83 (14.51)	ns
Full scale IQ	21	98.29 (11.82)	64	100.73 (13.29)	ns
Male	10	92.30 (12.46)	45	102.04 (13.21)	*
Female	11	103.73 (8.45)	19	97.63 (13.31)	ns

Notes: *$P < 0.05$, **$P < 0.01$. [a]Age at diagnosis of ADHD in the ADHD group and at diagnosis of PDD in the PDD group; [b]Age at answering the self-report questionnaire; [c]Chi-square test for "Number of subjects" or t-test for other items. Abbreviations: ADHD, attention-deficit/hyperactivity disorder; PDD, pervasive developmental disorder; M, mean; SD, standard deviation; ns, not significant; IQ, intelligence quotient.

cantly greater than that of subjects with ADHD ($\chi^2\{1, 85\} = 21.75$, $P < 0.01$). Overall, for men and women, the age at diagnosis was significantly higher in subjects with PDD than in subjects with ADHD (men: $t\{53\} = 2.93$, $P < 0.01$, women: $t\{28\} = 2.58$, $P < 0.05$). Overall, for women, subjects with ADHD were significantly older than subjects with PDD were ($t\{28\} = 3.22$, $P < 0.01$). The mean FIQ of subjects with PDD was 100.7 (range, 76 - 127), while the mean FIQ of subjects with ADHD was 98.3 (range, 75 - 120). For men, the FIQ scores were significantly higher in subjects with PDD than in subjects with ADHD ($t\{53\} = 2.13$, $P < 0.05$).

3.2. Diagnosis of ADHD and Perceived ADHD Symptoms

We calculated the ratio of subjects with PDD with ADHD and that of subjects with perceived ADHD among those with PDD in order to elucidate the exact frequencies or proportions of subjects who exhibited ADHD characteristics among subjects with PDD. Among the 64 subjects with PDD, 29 had PDD with ADHD (45.3% in all, 46.7% in men, and 42.1% in women) and 35 had PDD without ADHD (see **Table 3**).

In **Table 3**, we show the proportions of subjects with perceived ADHD in PDD. As shown in the table, 55.6% of subjects with PDD (52.3% of men, 63.2% of women) responded that they were aware of having ADHD symptoms at the level of the ADHD diagnostic criteria. In other words, our results suggest that a high percentage of subjects with PDD think they have ADHD. Note that while calculating the percentages, we excluded one subject who did not answer several of the questions related to inattention and hyperactivity-impulsivity in our questionnaire.

Among the 29 subjects with PDD with ADHD, 28 had inattention (96.6% in all, 95.2% in men, and 100% in women) and 19 had hyperactivity-impulsivity (65.5% in all, 71.4% in men, and 50.0% in women; see **Table 4**). Moreover, while it is not shown in the table, in terms of the psychiatrists' classifications of ADHD in subjects with PDD with ADHD, 18 (14 men and 4 women) had the combined type, 10 (6 men and 4 women) had the predominantly inattentive type, 1 (man) had the predominantly hyperactive-impulsive type, and none were in partial remission.

Table 3. The ratio of subjects with PDD and ADHD and the ratio of subjects with perceived ADHD among those with PDD.

	PDD with ADHD[a]	Perceived ADHD[b]
PDD		
Total (n = 64)	29/64 (45.3)[c]	35/63 (55.6)[d]
Male (n = 45)	21/45 (46.7)[c]	23/44 (52.3)[d]
Female (n = 19)	8/19 (42.1)[c]	12/19 (63.2)[d]

Notes: [a]Subjects diagnosed with ADHD using the DSM-IV-TR except for criterion E; [b]Subjects whose total score for inattention was ≥6 or whose score for hyperactivity-impulsivity was ≥6; [c]The proportion of subjects with a diagnosis of "PDD with ADHD" was calculated based on the total number of subjects in each group; [d]The proportion of subjects with "perceived ADHD" was calculated based on the number of subjects showing valid answers to the target questions. Abbreviations: PDD, pervasive developmental disorder; ADHD, attention-deficit/hyperactivity disorder; DSM-IV-TR, Diagnostic and Statistical Manual of Mental Disorders, Fourth Edition, Text Revision.

Table 4. The ratios of "inattentive PDD subjects" and "hyperactivity-impulsivity PDD subjects" among subjects with PDD and ADHD.

	Inattention PDD[a]	Hyperactivity-impulsivity PDD[b]
PDD with ADHD[c]		
Total (n = 29)	28 (96.6)[d]	19 (65.5)[d]
Male (n = 21)	20 (95.2)[d]	15 (71.4)[d]
Female (n = 8)	8 (100.0)[d]	4 (50.0)[d]

Notes: [a]Patients diagnosed as inattentive by psychiatrists. (Patients with predominantly inattentive type or combined type); [b]Patients diagnosed as hyperactive-impulsive subjects by psychiatrists. (Patients with predominantly hyperactive-impulsive type or combined type); [c]Patients who satisfied the diagnostic criteria for ADHD in the DSM-IV-TR except for criterion E; [d]The proportion of subjects was calculated based on the total number of subjects in each group. Abbreviations: PDD, pervasive developmental disorder; ADHD, attention-deficit/hyperactivity disorder; DSM-IV-TR, Diagnostic and Statistical Manual of Mental Disorders, Fourth Edition, Text Revision.

4. Discussion

The present study is the first to evaluate the frequency and characteristics of ADHD in Japanese adults with PDD. The results showed that PDD with ADHD is present in a high proportion of adults with high-functioning PDD. There are only a few reports that have investigated ADHD in adults with PDD [7]-[10], and they were all conducted in Sweden. Stahlberg, Soderstrom [10] investigated the prevalence of comorbid bipolar and psychotic disorder in adults with ADHD and/or autism spectrum disorders (ASD). They reported that out of 129 subjects with ASD, 14.8% had comorbid bipolar disorder with psychotic features, schizophrenia, or other psychotic disorders, and 38% had comorbid ADHD. Rydén and Bejerot [9] showed that out of 84 subjects with ASD, 37% had ADHD. Hofvander, Delorme [7] reported that 43% of subjects with ASD showed comorbid ADHD.

The proportion of adults with PDD with ADHD in our study was similar to or lower than the incidence of comorbid ADHD in children with PDD [3]-[6], but was similar to or slightly higher than the incidence of comorbid ADHD in Swedish adults with PDD [7]-[9]. The prevalence of PDD with ADHD (45.3%) in our study was remarkably higher than that for adult ADHD (3.4%) [12]. Our data suggest the need to examine the presence or absence of concomitant ADHD, not only in children, but also in adults with PDD.

Moreover, in terms of the presence of inattention or hyperactivity-impulsivity, inattention is more common in subjects with ADHD and subjects with PDD. In the present study, the proportion of subjects categorized as "inattention PDD subjects" in the PDD with ADHD group was 96.6%, replicating the high rates reported in the previously mentioned studies with adults (84.6% [7], 74.5% [8], ≥82% [9], and 75.5% [10]). In Japan, a study on children with PDD with ADHD by Yoshida and Uchiyama [6] reported that 88.9% of subjects with PDD with ADHD were diagnosed as having inattention, similar to the extent of inattention diagnosed in the aforementioned studies [7]-[10] of adults with PDD with ADHD. These findings suggest a high rate of inattention in children and adults with PDD.

Here, we found that the rate of subjects categorized as "hyperactivity-impulsivity PDD subjects" in the PDD with ADHD group was 65.5%; previous studies with adults have reported rates of 59.6% [7], 46.8% [8], and 46.9% [10]. Yoshida and Uchiyama [6] observed hyperactivity-impulsivity in 53.8% of subjects with PDD with ADHD ≤ 10 years old, but this figure decreased to 20% in subjects ≥ 11 years old. Although the rates of inattention exceed those of hyperactivity-impulsivity in adults with PDD with ADHD in both the present and previous studies [7] [8] [10], the rate of hyperactivity-impulsivity is considerable.

Implication of the Results in Terms of the Diagnostic Revisions in DSM-5

The present paper investigated ADHD symptoms in adults with PDD. As mentioned previously, PDD and ADHD comorbidity is not recognized in the DSM-IV-TR diagnostic criteria for ADHD; however, the DSM-5 does recognize this comorbidity [1]. The present study also showed that there are many cases of PDD with ADHD. Thus, the revision recognizing this comorbidity is considered very meaningful. In addition, for the diagnosis of ADHD under the DSM-IV-TR, patients were required to satisfy at least six of the nine criteria for inattention, or at least six of the nine criteria for hyperactivity-impulsivity. However, the DSM-5 changed this so that only five of the criteria are required for individuals 17 years of age or older. Similarly, diagnostic criteria in the past required that symptoms be recognized before 7 years of age; the age limit has been raised to 12 years in the DSM-5. These revisions will increase the number of adults with ADHD who fit the definitive diagnosis, resulting in an increase in the number of individuals with PDD with ADHD. This expected increase is thought to accurately reflect the true number of individuals with ADHD.

5. Limitations

This study had several limitations. First, it included a small number of subjects, and sufficient analysis could only be performed in men with PDD, and not in the other groups. The prevalence of PDD was higher in men than in women, and the male/female ratios of PDD in children were reported to be 3.3:1 [20], 4.8:1 [21], and 3.4 - 6.5:1 [22]. To ensure that these findings clearly reflect the gender differences in these disorders, future studies need to include a sufficient number of both genders. Second, although the questionnaire had symptom-related questions that were based on the diagnostic criteria, the reliability and validity of the questionnaire were not verified. However, no questionnaire about adult ADHD is currently available in Japan, whereas the number of adults requiring medical care and treatment for ADHD symptoms is increasing rapidly. Thus, the 18 questions regarding ADHD symptoms, based on the diagnostic criteria, were developed for self-evaluation.

6. Conclusion

To our knowledge, the present study is the first to examine the comorbidity of PDD and ADHD in adults in Asia. It is also the first to examine the frequency of ADHD in adults with PDD in Japan, as well as examine the perceived ADHD symptoms in adults with PDD. Our results showed that PDD with ADHD exists in a large number of adults with PDD in Japan. This suggests that it may be necessary to attend to concomitant ADHD symptoms in the medical care of adults with PDD.

Acknowledgements

This study was conducted as part of a junior study funded by a science research grant from the Ministry of Education, Culture, Sports, Science, and Technology for the "Preparation of the checklist of behavioral characteristics of attention-deficit/hyperactivity disorder and Asperger's disorder in adults" (2006 to 2008), and as part of a study approved by the ethics committee of Fukushima Medical University (approved on September 3, 2007). The authors do not have any conflicts of interest to declare.

References

[1] American Psychiatric Association (2013) The Diagnostic and Statistical Manual of Mental Disorders: DSM 5. 5th Edition, American Psychiatric Association, Washington, DC. http://dx.doi.org/10.1176/appi.books.9780890425596.910646

[2] American Psychiatric Association (2000) Diagnostic and Statistical Manual of Mental Disorders. American Psychiatric Association, Washington, DC. http://dx.doi.org/10.1176/appi.books.9780890423349

[3] Gadow, K.D., DeVincent, C.J. and Pomeroy, J. (2006) ADHD Symptom Subtypes in Children with Pervasive Developmental Disorder. *Journal of Autism and Developmental Disorders*, **36**, 271-283. http://dx.doi.org/10.1007/s10803-005-0060-3

[4] Goldstein, S. and Schwebach, A.J. (2004) The Comorbidity of Pervasive Developmental Disorder and Attention Deficit Hyperactivity Disorder: Results of a Retrospective Chart Review. *Journal of Autism and Developmental Disorders*, **34**, 329-339. http://dx.doi.org/10.1023/B:JADD.0000029554.46570.68

[5] Lee, D.O. and Ousley, O.Y. (2006) Attention-Deficit Hyperactivity Disorder Symptoms in a Clinic Sample of Children and Adolescents with Pervasive Developmental Disorders. *Journal of Child and Adolescent Psychopharmacology*, **16**, 737-746. http://dx.doi.org/10.1089/cap.2006.16.737

[6] Yoshida, Y. and Uchiyama, T. (2004) The Clinical Necessity for Assessing Attention Deficit/Hyperactivity Disorder (AD/HD) Symptoms in Children with High-Functioning Pervasive Developmental Disorder (PDD). *European Child & Adolescent Psychiatry*, **13**, 307-314. http://dx.doi.org/10.1007/s00787-004-0391-1

[7] Hofvander, B., Delorme, R., Chaste, P., Nydén, A., Wentz, E., Ståhlberg, O., et al. (2009) Psychiatric and Psychosocial Problems in Adults with Normal-Intelligence Autism Spectrum Disorders. *BMC Psychiatry*, **9**, 35. http://dx.doi.org/10.1186/1471-244X-9-35

[8] Anckarsä, H., Stahlberg, O., Larson, T., Hakansson, C., Jutblad, S.-B., Niklasson, L., et al. (2006) The Impact of ADHD and Autism Spectrum Disorders on Temperament, Character, and Personality Development. *American Journal of Psychiatry*, **163**, 1239-1244. http://dx.doi.org/10.1176/appi.ajp.163.7.1239

[9] Rydén, E. and Bejerot, S. (2008) Autism Spectrum Disorders in an Adult Psychiatric Population. A Naturalistic Cross-Sectional Controlled Study. *Clinical Neuropsychiatry*, **5**, 13-21. http://www.clinicalneuropsychiatry.org/pdf/03_ryden.pdf

[10] Stahlberg, O., Soderstrom, H., Rastam, M. and Gillberg, C. (2004) Bipolar Disorder, Schizophrenia, and Other Psychotic Disorders in Adults with Childhood Onset AD/HD and/or Autism Spectrum Disorders. *Journal of Neural Transmission*, **111**, 891-902. http://dx.doi.org/10.1007/s00702-004-0115-1

[11] Barkley, R.A., Fischer, M., Smallish, L. and Fletcher, K. (2006) Young Adult Outcome of Hyperactive Children: Adaptive Functioning in Major Life Activities. *Journal of the American Academy of Child & Adolescent Psychiatry*, **45**, 192-202. http://dx.doi.org/10.1097/01.chi.0000189134.97436.e2

[12] Fayyad, J., De Graaf, R., Kessler, R., Alonso, J., Angermeyer, M., Demyttenaere, K., et al. (2007) Cross-National Prevalence and Correlates of Adult Attention-Deficit Hyperactivity Disorder. *British Journal of Psychiatry*, **190**, 402-409. http://dx.doi.org/10.1192/bjp.bp.106.034389

[13] Holtmann, M., Boelte, S. and Poustka, F. (2007) Attention Deficit Hyperactivity Disorder Symptoms in Pervasive Developmental Disorders: Association with Autistic Behavior Domains and Coexisting Psychopathology. *Psychopathology*, **40**, 172-177. http://dx.doi.org/10.1159/000100007

[14] Gillberg, C. (2002) A Guide to Asperger Syndrome. Cambridge University Press, Cambridge. http://dx.doi.org/10.1017/CBO9780511543814

[15] Di Martino, A., Melis, G., Cianchetti, C. and Zuddas, A. (2004) Methylphenidate for Pervasive Developmental Disorders: Safety and Efficacy of Acute Single Dose Test and Ongoing Therapy: An Open-Pilot Study. *Journal of Child and Adolescent Psychopharmacology*, **14**, 207-218. http://dx.doi.org/10.1089/1044546041649011

[16] Posey, D.J., Aman, M.G., McCracken, J.T., Scahill, L., Tierney, E., Arnold, L.E., *et al.* (2007) Positive Effects of Methylphenidate on Inattention and Hyperactivity in Pervasive Developmental Disorders: An Analysis of Secondary Measures. *Biological Psychiatry*, **61**, 538-544. http://dx.doi.org/10.1016/j.biopsych.2006.09.028

[17] Posey, D.J., Wiegand, R.E., Wilkerson, J., Maynard, M., Stigler, K.A. and McDougle, C.J. (2006) Open-Label Atomoxetine for Attention-Deficit/Hyperactivity Disorder Symptoms Associated with High-Functioning Pervasive Developmental Disorders. *Journal of Child and Adolescent Psychopharmacology*, **16**, 599-610. http://dx.doi.org/10.1089/cap.2006.16.599

[18] Research Units on Pediatric Psychopharmacology Autism Network (2005) Randomized, Controlled, Crossover Trial of Methylphenidate in Pervasive Developmental Disorders with Hyperactivity. *JAMA Psychiatry*, **62**, 1266-1274. http://dx.doi.org/10.1001/archpsyc.62.11.1266

[19] Troost, P.W., Steenhuis, M.P., Tuynman Qua, H.G., Kalverdijk, L.J., Buitelaar, J.K., Minderaa, R.B. and Hoekstra, P.J. (2006) Atomoxetine for Attention-Deficit/Hyperactivity Disorder Symptoms in Children with Pervasive Developmental Disorders: A Pilot Study. *Journal of Child and Adolescent Psychopharmacology*, **16**, 611-619. http://dx.doi.org/10.1089/cap.2006.16.611

[20] Baird, G., Simonoff, E., Pickles, A., Chandler, S., Loucas, T., Meldrum, D. and Charman, T. (2006) Prevalence of Disorders of the Autism Spectrum in a Population Cohort of Children in South Thames: The Special Needs and Autism Project (SNAP). *The Lancet*, **368**, 210-215. http://dx.doi.org/10.1016/S0140-6736(06)69041-7

[21] Fombonne, E., Zakarian, R., Bennett, A., Meng, L. and McLean-Heywood, D. (2006) Pervasive Developmental Disorders in Montreal, Quebec, Canada: Prevalence and Links with Immunizations. *Pediatrics*, **118**, e139-e150. http://dx.doi.org/10.1542/peds.2005-2993

[22] Centers for Disease Control and Prevention (2007) Prevalence of Autism Spectrum Disorders—Autism and Developmental Disabilities Monitoring Network, 14 Sites, United States, 2002. *Morbidity and Mortality Weekly Report*, **56**, 12-22. http://www.cdc.gov/mmwr/preview/mmwrhtml/ss5601a2.htm

4

Difficult-to-Treat-Depression and GPs' Role: Perceptions of Psychiatry Registrars

4

4

Kay M. Jones, Leon Piterman

Office of the Pro Vice-Chancellor, Peninsula Campus, Monash University, Frankston, Australia
Email: *kay.jones@monash.edu

Abstract

Introduction: For patients, GPs are the most accessible medical resource in the community and are the gatekeepers to other community resources including psychiatrists. Qualifying as a psychiatrist in Australia involves completing a five-year training program that includes rotations in hospitals and community settings. The aims of this research were to 1) explore psychiatry registrars' perceptions of difficult-to-treat-depression (DTTD) and 2) what they thought about the GPs' role in this regard. Methods: A semi-structured interview schedule comprising six questions was used; 10 psychiatry registrars (6 females, 4 males) participated in a one-and-half-hour focus group. All were in their final year of training and undertaking a training post in a public hospital in Melbourne, Australia. Data were analysed using the Framework Method. Findings: Similar to GPs and GP trainees, psychiatry registrars' perceptions and understanding of DTTD varied. While acknowledging limited experience in diagnosis and management, issues important to them included the utility of labels such as DTTD; patients distressed because of another diagnosis, substance abuse and/or life problems, the importance of accurate histories and notes, cost and limited availability of services particularly in the private sector, prescribing regimens, referring to allied health professionals, and suggesting/prescribing non pharmacological and/or complementary treatment. Also what was of concern was communication, both between health professionals and between health professionals and patients. Consensus was that treating depression in general practice is one of the hardest things for GPs to manage but there was value in using mental health plans. Discussion and Conclusion: While this cohort was small in number with limited experience, this study is the first to contribute to the literature that provides some insight into psychiatry registrars' experiences and perceptions of DTTD. Outcomes may have implications for thepsychiatry training program and GPs who diagnose and manage patients with mental health problems.

Keywords

Depression, GP, Psychiatry

---

*Corresponding author.

1. Introduction

Against the background of researching GPs [1] and GP trainees' perceptions of difficult-to-treat depression [2] (DTTD), this research was undertaken to explore psychiatry registrars' perceptions of DTTD and what they think about the GPs' role. Since the endorsement of the National Mental Health Strategy in 1992, several initiatives have been introduced, including the Better Access program in 2007 [3]. Among other things, this initiative improved access to psychiatrists [3]. In the 2011-12 year, a conservative estimate of 1348 (full time equivalent) consultant psychiatrists and psychiatrists were employed in state and territory public hospitals, psychiatric units, community care mental care services and residential mental health services in Australia [4]. While the range of reform measures included greater emphasis on care within the community, resulting in an increase of service providers, linkages and communication pathways [5] [6], for some patients, access to psychiatrists remains limited because few psychiatrists work outside major cities and inner regional centres and those practising in the private sector are largely inaccessible due to cost [7].

At the end of 2013, there were 1442 psychiatry trainees at various stages of their training [8]. Qualifying as a psychiatrist in Australia involves joining and completing a five-year training program, which is based around rotations that cover ward rounds and case review in adult, child/adolescent and forensic psychiatry, consultation liaison, and experiences in rural psychiatry, indigenous mental health, psychiatry of old age, addiction, electroconvulsive therapy and psychotherapies [8] [9]. This training program provides the trainees with experiences and links to GPs and community services via their rotations in hospitals (public, remote public, private, not-for-profit hospitals) and community settings (public, private, not-for profit community settings, youth custodial facilities, residential facilities and Aboriginal Community Controlled Health Services) [9].

In Australia, GPs are often the patient's first contact point for health because they are the most accessible medical resource in the community and are the gatekeepers to other community resources [7]. In 2011-12 an estimated 12.1% of GP encounters were mental health-related with depression the most commonly managed problem by a GP [3]-[5] [10]. While it has been reported that GPs may fail to recognise depression in around half of cases, this degree of non-recognition is understandable because of the many barriers to recognition [11] including somatisation because of its relationship to depression and anxiety [12]. Although GPs can access services in both the private and public health sectors, as it is thought to be better for a person's mental health to treat them in the community rather than in a hospital, mental health services are increasingly provided in the community [13] [14]. However, health services and hospitals deliver their public specialist mental health services differently depending on the local environment and catchment area [15]. In addition, while based on the same set of symptoms, there may be differences in the GPs' and psychiatrists' diagnostic decision-making because of the emphasis accorded to different elements of the history [16]. Thus, partnerships in mental health care, particularly between public and private [17] and improved communication between health professionals and health services is extremely important and helps improve the quality of patient care [18].

While the Diagnostic and Statistical Manual of Mental Disorders, Fifth Edition (DSM V) provides information to diagnose, for example, depressive disorders, major depressive disorder and persistent depressive disorder (dysthymia) [19], no clear definition or information is provided for diagnosing and/or managing DTTD. Therefore, this paper uses the description of DTTD as "most often conceptualized in terms of repeated failures to ameliorate depressive symptoms" [20].

No literature could be found that described psychiatry registrars' perceptions of DTTD and what they think about the GPs' role in managing depression in Australia. Because of the absence of literature, it is important to undertake exploratory work to gain an understanding in this area.

The aims of this research were 1) to explore psychiatry registrars' perceptions of DTTD and 2) what they think about the GPs' role in this regard.

2. Methods

2.1. Sample Recruitment

A convenience sample was recruited via an email forwarded to registrars undertaking a training post in a public hospital in Melbourne, Australia. When potential participants responded and agreed to participate, they provided their contact details (email) for the purpose of the research team advising time, date and venue for the focus group [21] [22].

2.2. Data Collection and Analysis

A semi-structured interview schedule comprising six headings which had been previously developed and used when interviewing and/or conducting focus groups with GPs [1] and GP trainees [2] (**Table 1**).

All data were collected in Melbourne; a focus group was held with the psychiatry registrars (6 females, 4 males) which lasted approximately one-and-a-half-hours, was audio-taped and transcribed verbatim. At the time of the focus group, all participants were in their final year of training and undertaking a training post in a public hospital in Melbourne. No other demographic data were collected.

Data were analysed using the Framework Method [24] to understand participants' perspectives. Data were analysed manually and independently by investigators (KJ and LP). When there was a difference of opinion, the issues were discussed and agreement reached [24]. Findings, including discussion are reported under the interview schedule's six headings. Comments are reported as PR1-10.

Ethics approval to conduct the study was obtained from Monash University Human Research Ethics Committee (MUHREC).

3. Findings

Findings are reported under the interview schedule's six sub-headings.

Question 1: Understanding of difficult-to-treat depression (DTTD)?

Similar to GPs [1] and GP trainees [2], psychiatry registrars' (PRs) perceptions and understanding of DTTD varied. One thought of DTTD as "*being quite multi-factorial*" (PR5), another suggested "*it could be quite severe psycho-social stress*" (PR6).

"*So that's saying whether it's a difficult patient or a difficult depression*" (PR3).

"*That's right: the subjective experience, the symptoms of the depression would be exactly the same in difficult to treat depression. The difficult to treat part comes from something else. I mean, you know, outside. Which is the treatment or its lack of efficacy*" (PR8).

One considered the GPs' role:

"*I'm not sure [of the meaning of DTTD], but what might be important to GPs is looking at what makes it difficult to treat. I mean rather than maybe defining if it's this cluster of symptoms*" (PR5).

One suggested that DTTD may be misdiagnosed:

"*That the whole construct of depression has really been flawed and is invalid and non-viable and non-reproducible. There's no really well defined approach on the definition of depression. So difficult to treat depression is really just over-diagnosed non-depression that's been diagnosed as depression and doesn't respond to antidepressants*" (PR1).

Question 2: What is your understanding of other terms?

Registrars' understanding of other terms, viz treatment resistant depression, treatment-refractory depression, treatment-resistant major depressive disorder and major depressive disorder varied with around half indicating they had limited understanding of the terms:

"*I think we've got an enormous problem with semantics*" (PR2).

Table 1. Interview schedule.

1) What is your understanding of the term difficult-to-treat-depression (DTTD)?

2) What is your understanding of other terms; viz: treatment-resistant depression treatment-refractory depression, treatment-resistant major depressive disorder and major depressive disorder?

3) What are your experiences of diagnosing DTTD?

4) What are your experiences of managing DTTD?

5) Does your management of these patients include:
   a) using an illness management model or a chronic illness [23];
   b) communication with GPs;
   c) referring the patient to allied health professionals, and
   d) suggesting/prescribing non-pharmacological and/or complementary treatment?

6) If "no" to any of Question 5, have you ever considered using any of these options/other comments?

"For me, I see difficult to treat as where simple things like some psychiatrist trying antidepressants and CBT don't work. So there's definition by exclusions. And treatment resistant would be the next level. So you have second and third opinions that are multiple antidepressants, mood stabilisers, ECT and these things aren't working" (PR3).

"I still don't know what the difference is between treatment resistant and difficult to treat, or is there a difference, I don't know" (PR4).

"Yes, resistant is a strong word. It's heading more towards incurable in a way, whereas difficult-to-treat—it's a phrase laden with opportunity" (PR8).

The role of the GP and their knowledge of their patients were also discussed. The majority felt the GPs play a significant role in managing patients diagnosed with DTTD:

"I guess GPs who know people and build up that relationship and understanding of their life, their paths, their psycho-social stressors, and the way that the relationship, the way they relate" (PR6).

"I find that if I have been asked to see somebody by another member of the medical team and then I call the GP, the GP can often very clearly say look, they've [the patient] been like this for a long time, this is why this is happening. So I do think GPs have an understanding but I don't know if the system supports them in those areas" (PR5).

Question 3: What are your experiences of diagnosing DTTD?

While registrars' experience in diagnosing was limited compared to GPs, the registrars all agreed that GPs carry the majority of the burden of mental illness. All agreed that when diagnosing DTTD, the *"diagnosis is always loaded with management"* (PR9), and the utility of labels to describe an illness or management has positive and negative aspects:

"There are a lot of imprecise things in medicine, I feel we get bogged down getting the exact diagnosis or correct term, and maybe we just need to accept there is a degree of uncertainty and we are going to get our definitions wrong" (PR4).

"We've all [medical practitioners] signed up, psychiatry included, to this evidence based model of medicine and to have evidence you need labels; unfortunately with psychiatry, labelling reduces the infinite human complexity to a circumscribed area, and that circumscribed area is going to have boundaries, and the boundary is necessarily going to be arbitrary" (PR8).

Only one registrar raised using DSM to assist with diagnosis:

"Most psychiatrists don't vigorously use the DSM to make the diagnosis" (PR1).

Much of the discussion focussed on the role and input of the GP:

"I think particularly in general practice there's an enormous amount of good kind of non-billed for counselling/containing of people, because GPs know them for years and understand actually what it is that works and what it is that helps and that's a therapeutic relationship; perhaps it doesn't necessarily matter if it's your GP or your psychiatrist or psychiatry registrar, it's a therapeutic relationship" (PR2).

"I agree, it's the GPs that carry the majority of the burden of mental illness, I think the GPs provide a very holistic human relationship, like a long term human relationship that's vital in the treatment of depression" (PR6).

"We think of GPs generally as holistic practitioners. Some are extremely biological, as you have to acknowledge, but some of them are holistic" (PR7).

Question 4: What are your experiences of managing DTTD?

The registrars reported that in their experience, patients are a very heterogeneous group, some with other mental health disorders and others with substance abuse and/or life problems:

"Trying not to call something treatment resistant or treatment refractory, and also acknowledging that depression that is difficult to treat perhaps encompasses more than mere treatment resistance as defined by DSM depression" (PR10).

"Some of them [patient] have undiagnosed bipolar, lots of personality disorder, substance abuse, existential life problems. I mean it's very hard, all you know is it's basically a kind of 'heart-sink' patient, with low numbers of therapeutic optimism" (PR1).

Another felt that the depression may be difficult to manage because *"it isn't what we think that it is"* (PR2).

Regarding taking histories and making notes as part of management, all agreed that it is important to take an accurate developmental history:

"It is important to ensure that a developmental history is taken, rather than the psychiatrist saying 'I have not

had time to take a developmental history'" (PR1).

"Yes, the developmental history gets, you know, delegated to some other time" (PR4).

Management differences were also noted for patients in the public and private sector:

"I'm in outpatients clinic at the moment and being psych registrars in a public hospital we're the second line already, so perhaps you could say that all those that we're seeing depression, it's complicated in some way" (PR5).

While cost and availability were factors in the private sector, there was general consensus that the public sector is not really set up for these patients (PR4), *"which can result in these patients not getting a lot of treatment within the public system"* (PR1).

"So there is some utility in some of these labels from the perspective of accounting, planning, policy budgetary level" (PR10).

There was agreement that some patients presenting in the outpatient public sector may be distressed because of another diagnosis but aren't necessarily depressed, subsequently:

"You've got to find the right person. I mean, I think it's really quite difficult to do those things, although I'd like to think that I do address those. But I have to say it's much easier to consider medication first" (PR5).

Medication was described as part of management for most patients. Prescribing regiments were variously described:

"A friend of mine was a private psychiatrist, leaves a prescription pad at the reception desk, and it vastly reduces prescribing because she has to go outside to get it" (PR2).

"If I am treating someone with DTTD, I am more likely to perhaps follow an intense medication path if there's a risk... it is important to try as many medications as possible..." (PR6).

"... but not just reach for a prescribing pad"(PR1).

Question 5: Does your management of these patients include

a) using an illness management model [23];

b) communication with GPs;

c) referring to allied health professionals, and/or

d) suggesting/prescribing non pharmacological and/or complementary treatment?

1) Using an illness management model

Similar to the GP trainees, most of the psychiatry registrars were unsure what an illness management model was, one suggested:

"In the system that we work it becomes very much a medical model, you know" (PR4).

2) Communication with GPs

As psychiatry registrars who are in training posts in public hospitals work in teams, they communicate with a range of health professionals. They described the GPs' involvement with the patient's management as important:

"If it's looking for connectedness, then GPs are often actually a really good person for that. So that could be the GP... who gives them a call every week and listens to them on the phone. You know, if that could be the pathway if that we had mental health nurses that do the check-in all the time, that's the connectedness and that can help" (PR5).

"The GPs know the patients and within that relationship, understand the patient's life and stressors, the way they relate. I think we should also reflect on treatment resistant depression as a sociological problem in that it's the structure of our current modern day society in the west. And these GPs are; they're called upon to be, like a sort of connectedness to the community, and it must be so hard for them because they're so busy and they mean that for a lot of patients" (PR6).

Communication between health professionals was also raised, particularly when a GP refers a patient to a psychiatrist:

"Even if we don't agree with the definitions or they're not clear, we still need a quick way to communicate with our colleagues, and that's what they do in medicine; sometimes the diagnosis might not fit, but it's just a quick way to communicate if it gets through" (PR4).

"If a GP refers someone to you and says they are depressed, you come back with the answer, well what is depression?" (PR8).

3) Referring to allied health professionals

Whilst the majority had referred to allied health professionals, the majority thought that referring to allied health professionals would depend on the severity (PR1) and complexity of the patient's illness (PR2), and whether it will assist to preserve the patient's job and marriage (PR3) rather than the illness becoming their identity (PR6).

"*As well as social psychologists, we use other allied health professionals to manage these patients*" (PR9).

"*I think it comes down to resources, so if it's somebody that's really complex with a lot of risk, and can afford it, probably a psychiatrist. If it's somebody that's quite sever with a lot of risks, probably community mental health or GP*" (PR5).

4) Suggesting/prescribing non pharmacological and/or complementary treatment

Opinion varied; some felt these options may be problematic for a number of reasons, whereas others felt there is an increasing evidence base, thus some options have sufficient value to be considered as part of the management plan:

"*I think there is increasing evidence base for the variety of complementary medicines with which to treat depression and I think that we as professionals its incumbent upon us to be knowledgeable about them. I'm involved with a mob of GPs that use integrative medicine as a way of treating the patient so using the best evidence from complementary alternative therapies and from mainstream for treating somebody with depression… and there are some GPs who are extremely well trained in that, or some GPs who know very good naturopaths, or other complementary medical practitioners who they can refer to*" (PR2).

"*I'm thinking thinks like Mindfulness, yoga*" (PR4).

"*I went to St John's Wort*" (PR9).

"*Going back to whether you would have access to a good GP, you know, someone who is willing to spend the time to be broad minded to alternative treatments, all those things, you need a good GP*" (PR7).

"*And that's rarer than winning gold, a good GP!*" (PR2).

Question 6: If no to any of Question 5, have you ever considered using any of those options/other comments?

Participants felt that treating depression in general practice is one of the hardest things for GPs to manage, for example, time-pressure with the patient (PR7) and the patient expecting something concrete (PR7). The use of mental health plans (PR9) and resources such as education (PR2), papers published in journals (PR5) and guidelines (PR9, PR10) were described as important and valuable:

"*I think it's very hard for GPs, I think that if there could be a lot less sort of prescribing of SSRIs and a lot more capacity for GPs to feel confident and skilled to look at other ways in which to help manage mild to moderate is one thing about depression. Then that would be great*" (PR2).

4. Discussion and Conclusion

In response to the various questions, these registrars articulated their perceptions of DTTD and their thoughts about the GPs' role and relationship with the patient generally and with patients who experience depression that is difficult to treat [1] [2].

Rotations into various sectors of the mental health services provided this cohort of registrars with a range of experiences; all had rotated in the public sector, but few had in the private sector [8] [9]. These rotations provided insight into management differences both within the sectors, the various health professionals, and the impact on patients, but also highlighted gaps in the registrars' knowledge and experience. While Commonwealth government initiatives improved access to psychiatrists [3], major factors remain that impact on patients including cost, availability and access, because of limited personal resources and/or Medicare funding requirements [3]-[7].

General consensus was that GPs carry the majority of the burden of diagnosing, managing and treating patients with mental illness [3]-[7]. All had considered community options as part of their management plans; which included a range of treatment options including GPs, allied health professionals and complementary and alternative treatments [1] [2]. From the registrars' perspectives, the most important aspect of management was clear, effective communication regardless of whether it was between professionals or between professionals and patients, but as this did not always occur; possible changes to processes were discussed [11] [12] [15]-[18].

Few had referred to DSM V [19] or heard of a chronic disease management model [23], rather, significant emphasis was placed on the GPs' role and input, which was described as important, particularly for the patient [1] [7] [11] [12].

The generalisability of this study may be limited because of the small number of participants who were all from metropolitan Melbourne, with no input from the rural sector. Regardless, this study is the first to contribute to the literature by providing some insight into psychiatry registrars' experiences and perceptions of DTTD and what they think about the GPs' role in managing patients diagnosed with DTTD.

5. Implications for General Practice and Psychiatrist Registrar Training

- With the increasing number of trainee registrars [9], an increase in the number and/or duration of rotations to rural and remote rural locations would provide support in areas that have limited healthcare professionals.
- To enhance communication between health care professionals, discussion on team based care models and mental health care planning processes could be included in the training program, for example in the "consultation liaison" component [9].
- Where possible, GPs support community based rotations by having a trainee registrar in their practice as part of the psychiatry registrar rotation, to better understand each other's roles.
- Where relevant, analysis and report of trainee registrars' direct contact with GPs and allied health professionals, the role of DSM in training registrars to assist with diagnosis may need review.

References

[1]   Jones, K.M., Castle, D.J. and Piterman, L. (2012) Difficult-to-Treat-Depression: What Do General Practitioners Think? *MJA Open*, **1**, 6-8.

[2]   Jones, K.M., Piterman, L. and Spike, N. (2014) Difficult-to-Treat-Depression—Perceptions of GPs and GP Trainees. *Open Journal of Psychiatry*, **4**, 228-237. http://dx.doi.org/10.4236/ojpsych.2014.43029

[3]   Department of Health and Ageing (2013) National Mental Health Report 2013: Tracking Progress of Mental Health Reform in Australia 1993-2011. Commonwealth of Australia, Canberra.

[4]   AIHW: Mental Health Services in Australia (2012) Staffing of State and Territory Specialised Mental Health Care Facilities. https://mhsa.aihw.gov.au/resources/facilities/staffing/

[5]   Private Mental Health Alliance (PMHA) (2011) Principles for Collaboration, Communication and Cooperation between Private Mental Health Service Providers. Private Mental Health Alliance, Kingston.

[6]   Pirkis, J., Harris, M., Hall, W. and Ftanou, M. (2011) Evaluation of the Better Access to Psychiatrists, Psychologists and General Practitioners through the Medicare Benefits Schedule Initiative. Summative Evaluation, Final Report. Centre for Health Policy, Programs and Economics, The University of Melbourne.

[7]   Senate Select Committee Mental Health (2006) A National Approach to Mental Health—From Crisis to Community. Final Report. Senate Select Committee, Commonwealth of Australia, Canberra.

[8]   Royal Australian and New Zealand College of Psychiatrists (RANZCP) (2014) Quarterly Education Activities Report January-December 2013. RANZCP, Melbourne.

[9]   Royal Australian and New Zealand College of Psychiatrists (RANZCP) (2013) Education Activities Report for the 2012 Training Year. RANZCP, Melbourne.

[10] AIHW (2013) Mental Health Services—In Brief 2013 Cat.no.HSE 141. AIHW, Canberra.

[11] Clarke, D.M., Cook, K., Smith, G.C. and Piterman, L. (2008) What Do General Practitioners Think Depression Is? A Taxonomy of Distress and Depression for General Practitioners. *MJA*, **188**, S110-S113.

[12] Clarke, D.M., Piterman, L., Byrne, C.J. and Austin, D.W. (2008) Somatiac Symptoms, Hypochondriasis and Psychological Distress: A Study of Somatisation in Australian General Practice. *MJA*, **189**, 560-564.

[13] Better Health: The Roles of Psychiatrists and General Practitioners. http://www.betterhealth.vic.gov.au/bhcv2/bhcarticles.nsf/pages/Mental_illness_treatments

[14] Keks, N.A., Altson, M., Sacks, T.L., Hustig, H.H. and Tangahow, A. (1997) Collaboration between General Practice and Commkunity Psychiatric Services for People with Chronic Mental Illness. *The Medical Journal of Australia*, **167**, 266-271.

[15] Victorian Government (2011) Victorian Government Health Information: Adult Specialist Mental Health Services (16 - 64 Years). http://www.betterhealth.vic.gov.au/bhcv2/bhcarticles.nsf/pages/Mental_illness_treatments

[16] Lampe, L., Fritz, K., Boyce, P., Starcevic, V., Brakoulias, V., Walter, G., Shadbolt, N. and Harris, A. and Malhi, G. (2013) Psychiatrists and GPs: Diagnostic Decision Making, Personality Profiles and Attitudes toward Depression and Anxiety. *Australasian Psychiatry*, **21**, 231-237. http://dx.doi.org/10.1177/1039856213486210

[17] Yung, A., Gill, L., Somerville, E., Dowling, B., Simon, K., Pirkis, J., Livingston, J., Schweitzer, I., Tanaghow, A.,

Herrman, H., *et al.* (2005) Public and Private Psychiatry: Can They Work Together and Is It Worth the Effort? *Australian and New Zealand Journal of Psychiatry*, **39**, 67-73. http://dx.doi.org/10.1080/j.1440-1614.2005.01511.x

[18] Sain, K., Shah, N. and Hasan, S. (2012) GPs' Views on the Content and Quality of Psychiatrists' Clinic Letters. *Progress in Neurology and Psychiatry*, **16**, 6-10. http://dx.doi.org/10.1002/pnp.223

[19] American Psychiatric Association (2013) Diagnostic and Statistical Manual of Mental Disorders. 5th Edition (DSM-5), American Psychiatraic Publishing, Washington DC.

[20] Grote, N.K. and Frank, E. (2003) Difficult-to-Treat Depression: The Role of Contexts and Comorbidities. *Society of Biological Psychiatry*, **53**, 660-670. http://dx.doi.org/10.1016/S0006-3223(03)00006-4

[21] Liamputtong, P. and Ezzey, D. (2005) Qualitative Research Methods. Oxford University Press, Melbourne.

[22] Polgar, S. and Thomas, S. (2005) Introduction to Research in the Health Sciences. Elsevier Churchill Livingstone, Sydney.

[23] Wagner, E.H. (1998) Chronic Disease Management: What Will It Take to Improve Care for Chronic Illness? *Effective Clinical Practice*, **1**, 2-4.

[24] Ritchie, J. and Spencer, L. (1994) Qualitative Data Analysis for Applied Policy Research. In: Bryman, A. and Burgess, B., Eds., *Analyzing Qualitative Data*, Routledge, London, Chapter 9. http://dx.doi.org/10.4324/9780203413081

The Risk and Protective Factors of School Absenteeism

Rajeevan Rasasingham[1,2]

[1]University of Toronto, Toronto, Canada
[2]Harvard University, Cambridge, MA, USA
Email: rajrasas@hotmail.com

Abstract

Absenteeism from school in children and adolescents is a problem that impacts the social, emotional and educational development of the children (Haarman, 2011). While absenteeism can be seen as a short-term condition, prolonged absenteeism during childhood may be a predictor of lasting issues that may persist into adulthood (King, Ollendick and Tonge, 1995), such as "school dropout, delinquency and occupational and relationship problems" (Kearney and Bensaheb, 2006), and economic deprivation and social, marital, occupational and psychiatric problems (Kearney and Graczyk, 2014). Early absenteeism has been associated with school dropout, further disconnecting the children from school based health programs and leading the children into economic deprivation, and marital, social and psychiatric problems in adulthood (Kogan, Luo, Murry and Brody, 2005). Furthermore, absenteeism may be an indication of "suicide attempt, perilous sexual behaviour, teenage pregnancy, violence, unintentional injury, driving under the influence of alcohol, and alcohol, marijuana, tobacco, and other substance abuse" (Kearney, 2008). The purpose of this article is to provide a review of the literature on protective and risk factors for school absenteeism in youths aged 5 to 18 years old, with focus on articles published after 2004. First, the definition of absenteeism will be discussed, followed by the prevalence and demographic of this phenomenon, the protective and risk factors of school absenteeism, and a review of intervention strategies.

Keywords

School Absenteeism, Child and Adolescent Psychiatry and Review

1. Introduction

Absenteeism from school in children and adolescents is a problem that impacts the social, emotional and educational development of the children [1]. While absenteeism can be seen as a short-term condition, prolonged absenteeism during childhood may be a predictor of lasting issues that may persist into adulthood [2], such as "school dropout, delinquency and occupational and relationship problems" [3] and economic deprivation and social, marital, occupational and psychiatric problems (Kearney and Graczyk, 2014).

Early absenteeism has been associated with school dropout, further disconnecting the children from school based health programs and leading the children into economic deprivation, and marital, social and psychiatric problems in adulthood [4]. Furthermore, absenteeism may be an indication of "suicide attempt, perilous sexual behaviour, teenage pregnancy, violence, unintentional injury, driving under the influence of alcohol, and alcohol, marijuana, tobacco, and other substance abuse" [5].

The purpose of this article is to provide a review of the literature on protective and risk factors for school absenteeism in youths aged 5 to 18 years old with focus on articles published after 2004. First, the definition of absenteeism will be discussed, followed by the prevalence and demographic of this phenomenon, the protective and risk factors to school absenteeism, and a review of intervention strategies.

2. Definition

Literature on school absenteeism dates back to 1932 when Broadwin characterized some children to exhibit a set of behaviors in refusing school that "are an attempt to obtain love, or escape from real situations to which it is difficult to adjust" [6]. The early definitions of absenteeism were clinically driven, mostly anxiety and school-phobia based. Later on, *school phobia* was seen to be too psychopathological, so the alternative term *school refusal behavior* was used to describe the broader phenomena [7].

Absenteeism, defined by Kearny, refers to a legitimate or illegitimate absence from school or class. Legitimate reasons for missing school include illnesses, religious holidays, the need to attend a family funeral, hazardous weather conditions, and exemptions for college attendance or specific kinds of work [8].

School refusal behavior refers to a child-motivated refusal to attend school [9]. This is different from *truancy*, which is defined as unexcused and unlawful absence from school without parental knowledge and consent [10]. The truant child usually "conceals absences from his or her parents" [11].

This article focuses mainly on "absenteeism" as school refusal behavior, a parentally known behavior of the child. Occasionally, truancy will also be discussed where its risk and protective factors are similar to a child with school refusal behavior.

3. Prevalence

School absenteeism is prevalent. In 2012, the estimated American national rate for students missing 21 days of school is 10 percent [12]. This estimates to roughly 5 to 7.5 million students not attending school regularly in grades pre-kindergarten to grade 12 in America's public schools [12].

Absenteeism such as morning misbehaviors and school-based distress add up to 28% - 35% of students in America [8] [13]. A longitudinal study showed that 25% to 90% of youth aged 9 to 16 years old who were absent from school met the criteria for a diagnosis from the Diagnostic and Statistical Manual of Mental Disorders, Fourth Edition (DSM-IV; American Psychiatric Association, 1994) [14].

4. Risk and Protective Factors Related to Absenteeism

It is important to understand the risk and protective factors of school absenteeism in a contextual way by considering the co-occurrence of different factors [15]. The risk and protective factors related to absenteeism are discussed next.

4.1. Individual Psychiatric and Physical Conditions

Children and adolescents with school absenteeism are more likely to have anxiety disorders, affective disorders, disruptive disorders, substance abuse, or a combination of these compared to students without school absenteeism [5] [15]-[17]. However, there is also a number of youth having school refusal behavior or school absenteeism with no diagnosis of a psychiatric illness [5] [15].

Other somatic conditions that are linked to school absenteeism are asthma, headache, stomachache, nausea, vomiting, fatigue, sweating, lightheadedness, abdominal or back pain, heart palpitations, diarrhea, shortness of breath and menstruation symptoms [5].

Rumberger and Larson also suggested a pattern in which a student did worse academically when absent more from school. In return, the student felt less motivated to attend school because of the poor academic performance (1998). This cycle shows the beginning of academic disengagement [18].

4.2. School Climate

Perceptions of an unsafe school environment, inadequate peer and teacher support [19], inconsistent rules (Stickney and Miltenberger, 1998) and low school connectedness (Shochet et al., 2006) pose as risk factors to school absenteeism. On the other hand, a positive school climate with constructive student-teacher relationship is seen as protective factors against low attendance and drop-out rates [20].

A more recent study by Havik, Bru and Ertsevag shows similar findings. Havik et al.'s study suggests that noisy, disruptive and unpredictable classrooms pose as challenges to children (2013). In such environments, teachers spend more time calming the disruptions than in giving attention to more vulnerable students, which further increases the risk of school refusal [21]. Overall, students have a need for predictability and the feeling of being valued. Havik et al. argues that these are interconnected factors in creating a predictable learning situation (2013). To create such a predictable learning situation, Havik et al. emphasize for teachers to manage student behavior and provide emotional support, as well as the need in more knowledge of school refusal behavior to earlier identify the problem (2013).

4.3. Family Connectedness and Involvement

There has been well-established literature on family involvement as a protective factor from school truancy and absenteeism [22], with literature dating back to 1994 stating family-relationship factors having a positive correlation with truancy [23]. Variables include the family's socioeconomic status, the family's attitude towards education, parental knowledge of truancy, parental situations, parenting skills, child abuse and neglect [10].

Contrarily, risk factors of school absenteeism include crowded living conditions, weak parent-child relationships, frequent relocation, and low-income families [24]. One study shows that weak parental supervision poses as a key risk factor for problematic absenteeism [15] [25] [26].

Parental involvement for enhancing academic socialization has been supported more recently [27]. Hill and Tysons' study highlighted the significant role of families, family-school relations, and parental involvement in education to have positive associations with achievement in early adolescence. Their study also states that without effective parental involvement, the child's opportunities are limited, "leading to lost potential, unrealized talent, diminished educational and vocational attainment, and widening demographic gaps in achievement" [27].

4.4. Family Structure and Functioning

Children with teenage unmarried mothers are more likely to be chronically absent in elementary school [28]. As well, children who are homeless or have unstable housing situations are more likely to be absent from school [29]. McShane et al. shows that adolescents with school refusal behavior may be in separated families (21%) in families with conflicts (43%) (2001).

Adolescents with high levels of behavior problems and absenteeism were more likely to change schools [18].

School refusing adolescents may also have mothers (53%) or fathers (34%) with psychiatric illnesses in the family [17]. Other factors related to increased absenteeism are alcoholism in parents [30]. Children with parents who work nonstandard shifts (nights/weekends) may need to be more reliant on themselves, which may result in greater chance of absences [31].

4.5. Neighborhood and Community Factors

Wandersman and Nation's study shows that mental health outcomes are related to neighborhood characteristics such as the socioeconomic status, racial and ethnic composition, residential patterns and family disruption, social incivilities (public drunkenness, corner gangs, street harassment, drug trade) and physical incivilities (abandoned buildings, vandalism, litter, dilapidated housing) [1998]. In low-income neighborhoods, children may attend poorly funded schools, be exposed to acts of violence, experience maltreatment, and parents and teachers may have infrequent contact (Wandersman and Nation, 1998) [22].

More than a decade later, findings continue to support this by studying neighbor characteristics. Gottfried's study shows that higher levels of neighbor poverty, higher number of average neighbor household size, younger average neighbor age, neighbor home ownership, and greater percentage of Black neighbors in the student's residential block to be predictors of student absences [32] [33]. As students may not interact "on a sustained basis" with those employed, students exposed to areas of high levels of poverty may not see the value of education, resulting in a downward cycle of low expectations and low achievement [34].

Contrarily, youth and parents in affluent communities have more access to support systems and resources. Areas of greater neighbor homeownership have shown to have greater residential stability and larger neighbor social networks [35]. As well, increased homeownership may directly decrease neighborhood block crime, leading to improved schooling outcomes [36].

4.6. Ethnic Minority Status

In comparing White students with Black students, White students have been positively correlated with excused absences and negatively with unexcused absences [7]. Black students are more likely to have unexcused absences and less likely to have excused absences [7]. According to Gottfried, Asian students are less likely to have number of days absent (2009). As well, when compared to non-Asian children, White and Asian children are less often to be chronically absent in kindergarten and first grade children [37]. Children who missed more than 10 days of kindergarten and first grade were more likely to have English as a second language [37].

Benner and Graham also show that Latino adolescents report increased discrimination in the first two years of high school (2011). Perception of the school climate by the Latino adolescent indirectly affects the adolescents' grades and absences negatively [38].

Bayer and McMillian showed that neighborhoods with predominantly Black residents have less access to amenities and services (2005). Moreover, neighborhood sorting results in the decline of social capital, social services, and community resources (Bayer & McMillian, 2005).

The location of a neighborhood affects the youth's health, which in turn affects absenteeism. One example used is the rate of childhood asthma due to the environmental factors, further affecting absenteeism. Neighborhoods in chemically toxic areas or closer to hazardous waste sites are also neighborhoods with higher percentage of minority residents. In such neighborhoods, children are more exposed to the toxic environments [39]. Other studies have shown that stressors associated with poverty, family dysfunction, and neighborhood conditions may contribute to asthma, resulting in missed school days [40].

4.7. Sexual Minority Status

Burton, Marshal and Chisolm's study reported more excused and unexcused absences were found in sexual minority youth aged 14 to 19 compared to heterosexual youth (2014). This study also suggests that absences from school "may be an early warning sign for mental health issues, particularly in sexual minority youth" [41].

In Kosciw and Diazs' studies, sexual minority youth were youth who self-identified as a lesbian, gay, bisexual and transgender (LGBT) youth. Sexual minority youth often report experiencing violence and discrimination, resulting in higher rates of absenteeism, discipline problems, and low academic achievement [7] [42] due to feeling unsafe and uncomfortable at school [43] [44]. Violence includes experiences of verbal and physical harassment and assault [45], sexual harassment [46], social exclusion and isolation [47], and other interpersonal problems with peers [48] [49].

The most common reason youth reported for being bullied or harassed was because of the way they looked or their body size, followed by the self-identification or being perceived as lesbian, gay or bisexual [50]. Harris Interactive and GLSEN also reported that LGBT students (22%) were more likely than non-LGBT students (7%) to feel unsafe at school (2005). Supporting other previous studies, Harris Interactive and GLSEN's report also showed that experiences of violence and feeling unsafe at school were linked to poor academic performances, due to higher rates of absenteeism (missing classes and skipping school days) (2005).

Another study suggests that schools with low homophobic teasing and positive school climate reduce the prevalence of negative outcomes in LGB youth, such as drug use, depression, suicidality and truancy [51].

Unsafe school climates specific to sexual minority youth were more so in rural communities, whereas larger urban schools labeled as the most "dangerous" may actually provide safer environments for sexual minority youth [43]. Goodenow et al. [52] provides an explanation by suggesting that larger urban schools may have a more diverse climate, allowing for students to have a sense of belonging in identifying with more diverse social "niches" (2006).

5. Intervention

Intervention strategies for children and youth with absenteeism ranges from clinically and medically focused, school climate improvements, family based to systemic changes.

5.1. Clinically and Medically Focused: Cognitive Behavioral Therapy

Studies have shown the effectiveness of cognitive-behavioral therapy (CBT) for anxiety-based school refusal due to "the role of self-efficacy in mediating the outcome of CBT for school refusal" [53].

Aside from anxiety-based school absenteeism, Kearny also identified non-anxiety based cases of absenteeism for children aged 5 to 17 years old. Non-anxiety based cases are identified into two functions: refusing school to pursue attention from significant others, and refusing school to pursue tangible rewards outside of school. For cases of absenteeism based on non-anxiety cases, Kearney suggests more parent-based involvement by setting morning routines and providing attention-based consequences (Kearney and Graczyk, 2007). For those refusing school to pursue tangible rewards outside of school, Kearney suggests incentives for attendance and disincentives for nonattendance (Kearney and Graczyk, 2007)

Away from anxiety-based and non-anxiety based cases of absenteeism, other studies have shown interventions to target low self-esteem, social skills and medical conditions. A variety of interventions on the medical and individual level have been suggested, such as individual therapy, social-service referrals, hand-washing to prevent disease, and asthma prevention strategies [54].

5.2. School Climate Improvement

Feeling unsafe in the school environment has been a recurring issue for school absenteeism, especially for ethnic minority and sexual minority youth. Preliminary research has suggested that extracurricular clubs such as Gay Straight Alliances (GSAs) in schools have been successful in improving the school climate for sexual minority youth whether or not they participate in the club [55] [56].

Positive Behavioral Interventions and Supports (PBIS) is a whole-school prevention model that aims to modify school climate by promoting positive change in staff and student behaviors. Research has shown that school organizational health is positively associated with student performance and negatively associated with absenteeism and suspensions [57]. Kearney and Bates suggest that the homeroom or classroom teacher may be used to identify students at risk of absenteeism and to inform parents and other school officials of absences (2005).

5.3. Parental Involvement

Decades of studies show the powerful influence of parents and family members on student achievement (Galindo and Sheldon, 2012). Strategies have been developed to increase parental involvement in school, family, and community partnerships [22].

One study examined the significance of school partnership programs in helping families create supportive home environments, increase parent-school communication, recruit parents to help at school and serve on school committees, and provide information to families about how to help students with homework and integrate community-based resources to strengthen school programs [58]. This study showed that schools that had implemented this partnership program had significantly greater student attendance than schools that did not [58]. As well, schools' effort in engaging families have shown lower levels of chronic absenteeism and lower levels of student behavior problems [59].

As called to attention by Pina *et al.* [13], an important part of successfully implementing an intervention is the collaboration between school officials, parents, youth and others responsible for the youth's treatment to share a similar concept of the problem. In collaborating, the young person's chance of reversing to negative school refusal behavior is limited, with the help of the staff at school to monitor school attendance, and the youth to feel secure when at school [13]. As well, Schorr [60] states components of a successful program that successfully engages with parents to include "the ability to be comprehensive, responsive, and flexible; view children in their family context; understand that families are an integral part of neighborhoods and communities; operate and maintain long-term preventive measures; appoint highly trained staff and competent management with clearly identifiable skills; ensure ongoing training; and establish mutual trust and collaboration among practitioners" (1997).

5.4. Putting It All Together: A Holistic Approach

It is important to understand where each student stands in his or her severity in school absenteeism. Kearny and Graczyk (2013)'s Response to Intervention model distinguishes problematic school absenteeism into three tiers of increasing intervention intensity: universal intervention, targeted intervention (emerging absenteeism, 25% - 35% of students) and intensive intervention (severe absenteeism, 5% - 10% of students).

Intervention strategies are used differ based on the student's severity. In the tier 1 universal intervention approach, all students are involved in regular screening to promote attendance and to begin to identify students who may not be benefitting from the core strategies (Kearney and Graczyk, 2013). Such strategies include school climate strategies, safety-oriented strategies, health-based strategies, character education, parental involvement, orientation activities, summer bridge and school readiness programs, culturally responsive approaches and policy review may be used (Kearney and Graczyk, 2013).

Tier 2 intervention is a more targeted strategy, in which at-risk students are identified to begin setting goals, parent collaboration, and adjunctive supports (Kearney and Graczyk, 2013). Last but not least, Tier 3 interventions hone in on students with "complex or severe problems who require a concentrated approach and frequent progress monitoring" (Kearney and Graczyk, 2013), which may include a more innovative approach and an expansion from Tier 2 strategy. Tier 3 strategy may include alternative educational programs, legal strategies, or multisystemic therapy (Kearney and Graczyk, 2013).

6. Conclusion

This review of literature has shown development in more recent understanding of the risk and protective factors in children and adolescents with school absenteeism difficulties. What is important though is the early identification of at-risk students of absenteeism and school refusal behaviour in the school setting. Only one party cannot tackle school absenteeism. Rather, coordination and collaboration between different agencies, such as family members, school officials, social workers, mental health professionals, criminal justice and research, must happen to effectively work together to prevent and work with children and adolescents with school absenteeism.

References

[1]   Haarman, G.B. (2011) School Refusal Behaviour: Children Who Can't or Won't Go To School. Education and Consultation Press, Louisville.

[2]   King, N.J., Tonge, B.J. and Ollendic, T.H. (1995) School Refusal: Assessment and Treatment. Allyn & Bacon, Boston.

[3]   Kearney, C.A. and Bensaheb, A. (2006) School Absenteeism and School Refusal Behaviour: A Review and Suggestions for School-Based Health Professionals. *Journal of School Health*, **76**, 3-7. http://dx.doi.org/10.1111/j.1746-1561.2006.00060.x

[4]   Kogan, S.M., Luo, Z.P., Murry, V.M. and Brody, G.H. (2005) Risk and Protective Factors for Substance Use among African American High School Dropouts. *Psychology of Addictive Behaviors*, **19**, 382-391. http://dx.doi.org/10.1037/0893-164X.19.4.382

[5]   Kearney, C.A. (2008) School Absenteeism and School Refusal Behaviour in Youth: A Contemporary Review. *Clinical Psychology Review*, **28**, 451-471. http://dx.doi.org/10.1016/j.cpr.2007.07.012

[6]   Broadwin, I.T. (1932) A Contribution to the Study of Truancy. *American Journal of Orthopsychiatry*, **2**, 253-259. http://dx.doi.org/10.1111/j.1939-0025.1932.tb05183.x

[7]   Grossman, A.H., Haney, A.P., Edwards, P., Alessi, E.J., Ardon, M. and Howell, T.J. (2009) Lesbian, Gay, Bisexual and Transgender Youth Talk about Experiencing and Coping with School Violence: A Qualitative Study. *Journal of LGBT Youth*, **6**, 24-46. http://dx.doi.org/10.1080/19361650802379748

[8]   Kearney, C.A. (2001) School Refusal Behaviour in Youth: A Functional Approach to Assessment and Treatment. American Psychological Association, Washington DC. http://dx.doi.org/10.1037/10426-000

[9]   Kearney, C.A. (1996) The Evolution and Reconciliation of Taxonomic Strategies for School Refusal Behavior. *Clinical Psychology: Science and Practice*, **3**, 339-354. http://dx.doi.org/10.1111/j.1468-2850.1996.tb00087.x

[10] Bell, A.J., Rosen, L.A. and Dynlacht, D. (1994) Truancy Intervention. *Journal of Research and Development in Education*, **27**, 203-211.

[11] Lee, M.I. and Miltenberger, R.G. (1996) School Refusal Behaviour: Classification, Assessment, and Treatment Issues. *Education and Treatment of Children*, **19**, 474-486.

[12] Balfanz, R. and Byrnes, V. (2012) Chronic Absenteeism: Summarizing What We Know from Nationally Available Data. Johns Hopkins University, Baltimore.

[13] Pina, A.A., Zerr, A.A., Gonzales, N.A. and Ortiz, C.D. (2009) Psychosocial Interventions for School Refusal Behaviour in Children and Adolescents. *Child Development Perspectives*, **3**, 11-20.
http://dx.doi.org/10.1111/j.1750-8606.2008.00070.x

[14] Egger, H.L., Costello, E.J. and Angold, A. (2003) School Refusal and Psychiatric Disorders: A Community Study. *Journal of the American Academy of Child & Adolescent Psychiatry*, **42**, 797-807.
http://dx.doi.org/10.1097/01.CHI.0000046865.56865.79

[15] Ingul, J.M., Klockner, C.A., Silverman, W.K. and Nordahl, H.M. (2012) Adolescent School Absenteeism: Modelling Social and Individual Risk Factors. *Child and Adolescent Mental Health*, **17**, 93-100.
http://dx.doi.org/10.1111/j.1475-3588.2011.00615.x

[16] Kearney, C.A. and Albano, A.M. (2004) The Functional Profiles of School Refusal Behaviour: Diagnostic Aspects. *Behaviour Modification*, **28**, 147-161. http://dx.doi.org/10.1177/0145445503259263

[17] McShane, G., Walter, G. and Rey, J.M. (2001) Characteristics of Adolescents with School Refusal. *Australian and New Zealand Journal of Psychiatry*, **35**, 822-826. http://dx.doi.org/10.1046/j.1440-1614.2001.00955.x

[18] Rumberger, R.W. and Larson, K.A. (1998) Student Mobility and the Increased Risk of High School Dropout. *American Journal of Education*, **107**, 1-35. http://dx.doi.org/10.1086/444201

[19] Way, N., Reddy, R. and Rhodes, J. (2007) Students' Perceptions of School Climate during Middle School Years: Associations with Trajectories of Psychological and Behavioural Adjustment. *American Journal of Community Psychology*, **40**, 194-213. http://dx.doi.org/10.1007/s10464-007-9143-y

[20] Brookmeyer, K.A., Fanti, K.A. and Henrich, G.C. (2006) Schools, Parents, and Youth Violence: A Multilevel, Ecological Analysis. *Journal of Clinical Child and Adolescent Psychology*, **35**, 504-514.
http://dx.doi.org/10.1207/s15374424jccp3504_2

[21] Havik, T., Bru, E. and Ertesvag, S.K. (2013) Parental Perspectives of the Role of School Factors in School Refusal. *Emotional & Behavioural Difficulties*, **19**, 131-153. http://dx.doi.org/10.1080/13632752.2013.816199

[22] Teasley, M.L. (2004) Absenteeism and Truancy: Risk, Protection and Best Practice Implications for School Social Workers. *Children & Schools*, **26**, 117-126. http://dx.doi.org/10.1093/cs/26.2.117

[23] Kleine, P.A. (1994) Chronic Absenteeism: A Community Issue. National Centre for Research on Teacher Learning, East Lansing.

[24] Thornberry, T.P., Smith, C.A., Rivera, C., Huizinga, D. and Stouthamer-Loeber, M. (1999) Family Disruption and Delinquency. National Centre for Research on Teacher Learning, East Lansing.

[25] Reid, K. (2005) The Causes, Views and Traits of School Absenteeism and Truancy: An Analytical Review. *Research in Education*, **74**, 59-82. http://dx.doi.org/10.7227/RIE.74.6

[26] Kearney, C.A. (2008) An Interdisciplinary Model of School Absenteeism in Youth to Inform Professional Practice and Public policy. *Educational Psychology Review*, **20**, 257-282. http://dx.doi.org/10.1007/s10648-008-9078-3

[27] Hill, N.E. and Tyson, D.F. (2009) Parental Involvement in Middle School: A Meta-Analytic Assessment of the Strategies That Promote Achievement. *Developmental Psychology*, **45**, 740-763. http://dx.doi.org/10.1037/a0015362

[28] Romero, M. and Lee, Y. (2008) The Influence of Maternal and Family Risk on Chronic Absenteeism in Early Schooling. National Centre for Children in Poverty, Columbia University, New York.

[29] Rafferty, Y. (1995) The Legal Rights and Education Problems of Homeless Children and Youth. *Educational Evaluation and Policy Analysis*, **17**, 39-61. http://dx.doi.org/10.3102/01623737017001039

[30] Casas-Gil, M.J. and Navarro-Guzman, J.I. (2002) School Characteristics among Children of Alcoholic Parents. *Psychological Reports*, **90**, 341-348. http://dx.doi.org/10.2466/pr0.2002.90.1.341

[31] Han, W.-J. (2005) Maternal Nonstandard Work Schedules and Child Outcomes. *Child Development*, **76**, 137-154.
http://dx.doi.org/10.1111/j.1467-8624.2005.00835.x

[32] Gottfried, M.A. (2009) Excused versus Unexcused: How Student Absences in Elementary School Affect Academic Achievement. *Education Evaluation and Policy Analysis*, **31**, 392-415. http://dx.doi.org/10.3102/0162373709342467

[33] Gottfried, M.A. (2014) Can Neighbor Attributes Predict School Absences? *Urban Education*, **49**, 216-250.
http://dx.doi.org/10.1177/0042085913475634

[34] Jargowsky, P.A. and El Komi, M. (2009) Before or After the Bell? School Context and Neighborhood Effects on Student Achievement. Calder Working Paper No. 28, National Centre for Analysis of Longitudinal Data in Education Research, Washington DC.

[35] Dietz, R. and Haurin, D.R. (2003) The Private and Social Micro-Level Consequences of Homeownership. *Journal of Urban Economics*, **54**, 401-450. http://dx.doi.org/10.1016/S0094-1190(03)00080-9

[36] Sharkey, P. (2010) The Acute Effect of Local Homicides on Children's Cognitive Performance. *Proceedings of the National Academy of Sciences of the United States of America*, **107**, 11733-11738. http://dx.doi.org/10.1073/pnas.1000690107

[37] Ready, D.D. (2010) Socioeconomic Disadvantage, School Attendance, and Early Cognitive Development: The Differential Effects of School Exposure. *Sociology of Education*, **83**, 271-286. http://dx.doi.org/10.1177/0038040710383520

[38] Benner, A.D. and Graham, S. (2011) Latino Adolescents' Experiences of Discrimination Across the First 2 Years of High School: Correlates and Influences on Educational Outcomes. *Child Development*, **82**, 508-519. http://dx.doi.org/10.1111/j.1467-8624.2010.01524.x

[39] Berliner, D.C. (2009) Poverty and Potential: Out-of-School Factors and School Success. Education and the Public Interest Centre & Education Policy Research Unit, Boulder and Tempe.

[40] Bryant-Stephens, T. (2009) Asthama Disparities in Urban Environments. *Journal of Allergy and Clinical Immunology*, **123**, 1199-1206. http://dx.doi.org/10.1016/j.jaci.2009.04.030

[41] Burton, C.M., Marshal, M.P. and Chisolm, D.J. (2014) School Absenteeism and Mental Health among Sexual Minority Youth and Heterosexual Youth. *Journal of School Psychology*, **52**, 37-47. http://dx.doi.org/10.1016/j.jsp.2013.12.001

[42] Kosciw, J. and Diaz, E. (2006) 2005 National School Climate Survey: The Experiences of Lesbian, Gay, Bisexual and Transgender Youth in Our Nation's Schools. Gay, Lesbian and Straight Education Network, New York.

[43] Kosciw, J., Greytak, E. and Diaz, E. (2009) Who, What, Where, When and Why: Demographic and Ecological Factors Contributing to Hostile School Climate for Lesbian, Gay, Bisexual and Transgender Youth. *Journal of Youth and Adolescence*, **28**, 976-988. http://dx.doi.org/10.1007/s10964-009-9412-1

[44] McGuire, J.K., Anderson, C.R., Toomey, R.B. and Russell, S.T. (2010) School Climate for Transgender Youth: A Mixed Method Investigation of Student Experiences and School Responses. *Journal of Youth and Adolescence*, **39**, 1175-1188. http://dx.doi.org/10.1007/s10964-010-9540-7

[45] Bontempo, D.E. and D'Augelli, A.R. (2002). Effects of At-School Victimization and Sexual Orientation on Lesbian, Gay, or Bisexual Youths' Health Risk Behaviour. *The Journal of Adolescent Health*, **30**, 364-374. http://dx.doi.org/10.1016/S1054-139X(01)00415-3

[46] Bochenek, M. and Brown, A.W. (2001) Hatred in the Hallways: Violence and Discrimination against Lesbian, Gay, Bisexual, and Transgender Students in US Schools. Human Rights Watch, New York.

[47] Ueno, K. (2005) Sexual Orientation and Psychological Distress in Adolescence: Examining Interpersonal Stressors and Social Support Processes. *Social Psychology Quarterly*, **68**, 258-277. http://dx.doi.org/10.1177/019027250506800305

[48] Pearson, J., Muller, C. and Wilkinson, L. (2007) Adolescent Same-Sex Attraction and Academic Outcomes: The Role of School Attachment and Engagement. *Social Problems*, **54**, 523-542. http://dx.doi.org/10.1525/sp.2007.54.4.523

[49] Russell, S.T., McGuire, J.K., Laub, C., Manke, E., O'Shaughnessy, M., Heck, K. and Calhoun, C. (2006) Harassment in School Based on Actual or Perceived Sexual Orientation: Prevalence and Consequences. California Research Brief No. 2, California Safe Schools Coalition, San Francisco.

[50] Harris Interactive and GLSEN (2005) From Teasing to Torment: School Climate in America, a Survey of Students and Teachers. GLSEN, New York.

[51] Birkett, M., Espelage, D.L. and Koenig, B. (2009) LGB and Questioning Students in Schools: The Moderating Effects of Homophobic Bullying and School Climate on Negative Outcomes. *Journal of Youth and Adolescence*, **39**, 989-1000. http://dx.doi.org/10.1007/s10964-008-9389-1

[52] Goodenow, C., Szalacha, L. and Westheimer, K. (2006) School Support Groups, Other School Factors, and the Safety of Sexual Minority Adolescents. *Psychology in the Schools*, **43**, 573-589. http://dx.doi.org/10.1002/pits.20173

[53] Maric, M., Heyne, D.A., MacKinnon, D.P., van Widenfelt, B.M. and Westenburg, P.M. (2012) Cognitive Mediation of Cognitive-Behavioural Therapy Outcomes for Anxiety-Based School Refusal. *Behavioural and Cognitive Psychotherapy*, **41**, 549-564. http://dx.doi.org/10.1017/S1352465812000756

[54] Maynard, B.R., McCrea, K.T., Pigott, T.D. and Kelly, M.S. (2012) Indicated Truancy Interventions: Effects on School Attendance among Chronic Truant Students. *Campbell Systematic Reviews*, **8**, 8.

[55] Hatzenbuehler, M.L. (2011) The Social Environment and Suicide Attempts in Lesbian, Gay, and Bisexual Youth. *Pediatrics*, **127**, 896-903. http://dx.doi.org/10.1542/peds.2010-3020

[56] Walls, N.E., Kane, S.B. and Wisneski, H. (2010) Gay—Straight Alliances and School Experiences of Sexual Minority Youth. *Youth & Society*, **41**, 307-332. http://dx.doi.org/10.1177/0044118X09334957

[57] Bradshaw, C.O., Koth, C.W., Thornton, L.A. and Leaf, P.J. (2009) Altering School Climate through School-Wide Positive Behavioural Interventions and Supports: Findings from a Group-Randomizcd Effectiveness Trial. *Prevention Science*, **10**, 100-115. http://dx.doi.org/10.1007/s11121-008-0114-9

[58] Epstein, J.L. and Sheldon, S.B. (2002) Present and Accounted for: Improving Student Attendance through Family and Community Involvement. *Journal of Educational* Research, **95**, 308-318. http://dx.doi.org/10.1080/00220670209596604

[59] Sheldon, S.B. (2007) Improving Student Attendance with School, Family, and Community Partnerships. *The Journal of Educational Research*, **100**, 267-275. http://dx.doi.org/10.3200/JOER.100.5.267-275

[60] Schorr, L.B. (1997) Common Purpose: Strengthening Families and Neighborhoods to Rebuild America. Doubleday, New York.

6

Is the Walking Campaign Effective for Depressive Symptoms?

Setsuko Taneichi, Fumiharu Togo, Tsukasa Sasaki

Laboratory of Health Education, Graduate School of Education, Tokyo, Japan
Email: staneichi21@gmail.com, tougou@p.u-tokyo.ac.jp, psytokyo@yahoo.co.jp

Abstract

Aim: The aim of this study is to examine the effect of walking 10,000 steps per day on depressive symptoms for the company employees and their spouses in Japan. **Method:** Subjects were recruited from the participants of a walking campaign carried out by a Japanese company where the goal was to achieve 600,000 steps in 60 days. Among 221 subjects who participated in the campaign, 176 subjects (79.6%) agreed to participate in the present study. Sociodemographics and other information including depressive symptoms were assessed using a questionnaire. **Result:** Out of the 171 participants, 125 achieved the goal (73.1%). In the achiever's group, the GHQ-12 score was significantly reduced at the end of the campaign compared with the non-achiever's group. Exercise habit and the less overtime work (<45 hours past 1 month) at the baseline were significantly associated with the achievement of the goal. **Conclusion:** The achievement of 600,000 steps in 60 days is correlated with the improvement of depressive symptoms and the achievement of this goal might be related with the exercise habit and less overtime work before the campaign.

Keywords

Depressive Symptoms, 10,000 Steps, Physical Activity, Walking, Walking Campaign

1. Introduction

Depression is one of the most common diseases in developed countries and is predicted to become the world's second leading cause of disability by 2020 [1]. The pharmacotherapy is included in the popular management of depressive symptoms. However, physical activity is also effective to manage depressive symptoms. Several studies showed lower depressive symptoms among physically active people compared to non-active people [2] [3].

According to a review by Teychenne (2008) [4], physical activity of higher intensity was more strongly associated with effective treatment of depressive symptoms than those of lower intensities, but even a low dose of physical activity may bring about a positive result for treatment of depressive symptoms [4].

Although more intense physical activity may have a positive effect on the treatment of depressive symptoms, physical activity of vigorous intensity may be a challenge to continue for people without an exercise habit [5]. The portion of the people who can continue physical activity of vigorous intensity may be limited [6]. For those people, walking may be one of the most feasible and common physical activities. Walking is a physical activity of mild to moderate intensity and requires no financial cost and minimal risk of adverse effects [7]. According to a review by Robertson, walking has a statistically significant positive effect on treatment of depressive symptoms [1].

A number of Japanese companies are carrying out walking campaigns for the purpose of health promotion for their employees. The goal set for this campaign is 10,000 steps per day for 60 or 90 days at most of the companies connected with the same health insurance union in Japan.

The aim of the campaign has been focused on its effect on physical health. The effect of walking on mental health, including the treatment of depressive symptoms, is also covered by a review of Roberston et al. [2]. However their report doesn't describe the numbers of the steps of walking for the treatment of depressive symptoms.

In addition, few studies have investigated the effect of the walking campaign on depressive symptoms and several issues remain to be studied. The first issue is whether or not 10,000 steps per day, which is employed in most of the companies, is appropriate for the improvement of depressive symptoms. 10,000 steps is recommended by several guidelines [8] [9], because a number of studies showed the effect of the 10,000 steps to improve physical health [10] [11], while no study focused on the effect of 10,000 steps on depressive symptoms. The second issue is whether the 10,000 steps per day for several months is sustainable for the employees. Related with this issue, what factors are associated with the achievement of 10,000 steps per day may also be a question to be studied. Thus, the aims of this study are summarized as follows. 1) Whether or not the 10,000 steps per day walking campaign is effective for treatment of depressive symptoms. 2) What factors of the individuals are associated with the achievement of the 10,000 steps per day over several months?

2. Materials and Method

2.1. Method and Patient Selection

The walking campaign was carried out from April 2012 to May 2012 by a Japanese energy company with 2200 Japanese employees. The company advertised the campaign to the all employees and their spouses. 221 subjects participated in the walking campaign. Among the 221, 176 subjects (79.6%) agreed to participate in the presented research. The participants who did not answer the questionnaire at the end of the walking campaign were excluded from the analyses. Finally, 171 participants (100 males and 71 females, mean age 45.4 ± 10.4) who answered the questionnaires both at the baseline and at the end of the walking campaign were studied. All male participants were the company employees and the female participants consisted of 38 employees and 33 spouses of the male employees. These are not overlapping groups.

The pedometers (Yamasa mk-365, Japan Tokyo) were given to the participants before the start of the walking campaign (baseline). The participants were asked to complete the questionnaire with the following information: sociodemographic and other information including age, sex, job content (indoor or housework, outdoor), hours of overtime work (within the past 1 month; <45 hours, ≥45 hours) [12], sleep duration (within the past 1 month; 6 hours, ≥6 hours) [13], exercise habit as recreation (Yes, No). The goal of the campaign was 600,000 steps in 60 days (10,000 steps per day on average) during the period of the campaign. Depressive symptoms were also assessed using the Japanese version GHQ-12 (general health questionnaire-12) [14].

2.2. Statistical Analysis

A student's t-test was used to examine the difference of age and the GHQ-12 score between achiever's and non-achiever's groups. The changes of GHQ-12 score overtime between achiever's and non-achiever's group was assessed using analysis of covariance (repeated measures ANCOVA), with overtime work and exercise habit as covariates. All statistical analyses were carried out using SPSS 17.0 (IBM, New York, US).

3. Result

Table 1 shows the demographic characteristics between achiever's and non-achiever's group. 125 among the

171 participants achieved the goal (≥600,000 steps in 60 days; 10,000 steps per day for 60 days on average) (73.1%). At the baseline, the GHQ-12 score was not significantly different between the achiever's group and non-achiever's group. However, at the end of the campaign, the GHQ-12 score of the non-achiever's group was significantly higher than the achiever's group. Exercise habit and the less overtime work (<45 hours per month) at the baseline were significantly associated with the achievement.

Table 2 shows the changes of GHQ-12 score of achiever's and non-achiever's groups. *Post hoc* tests showed that the achiever's group at the end of the campaign exhibited reduced GHQ-12 score (1.42 ± 1.78) in comparison to the baseline (2.16 ± 2.41). *Post hoc* tests also showed that the achiever's group at the end of the campaign exhibited lower GHQ-12 score (1.42 ± 1.78) in comparison to non-achiever's group (2.72 ± 3.03). By using the analysis of repeated measures ANOVA, the difference of GHQ-12 score between achiever's and non-achiever's group was significant (main effect). However, adjusted for overtime work and exercise habit, there were no significant differences for time and group.

Table 1. Demographics and the other characteristics of the subjects at the baseline.

		Achiever	(%)	Non-achiever	(%)	p-value
Age (year)		45.60 ± 10.59		45.11 ± 9.65		NS
Sex	Male	75	(73.5)	27	(26.5)	NS
	Female	55	(74.3)	19	(25.7)	
Job content	Indoor or housework	50	(69.4)	22	(30.6)	NS
	Outdoor	77	(77.8)	22	(22.2)	
Overtime work	<45 hours	122	(77.2)	36	(22.8)	*
(past 1 month)	≥45 hours	9	(47.3)	10	(52.6)	
Sleep duration	<6 hours	67	(74.4)	23	(25.6)	NS
(past 1 month)	≥6 hours	64	(73.6)	23	(26.4)	
Exercise habit	No	47	(64.4)	26	(35.6)	*
	Yes	85	(81.0)	20	(19.0)	
GHQ-12 score	At the baseline	2.16 ± 2.41		2.89 ± 2.53		NS
	At the end of the campaign	1.43 ± 1.78		2.78 ± 3.03		*

Age and GHQ-12 score was analysed by student's t-test. Sex, job content, overtime work, sleep duartion, exercise habit were analysed by χ^2 test. Age and GHQ-12 score: mean ± SD. NS: not significant. *p < 0.05.

Table 2. The changes of GHQ-12 score over time achiever's and non-achiever's groups.

							Adjusted for overtime work		Adjusted for exercise habit	
All	Achiever's group		Non-achiever's group		Group × Time		Group × Time		Group × Time	
(n = 171)	(n = 125)		(n = 46)							
	Mean	SD	Mean	SD	F	p	F	p	F	p
GHQ-12 mean score										
At the baseline	2.16	2.41	2.89	2.53	8.97	**	1.24	0.27	0.545	0.462
At the end of the campaign	1.42†	1.78	2.72	3.03						

Repeated measures ANOVA was used to evaluated the changes in GHQ-12 scores. Repeated measures ANCOVA was used to evaluated the changes in GHQ-12 scores over time with overtime work and exercise habit as covariates. **p < 0.005. †*Post hoc* tests showed that the achiever's group at the end of the campaign exhibited reduced GHQ-12 score (1.42 ± 1.78) in comparison to the baseline (2.16 ± 2.41). *Post hoc* tests also showed that the achiever's group at the end of the campaign exhibited lower GHQ-12 score (1.42 ± 1.78) in comparison to non-achiever's group (2.72 ±3.03).

4. Discussion

At the baseline, the GHQ-12 score was not different between the achiever's group and non-achiever's group. At the end of the campaign, the GHQ-12 score was significantly reduced in the achiever's group. On the other hand, the GHQ-12 score did not change in the non-achiever's group. This suggests that the achievement of the 600,000 steps for 60 days may assist with treatment of depressive symptoms. Less overtime work (<45 hours per month) and exercise habits maintained before the start of the campaign were significantly associated with the achievement. The repeated measure ANOVA for GHQ-12 score revealed a significant main effect for time and group. This main effect means that GHQ-12 score significantly decreased from at the baseline to the end of the campaign in the achiever's group, but not in the non-achiever's group. Adjusted by overtime work or exercise habit, there were no significant differences for time and group. This result suggest that the subjects who work overtime within 45 hours and have exercise habit before campaign are the most effective to improve the depressive symptoms by participating in the campaign.

In the present study, 26.9% did not achieve the goal. Considering this rate of the achievement and that only 10% of the company employees participated in the campaign, whether the 10,000 steps is sustainable for company employees and their spouses may be also an important issue for the treatment of depressive symptoms. One of the factors associated with the non-achievement was overtime work. The association might be due to the lack of time for walking or exercise in subjects who have more overtime work. This should be noted because the workers who work overtime may have an increased risk of depressive symptoms [15] [16]. A considerable portion of the employees might not be able to participate in the campaigns due to the overtime work. In addition, this may be a major limitation of the walking campaigns in Japanese companies.

The present study has several limitations. First, the causal relation between the physical activity and depressive symptoms is not clear due to the study design. It is possible that improved mental health helped to facilitate walking. Second, the association between physical activity and improvement of depressive symptoms could be confounded by several unknown variables, but they were not controlled for in the present study. Third, the timing of the physical activity (during the working-time, commuting-time, housework-time, and leisure-time) is unknown. Several studies showed a stronger association between leisure-time physical activity and improvement of depressive symptoms than other timing physical activity [17]-[20]. Future studies may need the analyses of the optional timing of physical activity for decreasing depressive symptoms. Fourth, statistical power may be limited due to the number of the participants, especially in females. While the male participants consisted of employees only, the females consisted of both the employees and their spouses. Studies in larger sample size, especially in females are needed.

5. Conclusion

The achievement of 600,000 steps in 60 days may be associated with the improvement of depressive symptoms. The achievement of the goal might be related with the exercise habit and overtime work (below 45 hours before the start of the walking campaign). In the setting of the goal (the number of the walking steps per day), exercise habit and work condition (overtime work) might be considered.

Acknowledgements

This study was supported by a grant from National Federation of Workers and Consumers Insurance Cooperatives.

Declaration of Interest

No conflict of interest declared.

References

[1]   Robertson, R., Robertson, A., Jepson, R. and Maxwell, M. (2012) Walking for Depression or Depressive Symptoms: A Systematic Review and Meta-Analysis. *Mental Health and Physical Activity*, 6, 66-75.
      http://dx.doi.org/10.1016/j.mhpa.2012.03.002

[2]   Johnson, K.E. and Taliaferro, L.A. (2011) Relationships between Physical Activity and Depressive Symptoms among Middle and Older Adolescents: A Review of the Research Literature. *Journal for Specialists in Pediatric Nursing*, 16,

235-251. http://dx.doi.org/10.1111/j.1744-6155.2011.00301.x

[3] Brown, H.E., Pearson, N., Braithwaite, R.E., Brown, W.J. and Biddle, S.J. (2013) Physical Activity Interventions and Depression in Children and Adolescents: A Systematic Review and Meta-Analysis. *Sports Medicine*, **43**, 195-206. http://dx.doi.org/10.1007/s40279-012-0015-8

[4] Teychenne, M., Ball, K. and Salmon, J. (2008) Physical Activity and Likelihood of Depression in Adults: A Review. *Preventive Medicine*, **46**, 397-411. http://dx.doi.org/10.1016/j.ypmed.2008.01.009

[5] Sallis, J.F., Greenlee, L. and McKenzie, T.L. (2001). Changes and Tracking of Physical Activity across Seven Years in Mexican-American and European-American Mothers. *Women Health*, **34**, 1-14. http://dx.doi.org/10.1300/J013v34n04_01

[6] Sallis, J.F., Hovell, M.F. and Richard Hofstetter, C. (1992) Predictors of Adoption and Maintenance of Vigorous Physical Activity in Men and Women. *Preventive Medicine*, **3**, 237-251. http://dx.doi.org/10.1016/0091-7435(92)90022-A

[7] Craig, C.L., Tudor-Locke, C. and Bauman, A. (2007) Twelve-Month Effects of Canada on the Move: A Population-Wide Campaign to Promote Pedometer Use and Walking. *Health Education Research*, **22**, 406-413. http://dx.doi.org/10.1093/her/cyl093

[8] Tudor-Locke, C., Burkett, L., Reis, J.P., Ainsworth, B.E., Macera, C.A. and Wilson, D.K. (2005) How Many Days of Pedometer Monitoring Predict Weekly Physical Activity in Adults? *Preventive Medicine*, **40**, 293-298. http://dx.doi.org/10.1016/j.ypmed.2004.06.003

[9] Tudor-Locke, C., Craig, C.L., Aoyagi, Y., *et al.* (2011) How Many Steps/Day Are Enough? For Older Adults and Special Populations. *International Journal of Behavioral Nutrition and Physical Activity*, **28**, 80. http://dx.doi.org/10.1186/1479-5868-8-80

[10] Tudor-Locke, C., Craig, C.L., Brown, W.J., *et al.* (2011) How Many Steps/Day Are Enough? For Adults. *International Journal of Behavioral Nutrition and Physical Activity*, **28**, 79. http://dx.doi.org/10.1186/1479-5868-8-79

[11] Iwane, M., Arita, M., Tomimoto, S., Satani, O., Matsumoto, M., Miyashita, K. and Nishio, I. (2000) Walking 10,000 Steps/Day or More Reduces Blood Pressure and Sympathetic Nerve Activity in Mild Essential Hypertension. *Hypertension Research*, **23**, 573-580. http://dx.doi.org/10.1291/hypres.23.573

[12] Uchida, M., Kaneko, M. and Kawa, S. (2014) Effects of Personality on Overtime Work: A Cross-Sectional Pilot Study among Japanese White-Collar Workers. *BMC Research Notes*, **7**, 180.

[13] van Mill, J.G., Vogelzangs, N., van Someren, E.J., Hoogendijk, W.J. and Penninx, B.W. (2014) Sleep Duration, but Not Insomnia, Predicts the 2-Year Course of Depressive and Anxiety Disorders. *Journal of Clinical Psychiatry*, **75**, 119-126. http://dx.doi.org/10.4088/JCP.12m08047

[14] Armstrong, K. and Edwards, H. (2003) The Effects of Exercise and Social Support on Mothers Reporting Depressive Symptoms: A Pilot Randomized Controlled Trial. *International Journal of Mental Health Nursing*, **12**, 130-138. http://dx.doi.org/10.1046/j.1440-0979.2003.00229.x

[15] Proctor, S.P., White, R.F., Robins, T.G., Echeverria, D. and Rocskay, A.Z. (1996) Effect of Overtime Work on Cognitive Function in Automotive Workers. *Scandinavian Journal of Work, Environment & Health*, **22**, 124-132. http://dx.doi.org/10.5271/sjweh.120

[16] Chalupka, S. (2012) Overtime Work as a Predictor of a Major Depressive Episode. *Workplace Health Saf*, **60**, 192-20120328-26.

[17] Wise, L.A., Adams-Campbell, L.L., Palmer, J.R. and Rosenberg, L. (2006) Leisure Time Physical Activity in Relation to Depressive Symptoms in the Black Women's Health Study. *Annals of Behavioral Medicine*, **32**, 68-76. http://dx.doi.org/10.1207/s15324796abm3201_8

[18] Chen, L.J., Stevinson, C., Ku, P.W., Chang, Y.K. and Chu, D.C. (2012) Relationships of Leisure-Time and Non-Leisure-Time Physical Activity with Depressive Symptoms: A Population-Based Study of Taiwanese Older Adults. *International Journal of Behavioral Nutrition and Physical Activity*, **9**, 28.

[19] Torres, E.R., Sampselle, C.M., Ronis, D.L., Neighbors, H.W. and Gretebeck, K.A. (2013) Leisure-Time Physical Activity in Relation to Depressive Symptoms in African-Americans: Results from the National Survey of American Life. *Preventive Medicine*, **56**, 410-412. http://dx.doi.org/10.1016/j.ypmed.2013.02.013

[20] Yang, X., Telama, R., Hirvensalo, M., Hintsanen, M., Hintsa, T., Pulkki-Råback, L., *et al.* (2012) Moderating Effects of Leisure-Time Physical Activity on the Association between Job Strain and Depressive Symptoms: The Cardiovascular Risk in Young Finns Study. *Journal of Occupational & Environmental Medicine*, **54**, 303-309. http://dx.doi.org/10.1097/JOM.0b013e318240df39

7

Cultural Influences on the Presentation of Depression

Ahmed Mohamed Abdel Shafi[1], Reem Mohamed Abdel Shafi[2]

[1]Barts and The London School of Medicine and Dentistry, London, UK
[2]Fremantle Hospital, Fremantle, Australia
Email: a.m.a.shafi@smd10.qmul.ac.uk, Reem.Shafi@health.wa.gov.au

Abstract

Depression is predicted to become the second highest disease burden by 2020 as well as being a common mental health condition across the globe. Nevertheless, the presentation of depression varies depending on several factors with the patient's cultural background playing a significant role. Although depression is such a universal condition, the manner of how a patient presents not only affects the clinician's ability to make a diagnosis, but ultimately affects the wellbeing of the patient. It is therefore paramount that as clinicians we appreciate how culture not only affects the presentation of depression but also how cultural beliefs affect the patient's acceptance of such a diagnosis.

Keywords

Depression, Cultural Psychiatry, Affective Disorder

1. Introduction

Depression is an important diagnosis for doctors to make. Its prevalence is increasing and is a condition that some patients may not readily seek help for and suffer in silence. Due to advances in travel technology, there has been a worldwide phenomenon of cultural integration, leading to the phrase "multicultural". However, due to the vast number of cultures there are different beliefs and opinions on many aspects. The focus of this review will be on how culture affects the way suffering patients present with depression.

2. Epidemiology of Depression

It is important to appreciate just how common depression is before delving into the subject matter. It is estimated that one in four people will suffer with a mental disorder at some time in their life time. Depression is predicted to be the second highest disease burden by 2020 as per the World Health Organisation (WHO) [1].

Since the UK population is living longer psychiatric conditions will increase in prevalence. In 2002 depression was estimated to account for approximately around 4.5% of the total disease burden (in terms of disability) worldwide [2].

The prevalence of several psychiatric disorders were compared and published in 2009, looking at the incidence over a 14 years period, showing that depression was the most common, illustrated in the following graph [3] [4].

Prevalence of common mental health problems

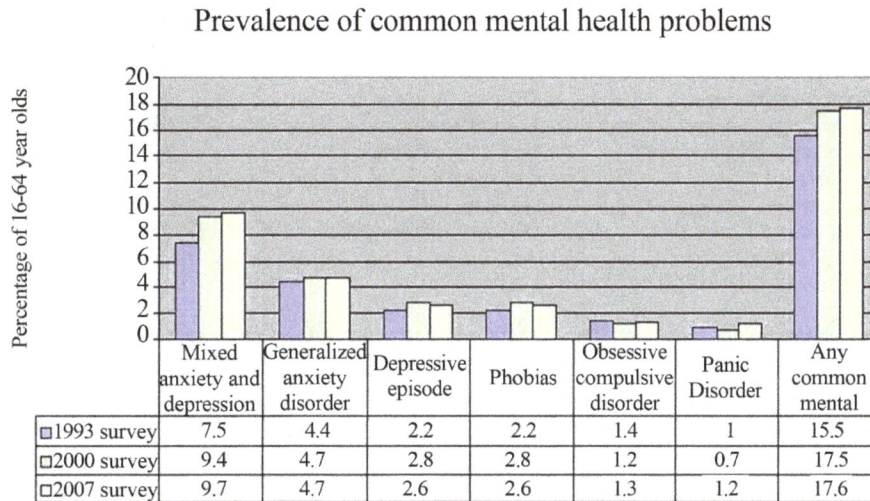

	Mixed anxiety and depression	Generalized anxiety disorder	Depressive episode	Phobias	Obsessive compulsive disorder	Panic Disorder	Any common mental
☐ 1993 survey	7.5	4.4	2.2	2.2	1.4	1	15.5
☐ 2000 survey	9.4	4.7	2.8	2.8	1.2	0.7	17.5
☐ 2007 survey	9.7	4.7	2.6	2.6	1.3	1.2	17.6

Graph shows the prevalence of common mental health problems since 1993 [3].

Depression is a condition which may worsen over a period of time and is commonly found in patients who already suffer with a chronic condition. In a study published in 2007 by Moussavi *et al.*, depression was found to produce the greatest decrement in the health of an individual when compared to other chronic conditions, illustrated in the following graph [5].

Mean health score by disease status, World health survey 2003

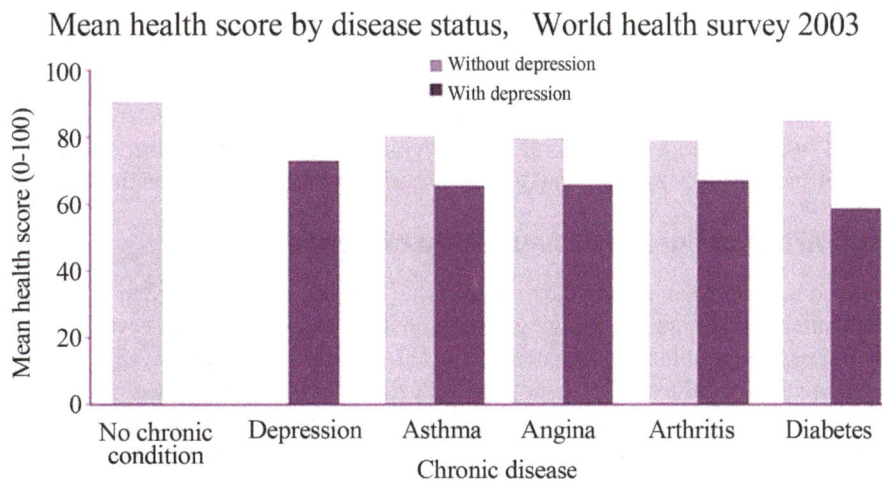

Graph illustrating the prevalence of depression in a number of chronic diseases [2].

3. Depression: Its Symptoms and Presentations

Depression is a mood disorder with three core features; low mood (excessive sadness), anhedonia and anergia. These should be present for over two weeks. Additional symptoms include negative thoughts and pessimistic views of oneself, the future and the present (Becks triad of depression). Cognitive, biological or psychotic symptoms may also be in attendance [6] [7].

Depression can be classified as mild, moderate, severe and severe with psychotic features. Some symptoms are more common than others as indicated in the following image [7]-[9].

Box 1.   Common clinical symptoms of major depression

Very common	*Common*	*Rare*
Low mood	Weight loss	Suicidal ideations
Irritability	Guilt feelings	Change in sexual activity
Anhedonia	Somatic complaints	Hallucinations
Decreased appetite	Self-injury	Delusions
Change in motor activity	Destruction of property	Eating disorder
Sleep disturbance	Diurnal variation in mood	Hysterical conversion
Fatigue	Loss of libido	Hypochondriasis
Decreased concentration	Loss of confidence	
Withdrawal	Constipation	
Aggression	Anxiety	
Tearfulness	Obsessions/compulsions	
Loss of interest		
Decline in social skills		

This summaries the very common, common and rare symptoms of major depression [9].

Depression is diagnosed using the ICD-10 criteria or the DSM-IV criteria, however there are no tests that can be carried out to confirm if a patient has depression. The diagnosis is based on the presenting complaints of a patient and is the physician's task to ask the relevant questions to make an accurate diagnosis.

Depression is not limited to a certain place or group of people and is therefore not confined by borders, racial background, age or wealth. The exact aetiology of depression remains unknown with multiple theories proposed. One of these is the monoamine theory, which hypothesises that depression may be due to a decrease in noradrenaline, serotonin or dopamine which explains why antidepressants work as a treatment by increasing the level of these neurotransmitters [8].

There are a number of risk factors that increase the likelihood of an individual developing depression e.g. female gender. A number of studies have shown that depression is more prevalent in women. Child-bearing women are also at risk of developing postpartum depression, with prevalence estimated to be 10% - 15% worldwide [10]. Other risk factors include (but are not limited to) suffering with a chronic condition, poverty, alcoholism, traumatic childhood experienced or bereavement, which may increase the chances of developing a stressful life.

In a study by McGirr *et al.*, individuals that suffered with depression had a greater risk of committing suicide, with the onset of insomnia being indicative of immediate suicide risk whereas other symptoms (loss of appetite, thoughts of death and feeling worthless) where characteristic for the predisposition for suicide [11].

4. Cultural Variations in the Presentation of Depression

Culture is defined as "the ideas, customs and social behaviour of a particular group of people or society", suggesting that culture is a dynamic and evolving process that varies over time. However the discussion of culture in Psychiatry focuses on minorities that are considered to be distinct in some way [12] [13].

The term culture can be influenced by your gender, age, race, religion, country of residence, country of origin and education. Globalisation has had a great effect on the integration of several cultures, with respect to cultural beliefs and ideology being accepted into other cultures. Several studies have looked into the variations in the presentation of depression, which could provide important clues as to why these variations occur.

A study by Kirmayer *et al.* (1993), found that the rate of diagnosis varied depending on how the patient presented. In some cultures visiting a doctor with depression is culturally unacceptable. It is therefore more common for these people to present with somatic symptoms, which is a frequently cited feature of depression. This may be viewed in some cultures to be a more appropriate reason to visit a doctor. This is referred to as "ticket behaviour" which may have less stigma associated with it, but can make it harder for the physician to diagnose depression and lead to unnecessary investigations as illustrated in the following graph [13] [14].

Styles of Clinical Presentation of Primary Care
Patients With Depression and Anxiety

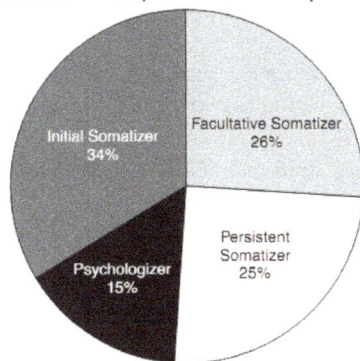

Rates of Primary Care Recognition of Depression
and Anxiety by Style of Clinical Presentation

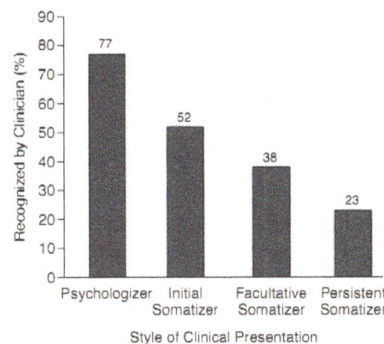

Pie chart shows the proportion of clinical presentation for patients with depression and anxiety. Bar chart shows the percentage of diagnosis of depression depending on the clinical presentation of the patient [13].

Another study by Bhugra *et al.*, concluded that the influence of culture and religion will lead to variation in presentation of depression, with somatic symptoms being the most common presenting compliant. This point is previously stated by Dejarlais *et al.*, when they thought that cultural background would determine whether or not depression was expressed in psychological or physical terms [15].

If we look at more specific studies we find different reasons for the variation in presentation. Looking at a study by Kleniman *et al.*, we find that in the mid 1980's only 1% of patients in a one week period who attend a psychiatric out patient's clinic in Hunan, China were diagnosed with depression. However 30% were diagnosed as "neurasthenic", which is commonly understood by the Chinese to mean "neurological weakness" which has become a common illness accepted by the public. Kleniman also noted that neurasthenia was a diagnosis more accepted by Chinese patients and their psychiatrists [16].

However a study by Yan *et al.*, noted that patients who were commonly diagnosed with neurasthenia presented with insomnia, headache and poor concentration [17]. Neurasthenia is therefore a non-stigmatising diagnosis which is distinct from any psychiatric label such as depression which can be perceived as degrading. In a study by Lee *et al.*, it described the popularity of the term "shenjongshuairuo" which is a translation of neurasthenia as "the indigenisation of a culture-friendly condition", unlike depression which has several meanings in Chinese including, "restrain" or "gloomy" thereby making it socially and morally unacceptable [17] [18]. From this we can appreciate that a term in a certain language may have a different meaning and interpretation in another.

In another study, Bhugra *et al.*, looked at Punjabi women of two generations, and found that pain was the most common symptom, which can be explained by understanding their culture. In Asian culture pain can mean suffering while at the same time disguising an underlying psychological disorder. The term depression was found to be recognised by the younger generation, whereas the older generation used terms such as "weight on my mind" or "pressure on the mind" [15].

On interviewing an Arab patient, he told me that in Arab culture "there is no depression as such" and made a distinction between depression and illness. He also believed that if you were a "good believer" you didn't deserve to be depressed and the solution is prayer rather than visiting a psychiatrist.

This view is reflected by other Arab patients as illustrated by Sulaiman *et al.*, who looked at opinions of Arab woman and men in Dubai. There were different opinions among woman in the importance of crying when depressed. The older generation viewed it as shameful, believing that their inner feelings should be hidden and kept to themselves. If the emotional burden became unbearable they should cry when alone, as highlighted in one quote, "we are Arabs, we never cry, we endure, but these new generations, they are so soft and weak, they cry for any reason". Whereas the young generations felt that expressing emotions through crying was more beneficial then hiding it, "a woman who cries feels better" [19].

The view of turning to God as an adequate cure to treat depression is shared among Arab men and women. The accepted coping resources are speaking to relatives, asking God for help, reading a religious scripture, praying or asking a religious leader for guidance. These are viewed more favourably compared with seeking help from a psychiatrist. When you feel depressed, "complaining to Allah is enough", "a psychiatrist cannot help the depressed patient if the problem which create this depression still exists" [19].

Both genders appreciated the fact that if treatment was not sought, depression could progress to madness "ji-noon", "it may increase suicidal ideas". This is interesting as although seeking treatment for depression from a psychiatrist was not a popular solution, there was an understanding that complications could arise without adequate treatment [19].

Another study also analysing Arab patients noted that they used metaphors and proverbs to describe their depression, such as "a dark life" in addition to describing physical symptoms, which are accepted as a legitimate and morally acceptable reason to go to the doctor. In a study by Bazzoui *et al.*, it states that the average Iraqi would come in with symptoms such as "oppression in the chest", or "hunger for air" to describe their depression [20].

5. The Issue of Stigma and Depression

Depression is considered in a number of cultures as degrading [18]. Patients may not readily seek help from a doctor instead turning to alternative means such as witch doctors or religious figures first. Stigma is therefore a barrier to treating depression and exacerbated by lack of public awareness and understanding of mental health [21].

There have been efforts in the past to combat stigma associated with depression. For example in 1992 an initiative entitled "defeat depression" was launched by the Royal College of Psychiatrists and Royal College of General Practitioners [22].

The role of stigma and depression is noted in Arab cultures, as a patient's resistance to report depression is usually associated with fear of embarrassment or shaming their family. As stated in the study by Sulaiman *et al.*, "our society looks at the person who visits the psychiatric clinic as though he is mad (majnoon) [19] [20].

The issue of stigma can be summed up by the fact that it is a label of infamy and social disgrace in which the individual's behaviour embarrasses family and friends. This can lead to fear of being disowned and brushed aside, leading patients to attempt concealing their true feelings as they don't have the confidence to confide in someone to share their burden. The unfortunate consequence then is that treatment is sometimes not sought until they find themselves in very desperate situations or several areas of their lives have been affected (e.g. employment, relationships). Stigma exacerbates a condition that already negatively impacts very vulnerable individuals and their families.

6. Conclusions

It is clear from available research studies of different cultures that the understanding, meaning and implications of depression for individuals vary across cultures and continents. Since integration of cultures has occurred in many countries, it is important for a doctor to have some appreciation as to how a patient's culture will affect their presentation, beliefs and acceptance of a diagnosis like depression.

In Western society the term depression is perhaps accepted more freely compared with other cultures. The term is readily used in everyday conversation, "I'm so depressed when we have exams". However despite this, stigma is still a significant factor that hinders presentation and the progress of depressed patients. It is a doctor's responsibility and duty to combat stigma by remaining open minded and facilitating clinical encounters with the aim of enabling the patient to confide in the doctor, safe in the knowledge that it is our aim to listen, treat and help without judgment.

It is therefore befitting to end with a statement by Skottowe, "The initial psychiatric interview is always important, but in no group of illnesses is it of greater importance as a first step in treatment than it is in the depressions. The gentle elucidation of all the symptoms is of the highest importance. Let the patient see that the doctor is thoroughly familiar with the kind of illness that confronts him; he knows the kind of feelings and thoughts that it brings the patient. This in itself is a most reassuring step" [23].

Acknowledgements

We would like to thank Professor Korzsun, Dr. Bains and Dr. Darwiche for their advice and help. We would also like to thank our family and friends for their support.

References

[1]   World Health Organisation. Mental Health, Disorders Management, Depression.
       http://www.who.int/mental_health/management/depression/en/

[2]   World Health Organisation (WHO). World Heath Statistics 2007: Part 1—Ten Statistical Highlights in Global Public
       Health, 16.

[3]   Mind.org.uk, for Better Mental Health, How Can We Help You, Mental Health Statistics, How Common Are Mental
       Health Problems.
       http://www.mind.org.uk/information-support/types-of-mental-health-problems/statistics-and-facts-about-mental-health/

[4]   McManus, S., Meltzer, H., Brugha, T.S., Bebbington, P.E. and Jenkins, R. (2009) Adult Psychiatric Morbidity in Eng-
       land, 2007: Results of a Household Survey.

[5]   Moussavi, S., Chatterji, S., Verdes, E., *et al.* (2007) Depression, Chronic Diseases, and Decrements in Health: Results
       from the World Health Surveys. *The Lancet*, **370**, 851-858.
       http://dx.doi.org/10.1016/S0140-6736(07)61415-9

[6]   Martin, E. (2007) Concise Medical Dictionary. 7th Edition, Oxford University Press, Oxford, 195.

[7]   Bourke, J., Castle, M. and Cameron, A.D. (2008) Crash Course: Psychiatry. 3rd Edition, MOSBY Elsevier, Amsterdam,
       xii and 99-102.

[8]   Stringer, S., Church, L., Davison, S. and Lipsedge, M. (2009) Psychiatry P.R.N.—Principles. Reality. Next Steps. Ox-
       ford University Press, Oxford, 32-40.

[9]   Prasher, V. (1999) Presentation and Management of Depression in People with Learning Disability. *Advances in Psy-
       chiatric Treatment*, **5**, 447-454.

[10]   Halbreich, U. and Karkun, S. (2006) Cross-Cultural and Social Diversity of Prevalence of Postpartum Depression and
       Depressive Symptoms. *Journal of Affective Disorders*, **9**, 97-111. http://dx.doi.org/10.1016/j.jad.2005.12.051

[11]   McGirr, A., Renaud, J., Seguin, M., Alda, M., Benkelfat, C., Lesage, A., *et al.* (2007) An Examination of DSM-IV De-
       pressive Symptoms and Risk for Suicide Completion in Major Depressive Disorder: A Psychological Autopsy Study.
       Journal of Affective Disorders, **97**, 203-209. http://dx.doi.org/10.1016/j.jad.2006.06.016

[12]   (2011) Oxford Dictionaries, Dictionary, Meaning of Culture. Oxford University Press, Oxford.

[13]   Kirmayer, L.J. (2001) Cultural Variations in the Clinical Presentation of Depression and Anxiety: Implications for Di-
       agnosis and Treatment. *Journal of Clinical Psychiatry*, **62**, 22-30

[14]   Kirmayer, L.J., Robbins, J.M., Dworkind, M. and Yaffe, M.J. (1993) Somatization and the Recognition of Depression
       and Anxiety in Primary Care. *American Journal of Psychiatry*, **150**, 734-741

[15]   Bhugra, D. and Mastrogianni, A. (2006) Globalisation and Mental Disorders: Overview with Relation to Depression.
       The British Journal of Psychiatry, **184**, 10-20. http://dx.doi.org/10.1192/bjp.184.1.10

[16]   Kleinman, A., Anderson, J.M., Finkler, K., Frankenberg, R.J. and Young, A. (1986) Social Origins of Distress and Di-
       sease: Depression, Neurasthenia, and Pain in Modern China. Yale University Press, New Haven.

[17]   Parker, G., Gladstone, G. and Chee, K.T. (2001) Depression in the Planet's Largest Ethnic Group: The Chinese. *Ame-
       rican Journal of Psychiatry*, **158**, 857-864. http://dx.doi.org/10.1176/appi.ajp.158.6.857

[18]   Lee, S. (1998) Estranged Bodies, Simulated Harmony, and Misplaced Cultures: Neurasthenia in Contemporary Chi-
       nese Society. Psychosomatic Medicine. *Journal of Behavioural Medicine*, **33**, 197-206.

[19]   Sulaiman, S.O.Y., Bhugra, D. and Da Silva, P. (2001) Perceptions of Depression in a Community Sample in Dubai.
       Transcultural Psychiatry, **38**, 201-218. http://dx.doi.org/10.1177/136346150103800204

[20]   Al-Krenawi, A. and Grham, J.R. (2000) Culturally Sensitive Social Work Practise with Arab Clients in Mental Health
       Settings. *Health and Social Work*, **25**, 9-22. http://dx.doi.org/10.1093/hsw/25.1.9

[21]   Givens, J.L., Katz, I.R., Bellamy, S., Holmes, W.C. (2007) Stigma and the Acceptability of Depression Treatments
       among African Americans and Whites. *Society of General Internal Medicine*, **22**, 1292-1297.
       http://dx.doi.org/10.1007/s11606-007-0276-3

[22]   Sims, A. (1993) Discussion Paper: The Scar That Is More than Skin Deep: The Stigma of Depression. *British Journal
       of General Practise*, **43**, 30-31.

[23]   Maj, M. and Sartorius, N. (2002) WPA Series Evidences and Experiences in Psychiatry: Depressive Disorders. 2nd
       Edition, Wiley, Hoboken, 115-116.

8

Antipsychotic Medication and Risk of QTc Prolongation: Focus on Multiple Medication and Role of Cytochrome P450 Isoforms

Takashi Ikeno[1,2*], Kiyotaka Kugiyama[2], Hiroto Ito[1,2]

[1]Department of Social Psychiatry, National Institute of Mental Health, National Center of Neurology and Psychiatry, Tokyo, Japan
[2]Faculty of Medicine, Graduate School of Medical Science, University of Yamanashi, Yamanashi, Japan
Email: *ikenot@ncnp.go.jp

Abstract

Objective: To identify the effects of antipsychotics on QTc prolongation in light of age, gender, antipsychotic combination pattern, antipsychotic doses and cytochrome P450 (CYP) mediation, using large database describing the antipsychotic treatment of patients with schizophrenia in Japan. Methods: Using database of 4176 patients with schizophrenia discharged between April 2004 and March 2005 and receiving outpatient treatment from 526 psychiatric hospitals in Japan. Of the patients, 1437 were included for the analysis. These patients were classified into three groups according to the antipsychotic CPZ-equivalent doses that they received (low, 1 - 299 mg; middle, 300 - 999 mg; and high, ≥1000 mg). QTc intervals ≥ 440 msec were considered prolonged. We reviewed all the package inserts of the antipsychotics used from the website of Pharmaceuticals and Medical Devices Agency. Results: The mean QTc interval of the total patient group was 410.4 ± 23.3 msec. The females had significantly higher QTc values than the males (414.5 ± 24.0 vs. 406.8 ± 22.2 msec, respectively; $p < 0.05$). Logistic regression analysis revealed that female gender (odds ratio [OR] = 1.83; 95% CI: 1.28 - 2.56), CYP3A4-metabolized drugs (OR 1.56; 95% CI: 1.05 - 2.30) were associated with an increased risk of QTc prolongation. Conclusion: The co-prescription of CYP3A4-mediated antipsychotic drugs should be carefully considered in females due to potential risk of QTc prolongation. Further studies of the cardiovascular safety of antipsychotics are warranted in patients receiving multiple medications.

Keywords

Antipsychotics, CYP, Drug Interaction, QTc Prolongation, Schizophrenia

---

*Corresponding author.

1. Introduction

Concern about cardiac safety is a leading cause for the withdrawal of several marketed drugs. The International Conference on Harmonisation of Technical Requirements for Registration of Pharmaceuticals for Human Use (ICH) has developed guidelines (E14) to assess corrected QT (QTc) prolongation, which can lead to life-threatening cardiac arrhythmia or torsade de pointes [1]. The QTc interval represents the duration of ventricular depolarization and subsequent repolarization, and a delay in cardiac repolarization can be measured as prolongation of the QTc interval by electrocardiography (ECG). The QTc interval is used as a surrogate marker for the prediction of serious adverse drug effects, syncope, or death due to torsade de pointes [2].

Drugs that cause prolongation of the QTc interval have been extensively studied in the past decade [3]-[13]. Antipsychotics have been known to be associated with QTc prolongation, as have drugs such as antidysrhythmics and antibiotics [6] [9]. The use of antipsychotics is a first-line treatment for psychotic disorders such as schizophrenia. Some of the typical antipsychotics that are in use today have been available since the 1950s, and atypical antipsychotics have been used since the 1990s as the second-generation medications for psychotic disorders [4]. Thioridazine (a typical antipsychotic) and ziprasidone (an atypical antipsychotic) were withdrawn from the market due to the increased risk of QTc prolongation and sudden death that they presented [14] [15]. Antipsychotic medications are commonly prescribed off-label for conditions such as delirium and autism spectrum disorder, in populations including the elderly and children [16]. The increased risk of death in elderly patients has been reported regarding both typical and atypical antipsychotics [17].

In clinical practice, more than one drug is often prescribed concurrently, and combination-drug treatment is a common prescription pattern of antipsychotics in psychiatry [18]-[20]. Although co-prescribing can be appropriate, the interaction of multiple drugs may increase the risk of adverse effects by pharmacokinetic and pharmacodynamic interactions. One drug may alter the other's absorption, distribution, metabolism, and/or excretion with a pharmacokinetic interaction, and two drugs may have additive, synergistic, and/or antagonistic effects with a pharmacodynamic interaction [21].

In efforts to predict clinically relevant drug interactions, the cytochrome P450 (CYP) system is important; the system's six enzymes (CYP 1A2, 2C9, 2C19, 2D6, 2E1 and 3A4) metabolize more than 90% of the existing drugs [22]. When two drugs sharing the same metabolic pathway compete for the same enzyme receptor site, enzyme inhibition occurs, and the plasma level of the unmetabolized drug is enhanced because the predominant inhibitor decreases the metabolism of the competing drug, leading to a greater potential for toxicity [23].

Adverse cardiovascular effects due to drug interactions are of great concern, but the effects of combined drugs on QTc prolongation have not been clarified. The objective of the present study was to identify the effects of antipsychotics on QTc prolongation in light of age, gender, antipsychotic combination pattern, antipsychotic doses and CYP mediation, using a large database of antipsychotic treatment of patients with schizophrenia in Japan.

2. Methods

2.1. Data Sources

A retrospective study was conducted using the database from a nationwide study conducted by the Japan Psychiatric Hospitals Association (JPHA) in 2007. Of the 1215 member hospitals of the JPHA, 526 hospitals (43.3%) participated in the original study to examine the effects of daycare services for patients with schizophrenia who were discharged between April 2004 and March 2005 and who continued to receive outpatient treatment at the hospitals [24] [25]. Using a systematic sampling technique, every fifth patient was selected from the medical records of the total 21,396 patients (n = 4176). QTc was measured during the patient's hospitalization at psychiatric hospitals. The database includes sociodemographics, diagnosis, and prescription drug and QTc information.

2.2. Study Population

In the present study, patients with following available data were included: 1) age, 2) gender, 3) QTc interval during hospitalization, and 4) prescription information of the antipsychotics used by the patients. Exclusion criteria were: 1) aged under 20 or over 99 years old, 2) history of myocardial infarction or angina, 3) patients whose QTc were monitored only at admission, 4) QTc under 360 msec or over 600 msec, 5) antipsychotic monotherapy, and 6) antipsychotics without any information on CYP. After 2598 patients were excluded based on these criteria, 1437 patients were included for the analysis.

QTc-interval measurements were generated by a computer algorithm at each participating hospital. In the present study, QTc intervals ≥ 440 msec were considered prolonged [26] [27]. All antipsychotic doses were converted to chlorpromazine equivalent (CPZ-equivalent) [28]. In general, 300 mg to 999 mg is known as the recommended dose of an antipsychotic CPZ-equivalent drug [19] [29]. In the present study, the patients were classified into three groups according to the CPZ-equivalent antipsychotic dose they had been prescribed: 1 - 299 mg as the low-dose group (n = 119), 300 - 999 mg as the middle-dose group (n = 789), and ≥1000 mg as the high-dose group (n = 529). QTc intervals were studied by drug combination patterns (typical + typical, typical + atypical, and atypical + atypical antipsychotics).

We examined the cardiac effects of combined antipsychotics that were metabolized by the same CYP system. We reviewed all of the package inserts of antipsychotics from the website of Japan's Pharmaceuticals and Medical Devices Agency (PMDA), and all of the relevant articles in scientific journals on CYP isoforms and QTc interval information of antipsychotics (**Table 1**) [3] [15] [22] [26] [30]-[50].

2.3. Statistical Analysis

Mean and standard deviation (SD) were used to represent distribution of continuous variables. We used Student's t-test and one-way analysis of variance (ANOVA) to compare QTc prolongation group (QTc ≥ 440 msec) and control group (QTc < 440 msec). Multiple logistic regression analysis was performed to assess factors that could contribute to QTc interval prolongation. Age, gender, and CYP groups (1A2, 2D6 and 3A4) were included in the forced entry method. Only the significant variables were included when comparing the dichotomized QTc intervals (≥ 440 msec vs. <440 msec). All statistical analyses were performed using SPSS version 18.0 for Windows (SPSS Inc., Chicago, IL). p-values < 0.05 were accepted as significant.

Table 1. CYP isoforms and QTc interval of antipsychotics.

Drug name	Antipsychotic class	CYP[a] isoform
Known to prolong the QTc interval		
Bromperidol [51]	Typical	3A4 [47]
Chlorpromazine [26] [52]	Typical	2D6 [38]
Fluphenazine decanoate [53] [54]	Typical	2D6 [50]
Haloperidol [55] [56]	Typical	2D6 [50]
Haloperidol decanoate [52] [57]	Typical	2D6 [34] [48]
Levomepromazine [52] [58]	Typical	2D6 [49]
Nemonapride [59]	Typical	2D6 [30]
Olanzapine [60] [61]	Atypical	1A2, 2D6 [45]
Perphenazine [8] [40]	Typical	2D6 [45]
Pimozide [41] [62]	Typical	1A2, 2D6, 3A4 [33]
Quetiapine [42] [60]	Atypical	3A4 [4] [35]
Risperidone [60] [63]	Atypical	2D6 [32]
Trifluoperazine [64]	Typical	1A2 [44]
No available information on QTc interval		
Perospirone	Atypical	1A2, 2C8, 2D6, 3A4 [5]
Zotepine	Atypical	1A2, 2B6, 2C9, 2C19, 2D6, 3A4, 3A5 [5]

[a]CYP: cytochrome P450.

2.4. Ethical Considerations

The study protocol was approved by the Institutional Review Boards of the JPHA and National Center of Neurology and Psychiatry (NCNP). The study protocol has been registered in the UMIN Clinical Trials Registry (UMIN-CTR) in Japan (UMIN000010473).

3. Results

The mean QTc interval of the total group of patients was 410.4 ± 23.3 msec (**Table 2**). The females (n = 670) had significantly longer than QTc intervals compared to the males (n = 767) (414.5 ± 24.0 vs. 406.8 ± 22.2 msec, respectively; $p < 0.05$). There were no significant differences in QTc intervals among the three dose groups or among the different drug combination patterns.

The results of the logistic regression analysis examining the risk factors of QTc interval prolongation are presented in **Table 3**. Females were more susceptible to QTc prolongation than men (odds ratio [OR] = 1.83; 95% CI: 1.28 - 2.56). CYP3A4-mediated antipsychotics were more likely to prolong the QTc interval compared to non-CYP3A4-mediated antipsychotics (OR 1.56; 95% CI: 1.05 - 2.30). CYP1A2-mediated antipsychotics were less likely to prolong the QTc interval compared to non-CYP1A2-mediated antipsychotics (OR 0.65; 95% CI: 0.44 - 0.97).

4. Discussion

The present study revealed that patients receiving combined antipsychotics that were metabolized by the CYP3A4 had longer QTc intervals than those receiving drugs that were metabolized by different pathways. The female patients were significantly more susceptible to QTc prolongation than the males. Antipsychotic dosing and typical/atypical combination patterns were not associated with QTc prolongation.

Although a recent study demonstrated that the use of combined antipsychotics did not increase the risk of sudden cardiac death or ventricular arrhythmia [12], the present analysis indicates that combined CYP3A4-mediated antipsychotics may be a risk factor for QTc prolongation. The results showed that the QTc interval was

Table 2. Mean QTc interval and patient characteristics.

	n (%)	Mean QTc ± SD (msec)
Overall	1437 (100)	410.4 ± 23.3
Gender		
Male	767 (53.4)	406.8 ± 22.2
Female	670 (46.6)	$414.5 \pm 24.0^*$
Age (years)		
<65	1290 (89.8)	409.9 ± 23.1
>65	147 (10.2)	414.7 ± 25.3
CPZeq[a]		
1 mg - 299 mg	119 (8.3)	406.2 ± 24.0
300 mg - 999 mg	789 (54.9)	411.2 ± 22.1
≥1000 mg	529 (36.8)	410.1 ± 24.9
Combination pattern		
Typical + typical	451 (31.4)	408.4 ± 23.2
Typical + atypical	880 (61.2)	411.3 ± 23.5
Atypical + atypical	106 (7.4)	411.3 ± 21.6

[a]CPZeq: chlorpromazine equivalent. $^*p < 0.05$.

Table 3. Risk factors of QTc prolongation by logistic regression.

	n (%)	QTc prolongation (%)[a]	Odds ratio (95% CI)	p value
Gender				
Female	670 (46.6)	89 (13.3)	1.83 (1.28 - 2.56)	0.001
Male	767 (53.4)	59 (7.7)	1.00	
Age (years)				
<65	1290 (89.8)	131 (10.2)	1.06 (0.61 - 1.83)	0.846
>65	147 (10.2)	17 (11.6)	1.00	
CYP 1A2				
CYP 1A2-mediated drugs	637 (44.3)	58 (9.1)	0.65 (0.44 - 0.97)	0.033
Non CYP 1A2-mediated drugs	800 (55.7)	90 (11.3)	1.00	
CYP 2D6				
CYP 2D6-mediated drugs	1414 (98.4)	145 (10.3)	0.94 (0.27 - 3.33)	0.925
Non CYP 2D6-mediated drugs	23 (1.6)	3 (13.0)	1.00	
CYP 3A4				
CYP 3A4-mediated drugs	574 (39.9)	68 (11.8)	1.56 (1.05 - 2.30)	0.026
Non CYP 3A4-mediated drugs	863 (60.1)	80 (9.3)	1.00	

[a]Number of patients with QTc $\geq$ 440 msec.

prolonged in patients receiving CYP3A4-mediated antipsychotic combinations. Ray *et al.* studied the potential relationship between macrolide antimicrobial agent and sudden death, and they concluded that the concurrent use of erythromycin and strong inhibitors of CYP3A4 should be avoided [43].

Several studies support the finding of a gender difference, *i.e.*, that female patients are at greater risk of QTc prolongation [7] [12]. The gender difference in QTc prolongation may be related to sex hormones [65] [66]. The QTc interval is similar in children aged younger than 15 years before puberty, but the QTc interval in males decreases after puberty, resulting in longer QTc intervals in females [67]. Testosterone may be related to the difference, and gender-specific medication therapy should be considered [36].

Also, the antipsychotic dosing and typical/atypical combinations were not associated with QTc prolongation in the present study. Regarding the dosing, the results of previous studies have been contradictory; one study reported that high doses presented a risk of QTc prolongation [7], whereas another suggested there was no association [12]. Ozeki *et al.* reported that the first-generation antipsychotics partly contributed to QTc prolongation, and the second-generation antipsychotics presented a relatively low risk of fatal arrhythmia [52].

Despite the documented abnormal QTc, the rate of serious cardiovascular effects is low [31]. QTc prolongation in a schizophrenic population cannot directly address clinically relevant issues of cardiovascular adverse effects due to acceptable small extensions, and the risk of sudden death is likely to be small in these data. The definitions of the QTc prolongation vary, and QTc intervals are different in males and females. When the QTc interval exceeds 500 msec, it implies clinical significance in both males and females [14]. Because the subjects of the present study were not patients with pre-existing cardiovascular conditions, 440 msec was used as the cutoff point of the QTc prolongation for both the males and females.

However, caution is needed when a drug is known to prolong the QTc interval due to potential inhibition of its metabolism by another drug. In clinical practice, the avoidance or the minimum use of co-prescribed CYP3A4-metabolized antipsychotics should be considered.

There are several limitations to the present study. First, the database did not include information on predisposing factors including congenital long QTc syndrome and comorbidity, or for prescriptions for comorbidity such as for the presence of diabetes and the prescription of antidiabetic drugs. Second, the effects of potential confounders cannot be excluded. The CYP pathway of antipsychotic drugs have not all been revealed, and thus further studies are required before the present results could be generalized. Third, QTc may be considerably affected by blood concentration of the antipsychotic drugs. The time points of the daily administration of the drugs and measurement of QTc was unknown because we used the secondary data from the multicenter study. More sophisticated study is needed. Fourth, context of the time the antipsychotics and the time of measurement of the QTc was prescribed is unknown. Fifth, the study design is a retrospective open cohort study, so the observed associations should be interpreted carefully. It is believed that the timing of the prescription blood levels to be involved, and further study. Despite these limitations, the present findings highlight the potential CYP-mediated drug-drug interactions in combined antipsychotics revealed by using a large database, and our results will contribute to the risk management of drug-induced QTc prolongation.

5. Conclusion

The co-prescription of CYP3A4-mediated antipsychotic drugs should be carefully considered in females due to potential risk of QTc prolongation. Further studies of the cardiovascular safety of antipsychotics are warranted in patients receiving multiple medications.

Acknowledgements

We thank Dr. Ken Mayahara, Mr. Yoshio Matsumoto, Dr. Junichi Hirakawa, and the Health-Economics Committee of the Japanese Association of Psychiatric Hospitals for allowing the analysis of the Committee's research data. This research was funded by the Health and Labour Sciences Research Grant for Comprehensive Research on Disability Health and Welfare from the Japanese Ministry of Health, Labour, and Welfare.

Competing Interests

The authors declare that they have no competing interests.

References

[1]   ICH Harmonized Tripartite Guideline E14 (2005) E14 Clinical Evaluation of QT/QTc Interval Prolongation and Proarrhythmic Potential for Non-Antiarrhythmic Drugs.
http://www.fda.gov/downloads/RegulatoryInformation/Guidances/ucm129357.pdf

[2]   Roden, D.M. (2004) Drug-Induced Prolongation of the QT Interval. *The New England Journal of Medicine*, **350**, 1013-1022. http://dx.doi.org/10.1056/NEJMra032426

[3]   Brown, C.S., Farmer, R.G., Soberman, J.E. and Eichner, S.F. (2004) Pharmacokinetic Factors in the Adverse Cardiovascular Effects of Antipsychotic Drugs. *Clinical Pharmacokinetics*, **43**, 33-56.
http://dx.doi.org/10.2165/00003088-200443010-00003

[4]   Glassman, A.H. and Bigger Jr., J.T., (2001) Antipsychotic Drugs: Prolonged QTc Interval, Torsade de Pointes, and Sudden Death. *American Journal of Psychiatry*, **158**, 1774-1782. http://dx.doi.org/10.1176/appi.ajp.158.11.1774

[5]   Mackin, P. and Young, A.H. (2005) QTc Interval Measurement and Metabolic Parameters in Psychiatric Patients Taking Typical or Atypical Antipsychotic Drugs: A Preliminary Study. *Journal of Clinical Psychiatry*, **66**, 1386-1391.
http://dx.doi.org/10.4088/JCP.v66n1107

[6]   Montanez, A., Ruskin, J.N., Hebert, P.R., Lamas, G.A. and Hennekens, C.H. (2004) Prolonged QTc Interval and Risks of Total and Cardiovascular Mortality and Sudden Death in the General Population: A Review and Qualitative Overview of the Prospective Cohort Studies. *Archives of Internal Medicine*, **164**, 943-948.
http://dx.doi.org/10.1001/archinte.164.9.943

[7]   Reilly, J.G., Ayis, S.A., Ferrier, I.N., Jones, S.J. and Thomas, S.H. (2000) QTc-Interval Abnormalities and Psychotropic Drug Therapy in Psychiatric Patients. *Lancet*, **355**, 1048-1052. http://dx.doi.org/10.1016/S0140-6736(00)02035-3

[8]   Stollberger, C., Huber, J.O. and Finsterer, J. (2005) Antipsychotic Drugs and QT Prolongation. *International Clinical Psychopharmacology*, **20**, 243-251. http://dx.doi.org/10.1097/01.yic.0000166405.49473.70

[9]   Taylor, D.M. (2003) Antipsychotics and QT Prolongation. *Acta Psychiatrica Scandinavica*, **107**, 85-95.
http://dx.doi.org/10.1034/j.1600-0447.2003.02078.x

[10] van Noord, C., Straus, S.M., Sturkenboom, M.C., Hofman, A., Aarnoudse, A.J., Bagnardi, V., *et al.* (2009) Psychotropic Drugs Associated with Corrected QT Interval Prolongation. *Journal of Clinical Psychopharmacology*, **29**, 9-15.
http://dx.doi.org/10.1097/JCP.0b013e318191c6a8

[11] Warner, J.P., Barnes, T.R. and Henry, J.A. (1996) Electrocardiographic Changes in Patients Receiving Neuroleptic Medication. *Acta Psychiatrica Scandinavica*, **93**, 311-313. http://dx.doi.org/10.1111/j.1600-0447.1996.tb10653.x

[12] Yang, F.D., Wang, X.Q., Liu, X.P., Zhao, K.X., Fu, W.H., Hao, X.R., *et al.* (2011) Sex Difference in QTc Prolongation in Chronic Institutionalized Patients with Schizophrenia on Long-Term Treatment with Typical and Atypical Antipsychotics. *Psychopharmacology*, **216**, 9-16. http://dx.doi.org/10.1007/s00213-011-2188-5

[13] Zemrak, W.R. and Kenna, G.A. (2008) Association of Antipsychotic and Antidepressant Drugs with Q-T Interval Prolongation. *American Journal of Health-System Pharmacy*, **65**, 1029-1038. http://dx.doi.org/10.2146/ajhp070279

[14] Haddad, P.M. and Anderson, I.M. (2002) Antipsychotic-Related QTc Prolongation, Torsade de Pointes and Sudden Death. *Drugs*, **62**, 1649-1671. http://dx.doi.org/10.2165/00003495-200262110-00006

[15] Khan, M.M., Logan, K.R., McComb, J.M. and Adgey, A.A. (1981) Management of Recurrent Ventricular Tachyarrhythmias Associated with Q-T Prolongation. *American Journal of Cardiology*, **47**, 1301-1308. http://dx.doi.org/10.1016/0002-9149(81)90263-0

[16] Leslie, D.L. and Rosenheck, R. (2012) Off-Label Use of Antipsychotic Medications in Medicaid. *The American Journal of Managed Care*, **18**, e109-e117.

[17] Wang, P.S., Schneeweiss, S., Avorn, J., Fischer, M.A., Mogun, H., Solomon, D.H., *et al.* (2005) Risk of Death in Elderly Users of Conventional vs. Atypical Antipsychotic Medications. *The New England Journal of Medicine*, **353**, 2335-2341. http://dx.doi.org/10.1056/NEJMoa052827

[18] Ito, H., Okumura, Y., Higuchi, T., Tan, C.H. and Shinfuku, N. (2012) International Variation in Antipsychotic Prescribing for Schizophrenia: Pooled Results from the Research on East Asia Psychotropic Prescription (Reap) Studies. *Open Journal of Psychiatry*, **2**, 340-346. http://dx.doi.org/10.4236/ojpsych.2012.224048

[19] Lelliott, P., Paton, C., Harrington, M., Konsolaki, M., Sensky, T. and Okocha, C. (2002) The Influence of Patient Variables on Polypharmacy and Combined High Dose of Antipsychotic Drugs Prescribed for In-Patients. *Psychiatric Bulletin*, **26**, 411-414. http://dx.doi.org/10.1192/pb.26.11.411

[20] Sim, K., Su, H.C., Fujii, S., Yang, S.Y., Chong, M.Y., Ungvari, G., *et al.* (2009) High-Dose Antipsychotic Use in Schizophrenia: A Comparison between the 2001 and 2004 Research on East Asia Psychotropic Prescription (REAP) Studies. *British Journal of Clinical Pharmacology*, **67**, 110-117. http://dx.doi.org/10.1111/j.1365-2125.2008.03304.x

[21] Scott, R.P. (2010) Drug Interactions. NIH. http://www.cc.nih.gov/training/training/principles/slides/DrugInteractions2010-2011_text.pdf

[22] Rendic, S. (2002) Summary of Information on Human CYP Enzymes: Human P450 Metabolism Data. *Drug Metabolism Reviews*, **34**, 83-448. http://dx.doi.org/10.1081/DMR-120001392

[23] Ogu, C.C. and Maxa, J.L. (2000) Drug Interactions Due to Cytochrome P450. *Baylor University Medical Center Proceedings*, **13**, 421-423.

[24] Kobayashi, M., Ito, H., Okumura, Y., Mayahara, K., Matsumoto, Y. and Hirakawa, J. (2010) Hospital Readmission in First-Time Admitted Patients with Schizophrenia: Smoking Patients Had Higher Hospital Readmission Rate than Non-Smoking Patients. *The International Journal of Psychiatry in Medicine*, **40**, 247-257. http://dx.doi.org/10.2190/PM.40.3.b

[25] Okumura, Y., Ito, H., Kobayashi, M., Mayahara, K., Matsumoto, Y. and Hirakawa, J. (2010) Prevalence of Diabetes and Antipsychotic Prescription Patterns in Patients with Schizophrenia: A Nationwide Retrospective Cohort Study. *Schizophrenia Research*, **119**, 145-152. http://dx.doi.org/10.1016/j.schres.2010.02.1061

[26] Christensen, P.K., Gall, M.A., Major-Pedersen, A., Sato, A., Rossing, P., Breum, L., *et al.* (2000) QTc Interval Length and QT Dispersion as Predictors of Mortality in Patients with Non-Insulin-Dependent Diabetes. *Scandinavian Journal of Clinical & Laboratory Investigation*, **60**, 323-332. http://dx.doi.org/10.1080/003655100750046486

[27] Saarnivaara, L., Klemola, U.M., Lindgren, L., Rautiainen, P. and Suvanto, A. (1990) QT Interval of the ECG, Heart Rate and Arterial Pressure Using Propofol, Methohexital or Midazolam for Induction of Anaesthesia. *Acta Anaesthesiologica Scandinavica*, **34**, 276-281. http://dx.doi.org/10.1111/j.1399-6576.1990.tb03085.x

[28] Inagaki, A. and Inada, T. (2006) Dose Equivalence of Psychotropic Drugs. Part 18: Dose Equivalence of Psychotropic Drugs: 2006-Version. *Japanese Journal of Clinical Psychopharmacology*, **9**, 1443-1447. (in Japanese)

[29] Bazett, H.C. (1920) The Time Relations of the Blood-Pressure Changes after Excision of the Adrenal Glands, with Some Observations on Blood Volume Changes. *The Journal of Physiology*, **53**, 320-339.

[30] Caccia, S. (2000) Biotransformation of Post-Clozapine Antipsychotics: Pharmacological Implications. *Clinical Pharmacokinetics*, **38**, 393-414. http://dx.doi.org/10.2165/00003088-200038050-00002

[31] Crouch, M.A., Limon, L. and Cassano, A.T. (2003) Clinical Relevance and Management of Drug-Related QT Interval Prolongation. *Pharmacotherapy*, **23**, 881-908. http://dx.doi.org/10.1592/phco.23.7.881.32730

[32] de Leon, J., Sandson, N.B. and Cozza, K.L. (2008) A Preliminary Attempt to Personalize Risperidone Dosing Using Drug-Drug Interactions and Genetics: Part II. *Psychosomatics*, **49**, 347-361. http://dx.doi.org/10.1176/appi.psy.49.4.347

[33] Desta, Z., Kerbusch, T., Soukhova, N., Richard, E., Ko, J.W. and Flockhart, D.A. (1998) Identification and Characterization of Human Cytochrome P450 Isoforms Interacting with Pimozide. *Journal of Pharmacology and Experimental Therapeutics*, **285**, 428-437.

[34] Fang, J., Baker, G.B., Silverstone, P.H. and Coutts, R.T. (1997) Involvement of CYP3A4 and CYP2D6 in the Metabolism of Haloperidol. *Cellular and Molecular Neurobiology*, **17**, 227-233.
http://dx.doi.org/10.1023/A:1026317929335

[35] Grimm, S.W., Richtand, N.M., Winter, H.R., Stams, K.R. and Reele, S.B. (2006) Effects of Cytochrome P450 3A Modulators Ketoconazole and Carbamazepine on Quetiapine Pharmacokinetics. *British Journal of Clinical Pharmacology*, **61**, 58-69. http://dx.doi.org/10.1111/j.1365-2125.2005.02507.x

[36] Lazarus, G.M. (2001) Gender-Specific Medicine in Pediatrics. *The Journal of Gender-Specific Medicine*, **4**, 50-53.

[37] Mizuno, Y., Tani, N., Komuro, S., Kanamaru, H. and Nakatsuka, I. (2003) *In Vitro* Metabolism of Perospirone in Rat, Monkey and Human Liver Microsomes. *European Journal of Drug Metabolism and Pharmacokinetics*, **28**, 59-65.
http://dx.doi.org/10.1007/BF03190868

[38] Muralidharan, G., Cooper, J.K., Hawes, E.M., Korchinski, E.D. and Midha, K.K. (1996) Quinidine Inhibits the 7-Hydroxylation of Chlorpromazine in Extensive Metabolisers of Debrisoquine. *European Journal of Clinical Pharmacology*, **50**, 121-128. http://dx.doi.org/10.1007/s002280050079

[39] Olesen, O.V. and Linnet, K. (2000) Identification of the Human Cytochrome P450 Isoforms Mediating *in Vitro* N-Dealkylation of Perphenazine. *British Journal of Clinical Pharmacology*, **50**, 563-571.
http://dx.doi.org/10.1046/j.1365-2125.2000.00298.x

[40] Perphenazine Package Insert (2013) http://www.info.pmda.go.jp/go/pack/1172006F1030_1_07/

[41] Pimozide Package Insert (2013) http://www.info.pmda.go.jp/go/pack/1179022C1034_1_07/

[42] Quetiapine Package Insert (2013) http://www.info.pmda.go.jp/go/pack/1179042C1023_2_14/

[43] Ray, W.A., Murray, K.T., Meredith, S., Narasimhulu, S.S., Hall, K. and Stein, C.M. (2004) Oral Erythromycin and the Risk of Sudden Death from Cardiac Causes. *The New England Journal of Medicine*, **351**, 1089-1096.
http://dx.doi.org/10.1056/NEJMoa040582

[44] Semla, T.P., Beizer, J.L. and Higbee, M.D. (2005) Geriatric Dosage Handbook. 10th Edition, Lexi Comp Inc, Hudson, 1286-1290.

[45] Sharif, Z.A. (2003) Pharmacokinetics, Metabolism and Drug-Drug Interactions of Atypical Antipsychotics in Special Populations. *Journal of Clinical Psychiatry*, **5**, 22-25.

[46] Shiraga, T., Kaneko, H., Iwasaki, K., Tozuka, Z., Suzuki, A. and Hata, T. (1999) Identification of Cytochrome P450 Enzymes Involved in the Metabolism of Zotepine, an Antipsychotic Drug, in Human Liver Microsomes. *Xenobiotica*, **29**, 217-229. http://dx.doi.org/10.1080/004982599238623

[47] Tateishi, T., Watanabe, M., Kumai, T., Tanaka, M., Moriya, H., Yamaguchi, S., *et al.* (2000) CYP3A Is Responsible for N-Dealkylation of Haloperidol and Bromperidol and Oxidation of Their Reduced Forms by Human Liver Microsomes. *Life Sciences*, **67**, 2913-2920. http://dx.doi.org/10.1016/S0024-3205(00)00874-2

[48] Tyndale, R.F., Kalow, W. and Inaba, T. (1991) Oxidation of Reduced Haloperidol to Haloperidol: Involvement of Human P450IID6 (Sparteine/Debrisoquine Monooxygenase). *British Journal of Clinical Pharmacology*, **31**, 655-660.
http://dx.doi.org/10.1111/j.1365-2125.1991.tb05588.x

[49] Yukawa, E., Hokazono, T., Yukawa, M., Ichimaru, R., Maki, T., Matsunaga, K., *et al.* (2002) Population Pharmacokinetics of Haloperidol Using Routine Clinical Pharmacokinetic Data in Japanese Patients. *Clinical Pharmacokinetics*, **41**, 153-159. http://dx.doi.org/10.2165/00003088-200241020-00006

[50] Zhou, S.F. (2009) Polymorphism of Human Cytochrome P450 2D6 and Its Clinical Significance: Part II. *Clinical Pharmacokinetics*, **48**, 761-804. http://dx.doi.org/10.2165/11318070-000000000-00000

[51] Bromperidol Package Insert (2013) http://www.info.pmda.go.jp/go/pack/1179028C1066_2_11/

[52] Ozeki, Y., Fujii, K., Kurimoto, N., Yamada, N., Okawa, M., Aoki, T., *et al.* (2010) QTc Prolongation and Antipsychotic Medications in a Sample of 1017 Patients with Schizophrenia. *Progress in Neuro-Psychopharmacology & Biological Psychiatry*, **34**, 401-405. http://dx.doi.org/10.1016/j.pnpbp.2010.01.008

[53] Chong, S.A., Mythily, Lum, A., Goh, H.Y. and Chan, Y.H. (2003) Prolonged QTc Intervals in Medicated Patients with Schizophrenia. *Human Psychopharmacology*, **18**, 647-649. http://dx.doi.org/10.1002/hup.540

[54] Fluphenazine Decanoate Package Insert (2013) http://www.info.pmda.go.jp/go/pack/1172405A1031_2_07/

[55] Beach, S.R., Celano, C.M., Noseworthy, P.A., Januzzi, J.L. and Huffman, J.C. (2013) QTc Prolongation, Torsades de Pointes and Psychotropic Medications. *Psychosomatics*, **54**, 1-13. http://dx.doi.org/10.1016/j.psym.2012.11.001

[56] Haloperidol Package Insert (2013) http://www.info.pmda.go.jp/go/pack/1179020C1191_1_11/

[57] Haloperidol Decanoate Package Insert (2013) http://www.info.pmda.go.jp/go/pack/1179406A1037_2_09/

[58] Levomepromazine Package Insert (2013) http://www.info.pmda.go.jp/go/pack/1172014B2056_1_13/

[59] Nemonapride Package Insert (2013) http://www.info.pmda.go.jp/go/pack/1179036F1024_1_01/

[60] Harrigan, E.P., Miceli, J.J., Anziano, R., Watsky, E., Reeves, K.R., Cutler, N.R., *et al.* (2004) A Randomized Evaluation of the Effects of Six Antipsychotic Agents on QTc, in the Absence and Presence of Metabolic Inhibition. *Journal of Clinical Psychopharmacology*, **24**, 62-69. http://dx.doi.org/10.1097/01.jcp.0000104913.75206.62

[61] Olanzapine Package Insert (2013) http://www.info.pmda.go.jp/go/pack/1179044F4028_1_18/

[62] Desta, Z., Kerbusch, T. and Flockhart, D.A. (1999) Effect of Clarithromycin on the Pharmacokinetics and Pharmacodynamics of Pimozide in Healthy Poor and Extensive Metabolizers of Cytochrome P450 2D6 (CYP2D6). *Clinical Pharmacology & Therapeutics*, **65**, 10-20. http://dx.doi.org/10.1016/S0009-9236(99)70117-7

[63] Risperidone Package Insert (2013) http://www.info.pmda.go.jp/go/pack/1179038C1027_1_27/

[64] Trifluoperazine Package Insert (2013) http://www.info.pmda.go.jp/go/pack/1172008F1021_2_07/

[65] Bai, C.X., Kurokawa, J., Tamagawa, M., Nakaya, H. and Furukawa, T. (2005) Nontranscriptional Regulation of Cardiac Repolarization Currents by Testosterone. *Circulation*, **112**, 1701-1710. http://dx.doi.org/10.1161/CIRCULATIONAHA.104.523217

[66] Shuba, Y.M., Degtiar, V.E., Osipenko, V.N., Naidenov, V.G. and Woosley, R.L. (2001) Testosterone-Mediated Modulation of HERG Blockade by Proarrhythmic Agents. *Biochemical Pharmacology*, **62**, 41-49. http://dx.doi.org/10.1016/S0006-2952(01)00611-6

[67] Ramirez, A.H., Schildcrout, J.S., Blakemore, D.L., Masys, D.R., Pulley, J.M., Basford, M.A., *et al.* (2011) Modulators of Normal Electrocardiographic Intervals Identified in a Large Electronic Medical Record. *Heart Rhythm*, **8**, 271-277. http://dx.doi.org/10.1016/j.hrthm.2010.10.034

9

Problems with Double Blind in Medicine

Yngvar Reichelt[1], Karl L. Reichelt[2]

[1]Department of Mathematics, University of Oslo, Oslo, Norway
[2]Lab 1, No 1337, Sandvika, Norway and Kleve 4541 m, University of Oslo, Oslo, Norway
Email: karlr@ulrik.uio.no

Abstract

Double blind tests of drugs and procedures depend on obtaining two equal and randomly assigned groups to be compared. With a diagnosis based only on symptoms, but with different etiologies, this is not very likely. We here show the probability of obtaining two equal groups with one diagnosis but three etiologies. The mathematical name for such a problem is multivariate hypergeometric distribution. We find that increasing the group size decreases the probability.

Keywords

Diagnosis, Difference, Etiologies, Distribution, Groups

1. Introduction

Randomly assigned double blind is the gold standard for therapeutic interventions and procedures in medicine. However, one of the conditions for using this method is that the two compared, randomly assigned groups are equal. Many diagnoses are symptom based, and there is every possibility that a diagnostic entity may have several different causes. This is problematic. We have tried to calculate the chance that a group of patients divided into two groups randomly assigned would be equal, if three different etiologies were subsumed under the same diagnosis.

As an example, decreased serotoninergic activity in the brain can have many different causes. In **Figure 1** we can have 1) Decreased release of transmitter into the synaptic cleft; 2) Increased re-uptake from the synaptic cleft; 3) Increased uptake into astroglia from the synaptic cleft; 4) Decreased number of receptors in the post synaptic structure; 5) Decreased receptor sensitivity or inhibition of the same; 6) Inhibition of secondary signals coupled to the receptors such as cyclic AMP and, or cyclic GMP formation; 7) Increased monoamine oxidase activity; 8) Long-term effects of decreased serotonin synthesis [1]. The list can be extended, but it is clear that a decreased serotoninergic state may have several causes. A set of symptoms subsumed under a diagnostic label may well need different interventions. Strongly suspected of having several etiologies are depressions and schizophrenia. This is so because no finding or treatment is found adequate in all individuals in each diagnostic group.

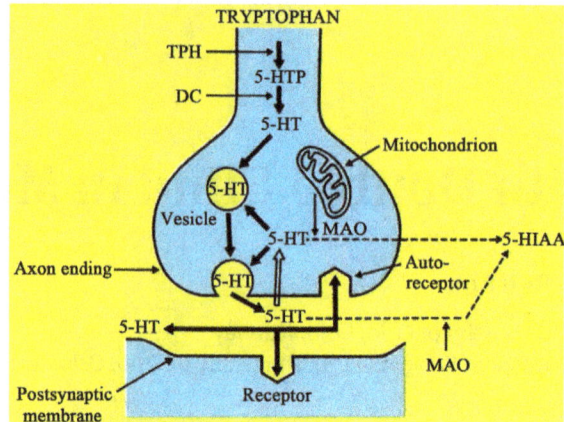

Figure 1. A simplified serotoninergic synapse. 5HT = serotonin; MAO = monoamineoxidase; TpH is Tryptophan hydroxylase; 5HTP = 5 hydroxytryptophan; DC = 5-hydroxytryptophan decarboxylase.

If we randomly pick two and two persons in a group with three different etiologies subsumed under one diagnosis. We remove these two each time to two groups (control and experimental group)—What are the chances of picking two of the same each time? In mathematics this is known as multivariate hypergeometric distribution.

Here we let different colored beads represent the different etiologies.

A: We then have four red, four white and four blue beads with a total of $n = 12$.

Then

$$P(\text{probability}) = P(2 \text{ red, } 2 \text{ white, } 2 \text{ blue}) = \frac{\binom{4}{2}\binom{4}{2}\binom{4}{2}}{\binom{12}{6}} = 0.2338$$

where the binomial coefficient is $\binom{n}{k} = \frac{n!}{(n-k)!k!}$.

B. If $n = 60$ with 20 of each red, white and blue, or

Red = 20, white = 20, blue = 20 then

$P(10 \text{ r, } 10 \text{ h, } 10 \text{ b}) \approx 0.0533$

C. If red = 50, white = 50 and blue = 50 and total $n = 150$

Then

$P(25 \text{ red, } 25 \text{ white and } 25 \text{ blue}) = 0.0218$

C. In general

if n = numbers of marbles; $n/3$ = numbers of each color (etiologies); $n/2$ number of marbles to be distributed to each of the random groups

$$P = \frac{\binom{n/3}{n/6}^3}{\binom{n}{n/2}}$$

D. Other distributions. In case the frequency of each etiology (here beads) is different.

Red = 12, white = 6, blue = 2 and total $n = 20$

$$P = \frac{\binom{12}{6}\binom{6}{3}\binom{2}{1}}{\binom{20}{10}} \approx 0.2000$$

E-increasing the total to $n = 60$
Red = 36, white = 18, blue = 6

$$P = \frac{\binom{36}{18}\binom{18}{6}\binom{6}{3}}{\binom{60}{30}} \approx 0.0746$$

2. Discussion

Mathematically it is clear that with different etiologies (here beads) subsumed under one diagnosis, then the random distribution into two equal groups is improbable. It is also clear from the calculations done that increasing the numbers, decreases the probability of getting two equal groups with the same distribution.

Based on symptoms alone without a common marker this is hazardous at best. Pneumonia has very many different etiologies, but with microbial diagnosis (markers) this fairly large group can now be divided into etiological sub-groups. Specific treatment is hence more likely to be successful.

Author Contributions

a) Mathematics written by Yngvar Reichelt;
b) Neurochemical example and final Ms by Karl L. Reichelt.

Funding

No funding.

Conflict of Interest

None.

References

[1]   Lehman, J. (1972) Mental and Neuromuscular Symptoms in Tryptophan Deficiency. *Acta Psychiatrica Scandinavica*, **Suppl. 237**.

10

Long-Term, Open-Label, Safety Study of Edivoxetine as Adjunctive Treatment for Adult Patients with Major Depressive Disorder Who Were Partial Responders to Selective Serotonin Reuptake Inhibitor Treatment in Japan

Emel Serap Monkul[1], Mark Bangs[1], Keita Asato[2], Masashi Takahashi[2], Yasushi Takita[2], Mary Anne Dellva[1], Jonna Ahl[1], Celine Goldberger[1]

[1]Eli Lilly and Company, Indianapolis, IN, USA
[2]Eli Lilly Japan K.K. Office, Kobe, Japan
Email: nery_emel_serap_monkul@lilly.com

Abstract

Edivoxetine is a highly selective norepinephrine reuptake inhibitor (NRI) that has been investigated in short-term studies as adjunctive therapy to selective serotonin reuptake inhibitor antidepressants (SSRIs) in patients with major depressive disorder (MDD) who were partial responders to their SSRIs. This 52-week open-label study investigated the safety and tolerability of longer-term treatment with adjunctive edivoxetine in patients with MDD in Japan, who had completed one of two placebo-controlled acute studies of edivoxetine as adjunctive therapy to SSRIs. All patients continued on their stable dose of SSRI. Two hundred eighty-eight patients were enrolled and assessed for up to 1 year using standard safety and tolerability measures. Of these, 195 patients previously received only placebo in the parent study and, therefore, were first exposed to edivoxetine in this study. Approximately 46% of patients completed the study. The most frequently cited (>5%) reasons for discontinuation were sponsor decision (19.4%, which included patients discontinued due to early study termination), adverse event (17.4%) and subject decision (8.7%). Adverse events leading to discontinuation in more than 2 patients (>1%) were palpitations, vomiting, hepatic function abnormal, hypertension, nausea, and tachycardia. Treatment-emergent elevations in diastolic blood pressure and pulse were at least twice that reported in the literature for non-Asian patients. Twenty percent of patients had sustained elevations in pulse. Treatment-

emergent changes in laboratory measures were small and not clinically meaningful. Assessment across all safety measures in this study indicated that the safety profile of edivoxetine was consistent with that expected for a selective NRI.

Keywords

Edivoxetine, Depression, SSRI, NRI, Japan, Adjunctive Therapy

1. Introduction

Major depressive disorder (MDD) is a chronic illness that is estimated to have 2.9% lifetime prevalence in Japan [1]. Although the prevalence rates for MDD are lower in Japan than those reported in western countries, suicide rates in Japan are among the highest in the world with 24.4 per 100,000 inhabitants [2]. In a psychological autopsy case-control study of suicide in Japan, MDD was the disorder that was the most strongly associated with suicide, as well as anxiety disorder, alcohol-related disorders, and brief psychotic disorder [1]. As in other countries, the societal cost of depression in Japan is enormous, and was estimated to be ¥2.0 trillion in 2005 [3].

Complete remission of symptoms is the treatment goal in MDD, but is unattainable for many patients, which puts them at risk for relapse [4] and suicide [5]. First-line therapy for MDD is the most frequent monotherapy with a selective serotonin reuptake inhibitor (SSRI), though individual differences in response to treatment can contribute to incomplete symptom resolution. One second-step treatment option would be to switch to or add on another antidepressant with a different mode of action [6], and the addition of an agent with selective norepinephrine reuptake inhibition (NRI) to an SSRI antidepressant may provide additional benefit [7].

Edivoxetine is a highly selective NRI that has been investigated as adjunctive therapy to SSRI antidepressants in several acute placebo-controlled trials [8]-[10] and one open-label long-term safety trial [11] in patients with MDD who were partial responders to SSRI treatment. However, these studies were conducted in predominantly white populations. Since racial/genetic variations can contribute to differences in metabolism of psychiatric medications, which can ultimately impact efficacy and safety outcomes [12], it is important to conduct analyses in specific racial/genetic populations [13]. Herein we report on the tolerability and safety of edivoxetine as adjunctive treatment to SSRI antidepressants in a year-long, open-label trial conducted in Japan in patients with MDD who were partial responders to SSRI treatment.

2. Methods

This was a phase III, multicenter, open-label investigation of the long-term tolerability and safety of edivoxetine as adjunctive treatment in patients with MDD in Japan. The study was conducted at 27 sites in accordance with ethical principles that had their origin in the Declaration of Helsinki, and were consistent with Good Clinical Practices and applicable laws and regulations. The institutional review boards for each site approved the protocol and all patients provided written informed consent.

Enrollment began 2 August 2011 and the final visit occurred on 16 January 2014 (Clinical Trials.gov identifier: NCT01370499). The study planned to enroll approximately 320 patients, but was closed early because the parent studies, H9P-MC-LNBQ (NCT01187407) and H9P-MC-LNBM (NCT01173601), did not meet the primary efficacy endpoint of a statistically significant difference between adjunctive edivoxetine and adjunctive placebo on the mean change from baseline to Week 8 in the Montgomery-Asberg Depression Rating Scale (MADRS) [14] total score. At the time of study closure, 288 patients had been enrolled and assessed for up to one year from baseline.

Patients were eligible to enter the parent studies if they had been taking an SSRI that had been approved for MDD at a dose within the labeling guidelines for Japan. Duration of SSRI treatment had to be ≥6 weeks before visit 2, with at least the last 4 weeks at a stable, optimized dose as determined by the investigator. Eligible patients were required to meet criteria for partial response at visits 1 and 2, as defined by the investigator's opinion that the patient had experienced at least a minimally clinically meaningful improvement with the SSRI treatment. Additionally, patients had to score ≥16 on the GRID 17-Item Hamilton Depression Rating Scale total score [15] and to rate ≤75% improvement for their current SSRI by using the patient-rated Massachusetts General Hospital

Antidepressant Treatment Response Questionnaire-Modified Version [16] at visit 1.

Both parent studies included three periods: screening, an 11-week double-blind treatment period [3-week placebo lead-in and 8 weeks of acute therapy for randomized patients], and a discontinuation period of 1 - 2 weeks. Throughout all study periods, patients were required to take their SSRI at a stable dose. During the double-blind placebo lead-in, those patients who had <25% improvement on the MADRS total score and a MADRS total score ≥14 at the end of the 3 weeks were randomly assigned to receive adjunctive edivoxetine or adjunctive placebo for 8 weeks. Patients who did not meet randomization criteria were kept on adjunctive placebo plus their SSRI, and were continued in the study to maintain the blind.

The studies differed with respect to dosing and discontinuation of adjunctive edivoxetine. In the LNBQ study, patients meeting randomization criteria were randomly assigned to once daily (QD) doses of adjunctive edivoxetine 6 mg fixed-dose, adjunctive edivoxetine 12 - 18 mg flexible dose, or adjunctive placebo. At the end of the double-blind treatment period, patients were abruptly discontinued from adjunctive edivoxetine and received adjunctive placebo for one week. In the LNBM study, patients meeting randomization criteria were randomly assigned to receive fixed doses of adjunctive edivoxetine 12 mg QD or 18 mg QD or placebo. At the end of double-blind treatment, study medication was discontinued over a 2-week period. Patients in both adjunctive edivoxetine groups were randomized to an abrupt or tapered discontinuation. The taper schedule was 12 mg for 4 days, 6 mg for 4 days, and placebo for 6 days. Patients randomly assigned to abrupt discontinuation received placebo for the entire 2 weeks. Patients who received placebo during the acute adjunctive treatment phase continued to receive placebo during the discontinuation period.

To be eligible for the current study, patients in Japan were to have completed one of the two acute phase III parent studies (including the discontinuation period and were no longer taking adjunctive medication), and were still taking the same SSRI at the optimized and stable dose as in the parent study. Since these patients had already met the inclusion and exclusion criteria at entry to the parent studies, they were not re-assessed prior to enrollment in this study. Both non-randomized and randomized patients from the parent studies were eligible.

At enrollment, all patients began treatment with oral adjunctive edivoxetine 12 mg QD. After 1 week, the dose could be adjusted up to 18 mg/day and then back down to 12 mg/day if needed, based on tolerability and efficacy. At week 12, the dose could not be adjusted for the remainder of the study. At week 52 or at early discontinuation, adjunctive edivoxetine was discontinued abruptly and patients were followed up one week later. All patients were maintained on their stable dose of SSRI throughout the study including follow up after abrupt discontinuation of adjunctive edivoxetine.

The primary safety and tolerability assessments included: discontinuation rates, treatment-emergent adverse events (TEAEs), vital signs, weight, electrocardiograms (ECGs), and laboratory analysis. Secondary safety and tolerability measures included serious adverse events, adverse events that were reported as a reason for discontinuation, dose reduction, or were associated with discontinuation of adjunctive edivoxetine; suicidal ideation/behavior assessed with the Columbia-Suicide Severity Rating Scale (CSSR-S) [17], changes in sexual function assessed with the Arizona Sexual Experiences (ASEX) scale [18]; and cognitive and physical function assessed using the Massachusetts General Hospital Cognitive and Physical Functioning Questionnaire (MGH-CPFQ) [19].

The C-SSRS [17] captures the occurrence, severity, and frequency of suicide-related thoughts and behaviors during the assessment period. The scale includes suggested questions to solicit the type of information needed to determine if a suicide-related thought or behavior occurred.

The ASEX [18] is a patient-rated assessment of sexual interest, arousal, response, ability to achieve orgasm, and satisfaction with orgasm that uses a 6-point scale, ranging from "extremely" (score = 1) to "never" or "no" (score = 6). Patients were categorized as having sexual dysfunction if they had an ASEX total score of ≥19, a score of ≥5 on any item; or a score of ≥4 on any 3 items.

The MGH-CPFQ [19] is a patient-rated questionnaire consisting of 7 questions pertaining to a patient's cognitive and physical well-being in which each question is rated on a 6-point scale, with scores ranging from "greater than normal" (score = 1) to "normal" (score = 2), to "totally absent" (score = 6). The MGH-CPFQ total score ranges from 7 to 42, and higher scores were associated with less cognitive and physical well-being. The scale assesses symptoms that may be either residual to the depressive illness or associated with TEAEs of antidepressant therapies for the previous month.

Triplicate measures of blood pressure and single measures of pulse were taken at each study visit in the sitting position. The three blood pressure measures were averaged for use in the analyses. Elevated blood pressure was defined as: systolic blood pressure (SBP) ≥140 mm Hg and an increase of ≥20 mm Hg from baseline; or diastolic blood pressure (DBP) ≥90 mm Hg and an increase of ≥10 mm Hg from baseline. Elevated pulse was defined as >100 beats per minute (bpm) and an increase of ≥15 bpm from baseline. Sustained elevations in blood pressure and pulse were defined by the above criteria that occurred at three consecutive visits. Potentially clinically significant changes in blood pressure were defined as: SBP ≥180 mm Hg and an increase ≥20 mm Hg from baseline; or DBP ≥105 mm Hg and an increase ≥15 mm Hg from baseline.

The safety analyses were conducted on all enrolled patients who took at least one dose of adjunctive edivoxetine. For those patients who received placebo in the parent studies, this study was the first time that they received adjunctive edivoxetine, so the safety results were summarized for all patients and by the adjunctive treatment assignments in the parent studies. Patients who received adjunctive placebo in the parent studies comprised the placebo/edivoxetine (PBO/EDX) group, and those patients who received adjunctive edivoxetine in the parent studies comprised the edivoxetine/edivoxetine (EDX/EDX) group. Safety outcomes were evaluated based on adjunctive treatment assignment in the parent study. There were baseline differences between patients with prior exposure to edivoxetine (EDX/EDX) and those who had no prior exposure (PBO/EDX); however, no statistical comparisons were made between these two groups. Categorical variables were summarized with counts and percentages. Analyses of covariance (ANCOVA) models were used to analyze continuous variables, and the model contained the main effect of pooled investigative site and the baseline value as a covariate. Type III sum-of-squares were used to calculate the least-squares (LS) means from the ANCOVA model. For continuous analyses, a separate model was fit for each group defined by the adjunctive treatment phase assignments from the parent studies.

3. Results

Patient characteristics, illness severity, and SSRI treatment are summarized in **Table 1**. Twice as many patients comprised the PBO/EDX group because it included patients from the parent study lead-in period who remained on placebo, in addition to those patients who were randomized to adjunctive placebo. Approximately 46% of the patients completed the study. The most frequently cited (>5%) reasons for discontinuation were sponsor decision (19.4%, which included patients discontinued due to early study termination), adverse event (17.4%) and subject decision (8.7%).

Over the course of the study, 88.9% of all patients reported at least one TEAE and there were no deaths. The most common (>5% frequency) TEAEs are summarized in **Table 2**. Most of the TEAEs were mild or moderate in severity.

SAEs were reported by 2 patients in the EDX/EDX group (contusion and hyperglycemia) and 1 patient in the PBO/EDX group reported an SAE of subdural hygroma. None of these events were considered by the investigator to be associated with the investigational product or study procedure.

Table 1. Patient demographics, baseline illness severity, and selective serotonin reuptake inhibitor treatment.

Variable	PBO/EDX N = 195	EDX/EDX N = 93	All Patients N = 288
Age (years), mean (SD), range	39.3, (9.4), 21.2 - 77.8	37.4, (9.2), 20.6 - 64.9	38.7, (9.4), 20.6 - 77.8
Males, n (%)	107 (54.9)	48 (51.6)	155 (53.8)
Females, n (%)	88 (45.1)	45 (48.4)	133 (46.2)
Japanese, n (%)	195 (100)	93 (100)	288 (100)
Weight (kg), mean (SD)	66.3, (15.5)	64.5, (14.4)	65.7, (15.1)
SSRI, n (%)			
Sertraline	80 (41.0)	36 (38.7)	116 (40.3)
Paroxetine	57 (29.2)	21 (22.6)	78 (27.1)
Fluvoxamine	35 (18.0)	20 (21.5)	55 (19.1)
Escitalopram	23 (11.8)	16 (17.2)	39 (13.5)

Abbreviations: PBO = placebo; EDX = edivoxetine; SD = standard deviation; SSRI = selective serotonin reuptake inhibitor.

Table 2. Treatment-emergent adverse events that were reported by at least 5% of all patients.

Variable, n (%)	Placebo/Edivoxetine N = 195	Edivoxetine/Edivoxetine N = 93	All Patients N = 288
Patients with at least one TEAE	176 (90.3)	79 (85.9)	255 (88.9)
Nasopharyngitis	56 (28.7)	29 (31.5)	85 (29.6)
Tachycardia	62 (31.8)	17 (18.5)	79 (27.5)
Hyperhidrosis	33 (16.9)	16 (17.4)	49 (17.1)
Palpitations	36 (18.5)	12 (13.0)	48 (16.7)
Nausea	26 (13.3)	8 (8.7)	34 (11.9)
Heart rate increased	25 (12.8)	7 (7.6)	32 (11.2)
Constipation	19 (9.7)	7 (7.6)	26 (9.1)
Dizziness	21 (10.8)	4 (4.4)	25 (8.7)
Headache	17 (8.7)	7 (7.6)	24 (8.4)
Vomiting	14 (7.2)	3 (3.3)	17 (5.9)

Abbreviation: TEAE = treatment-emergent adverse event.

Adverse events leading to study discontinuation in ≥2% patients in the PBO/EDX group were palpitations (n = 6, 3.1%), vomiting (n = 5, 2.6%), and hypertension (n = 4, 2.1%); in the EDX/EDX group only palpitations was reported by at least 2% of the patients.

Longitudinal changes in blood pressure and pulse are shown in **Figure 1**. Across the study, changes in blood pressure and pulse were numerically greater in the PBO/EDX group. At the end of 52 weeks of adjunctive treatment, LS mean (SE) changes from baseline in blood pressure and pulse measures in the PBO/EDX and EDX/EDX groups, respectively, were: 6.7 (0.9) mm Hg and 3.7 (1.3) mm Hg for SBP; 7.6 (5.9) mm Hg and 6.3 (1.0) mm Hg for DBP; and 17.0 (1.2) bpm and 11.0 (1.5) bpm for pulse. A week after abrupt discontinuation of adjunctive edivoxetine LS mean (SE) changes in blood pressure and pulse measures in the PBO/EDX and EDX/EDX groups (respectively) were 0.9 (0.7) mm Hg and 0.3 (1.0) mm Hg for SBP; −2.2 (0.6) mm Hg and −2.7 (0.9) mm Hg for DBP; and −8.1 (0.7) bpm and −8.3 (1.0) bpm for pulse.

Categorical treatment-emergent changes in blood pressure and pulse are summarized in **Table 3**. These changes were more frequently noticed in DBP and pulse. The percentage of patients who met criteria for an elevation in these measures at any time was higher (27% and 50%, respectively), than that observed for sustained elevations (11% and 20%). Potentially clinically significant elevations were only noted for DBP in 3% of the patients.

The percentage of patients with treatment-emergent changes in weight (≥7% loss at any time) was 15% (17% and 10% in the PBO/EDX and EDX/EDX groups, respectively). The overall frequency of treatment-emergent weight gain ≥7% was 6% (5% and 9%, respectively).

Treatment-emergent changes in ECG parameters included rates of PR < 120 ms in 2.1% of patients overall (1.6% of PBO/EDX and 3.3% of EDX/EDX patients); the overall rate was 1.1% for QTC Fridericia changes that were >450 ms in males and >470 ms in females (1.0% of PBO/EDX and 1.1% of EDX/EDX patients), and none of the patients had QTc > 500 ms. Changes in heart rate >100 bpm and an increase ≥15 bpm from baseline were observed in 29.0% of patients overall (32.5% of PBO/EDX and 21.7% of EDX/EDX patients). No clinically significant changes from baseline were observed in any of the other ECG parameters in either adjunctive treatment group.

Mean changes from baseline to each visit during the open-label adjunctive treatment phase were statistically significant for various chemistry, hematology, and urinalysis analytes. However, the mean changes were small and not considered clinically meaningful. During the study, 15% of the patients overall reported an adverse event as a reason for a dose reduction, and the most common events (≥5 patients) were tachycardia (n = 11, 3.8%) and palpitations (n = 5, 1.7%), both of which occurred more frequently in the PBO/EDX group (n = 9, 4.6%; and n = 4, 2.1%).

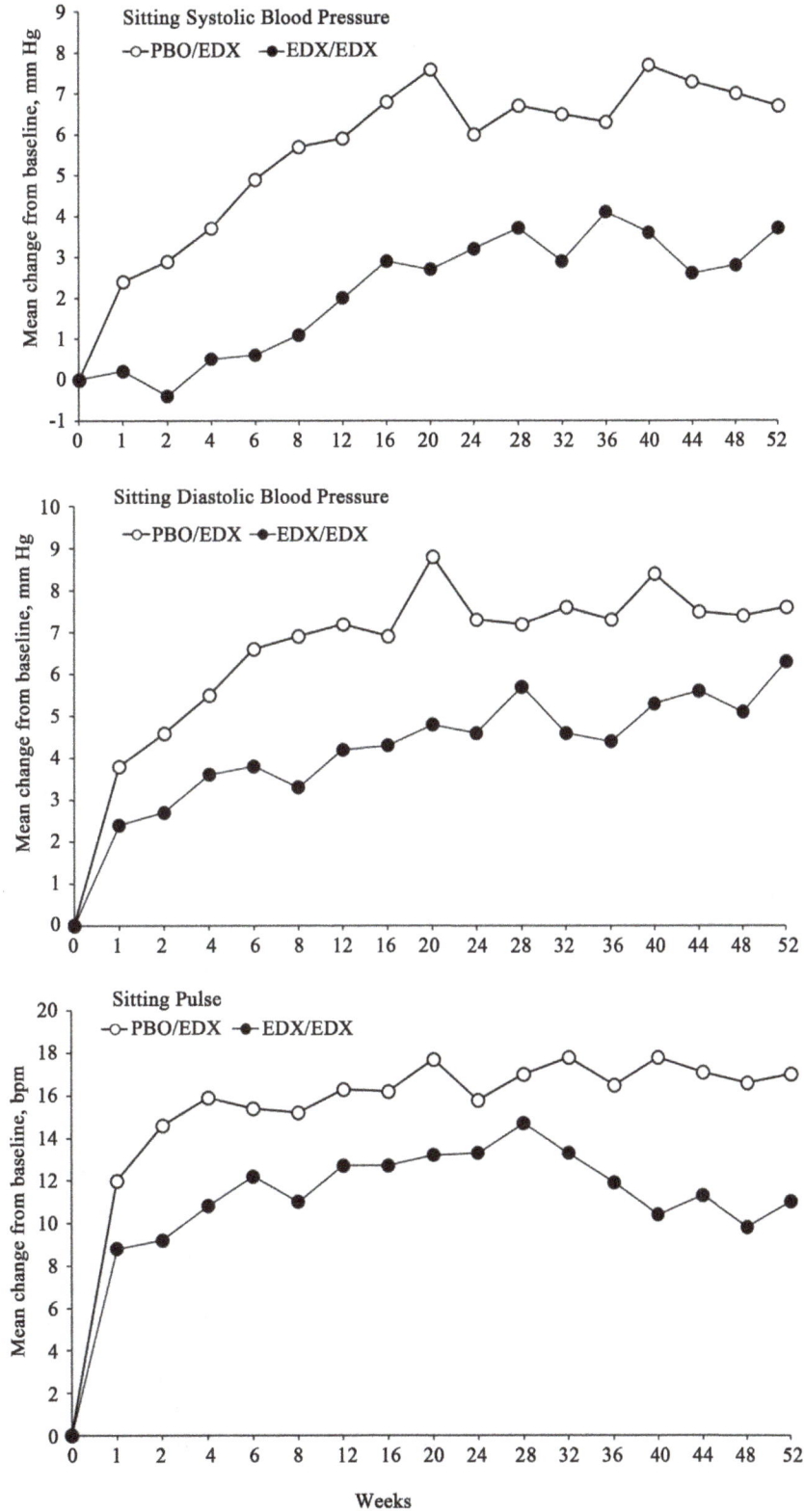

Figure 1. Least-squares mean changes from baseline in systolic blood pressure (top), di-astolic blood pressure (middle) and pulse (bottom) taken while sitting at each study visit. Abbreviations: PBO = placebo; EDX = edivoxetine; mm Hg = millimeters of mercury; bpm = beats per minutes.

Table 3. Treatment-emergent elevations in sitting blood pressure and pulse.

Measure (Unit)/Criteria	Placebo/Edivoxetine		Edivoxetine/Edivoxetine		All Patients	
	N	n (%)	N	n (%)	N	n (%)
Elevated Any Time						
SDP of ≥140 mm Hg and an increase of ≥20 mm Hg from baseline	195	20 (10.3)	92	4 (4.4)	287	24 (8.4)
DBP of ≥90 mm Hg and an increase of ≥10 mm Hg from baseline	195	54 (27.7)	92	24 (26.1)	287	78 (27.2)
Pulse > 100 beats per minute (bpm) and an increase of ≥15 bpm from baseline.	195	109 (55.9)	92	35 (38.0)	287	144 (50.2)
Sustained Elevation at 3 Consecutive Visits						
SDP of ≥140 mm Hg and an increase of ≥20 mm Hg from baseline	185	2 (1.1)	86	0	271	1 (0.7)
DBP of ≥90 mm Hg and an increase of ≥10 mm Hg from baseline	185	22 (11.9)	86	8 (9.3)	271	30 (11.1)
Pulse >100 beats per minute (bpm) and an increase of ≥15 bpm from baseline	185	46 (24.9)	86	8 (9.3)	271	54 (20.0)
Potentially Clinically Significant, Any Time						
SDP of ≥180 mm Hg and an increase of ≥20 mm Hg from baseline	195	0	92	0	287	0
DBP of ≥105 mm Hg and an increase of ≥15 mm Hg from baseline	195	6 (3.1)	92	2 (2.2)	287	2 (2.8)

Abbreviations: SDP = systolic blood pressures; DBP = diastolic blood pressure; mm Hg = millimeters of mercury; bpm = beats per minute.

Treatment-emergent suicidal ideation or behavior as assessed by the C-SSRS was reported by 9.8% of patients overall and there was one interrupted suicide attempt in the PBO/EDX group.

The majority of patients met criteria for sexual dysfunction at baseline based on the ASEX scores: 79.6% (121/152) of male patients and 90.2% of female patients (119/132). For patients who met criteria for sexual dysfunction at baseline, most continued to meet criteria at endpoint (88.4% of males and 90.8% of females). For patients who did not meet sexual dysfunction at baseline, 35.5% of male patients and 61.5% of female patients worsened and met dysfunction criteria at endpoint.

At baseline, the mean (SD) MGH-CPFQ total score was 23.8 (6.6) in the PBO/EDX group and was 25.2 (6.0) in the EDX/EDX group. At the end of the study, cognitive and physical well-being was improved with LS mean changes (SE) from baseline that were statistically significant (p ≤ 0.001) from zero in both groups: −4.02 (0.5) and −2.53 (0.8), respectively.

4. Discussion

This is the first long-term safety study of edivoxetine as adjunctive therapy to SSRI antidepressants inpatients with MDD in Japan, who were partial responders to their SSRI treatment. Long-term treatment with adjunctive edivoxetine in Japanese patients with MDD did not reveal safety and tolerability concerns that differed substantially from the outcomes of short-term (1 phase II and 3 phase III) adjunctive edivoxetine trials [8] [10] and a1-year open-label safety and tolerability study [11]. In addition, there were no deaths during this study.

Discontinuation due to adverse events in this study (17.4%) was higher than in the short-term adjunctive edivoxetine studies (4.9% - 5.4%) [8] [10], but was similar to the rate reported in the other long-term study of adjunctive edivoxetine (17.0%) [11]. The most common adverse events (≥2% frequency) leading to early discontinuation were palpitations, vomiting and hypertension in this study; the other long-term study reported hypertension (2.0%) [11]. The most common (≥5%) TEAEs reported in this study were similar to those reported in the previous studies: nasopharyngitis, tachycardia, hyperhidrosis, nausea, palpitations, and increased heart rate [8] [10]. Adverse events (≥5 patients) that led to a dose reduction were palpitations and tachycardia in this study; and erectile dysfunction, nausea, and hyperhidrosis in the other long-term study [11].

Mean increases in blood pressure and pulse were observed across visits during this study. These increases were observed in the previous adjunctive edivoxetine studies [8] [10], and were expected given the mechanism of action of edivoxetine as a norepinephrine reuptake inhibitor. However, the mean increases in pulse rate and DBP was higher in this study as compared with the previous short- and long-term studies of adjunctive edivoxetine [8] [10] [11]. In a pooled analysis of the three phase III trials [10], there was a significant treatment-by-geographic region interaction (across Japan, the UK and the US) with adjunctive edivoxetine that was observed with changes in DBP and pulse. The interaction suggested that the hemodynamic response to NRIs as adjunctive treatment to SSRIs in Japanese patients may be different from that in non-Japanese. However, in the 1-year open-label safety study, ethnic differences in vital sign changes were not observed probably because the study population was mostly comprised of Caucasian patients [11].

It is unclear why treatment with edivoxetine as adjunctive treatment to SSRI antidepressants would be associated with higher increases in DBP and pulse in Japanese patients than that observed in Caucasian patients. In a short-term safety study of edivoxetine given as single or multiple doses that was conducted in healthy adult male Japanese and Caucasian patients (unpublished), greater increases in pulse and blood pressure were observed in the Japanese patients relative to the Caucasian patients. However, the trends of the changes were similar between the groups, and there were no significant differences between the Japanese and Caucasian patients in pharmacokinetics (PK) or pharmacodynamic (PD) evaluations (unpublished). However, PK and PD evaluations were not done in this study, so it was not known if the outcome of these measures would be different when edivoxetine was given with SSRI antidepressants.

There are few long-term studies of treatment with NRI drugs in Japan. However, there is one long-term (58 weeks) safety study of treatment with the NRI atomoxetine that is conducted in adult Japanese patients with attention deficit hyperactivity disorder (ADHD) [20]. Similarly, this study reported treatment-emergent increases in pulse (9 bpm), and systolic and diastolic blood pressure (4 mm Hg and 5 mm Hg, respectively). Because these vital sign changes were similar to those reported in long-term studies in North American adults with ADHD [21]-[23], they were considered to be consistent with the known NRI mode of action.

The open-label study design and lack of control group limit the interpretation of observed changes that may have been associated with non-treatment effects. In addition, there were no statistical comparisons performed between groups and only categorical variables were summarized with counts and percentages. However, the open-label design mirrored clinical practice and provided a description of key clinically relevant safety outcomes in Japanese patients.

In conclusion, the assessment across all safety measures in the long-term treatment with edivoxetine as adjunctive therapy to SSRI antidepressants in Japanese patients with MDD indicated that the safety profile of edivoxetine was consistent with that expected for a selective NRI.

Acknowledgements

This work was supported by Eli Lilly and Company, Indianapolis, IN, USA.

References

[1] Kawakami, N., Takeshima, T., Ono, Y., Uda, H., Hata, Y., Nakane, Y., *et al.* (2005) Twelve-Month Prevalence, Severity, and Treatment of Common Mental Disorders in Communities in Japan: Preliminary Finding from the World Mental Health Japan Survey 2002-2003. *Psychiatry and Clinical Neuroscience*, **59**, 441-452. http://dx.doi.org/10.1111/j.1440-1819.2005.01397.x

[2] Värnik, P. (2012) Suicide in the World. *International Journal of Environmental Research and Public Health*, **9**, 760-771. http://dx.doi.org/10.3390/ijerph9030760

[3] Sado, M., Yamauchi, K., Kawakami, N., Ono, Y., Furukawa, T.A., Tsuchiya, M., *et al.* (2011) Cost of Depression among Adults in Japan in 2005. *Psychiatry and Clinical Neuroscience*, **65**, 442-450. http://dx.doi.org/10.1111/j.1440-1819.2011.02237.x

[4] Bakish, D. (2001) New Standard of Depression Treatment: Remission and Full Recovery. *The Journal of Clinical Psychiatry*, **62**, S5-S9.

[5] McGirr, A., Séguin, M., Renaud, J., Benkelfat, C., Alda, M. and Turecki, C. (2006) Gender and Risk Factors for Suicide: Evidence for Heterogeneity in Predisposing Mechanisms in a Psychological Autopsy Study. *Journal of Clinical Psychiatry*, **67**, 1612-1617. http://dx.doi.org/10.4088/JCP.v67n1018

[6] Trivedi, M.H., Rush, A.J., Wisniewski, S.R., Nierenberg, A.A., Warden, D., Ritz, L., *et al.* (2006) Evaluation of Outcomes with Citalopram for Depression Using Measurement-Based Care in STAR*D: Implications for Clinical Practice. *The American Journal of Psychiatry*, **163**, 28-40. http://dx.doi.org/10.1176/appi.ajp.163.1.28

[7] Lucca, A., Serretti, A. and Smeraldi, E. (2000) Effect of Reboxetine Augmentation in SSRI Resistant Patients. *Human Psychopharmacology: Clinical and Experimental*, **15**, 143-145.

http://dx.doi.org/10.1002/(SICI)1099-1077(200003)15:2<143::AID-HUP152>3.0.CO;2-N

[8]   Ball, S., Dellva, M.A., D'Souza, D.N., Marangell, L.B., Russell, J.M. and Goldberger, C. (2014) A Double-Blind, Place-bo-Controlled Study of Edivoxetine as an Adjunctive Treatment for Patients with Major Depressive Disorder Who Are Partial Responders to Selective Serotonin Reuptake Inhibitor Treatment. *Journal of Affective Disorders*, **167**, 215-223. http://dx.doi.org/10.1016/j.jad.2014.06.006

[9]   Ball, S.G., Ferguson, M.B., Martinez, J.M., Pangallo, B.A., Nery, E.S., Dellva, M.A., Sparks, J., Liu, P., Zhang, Q. and Bangs, M. (in Press) Efficacy Outcomes from 3 Clinical Trials of Edivoxetine as Adjunctive Treatment for Patients with Major Depressive Disorder who are Partial Responders to Selective Serotonin Reuptake Inhibitor Treatment. Un-published. *Journal of Clinical Psychiatry*.

[10] Martinez, J.M., Ferguson, M.B., Pangallo, B.A., Oakes, T.M., Sparks, J., Dellva, M.A., Zhang, Q., Liu, P., Bangs, M.E., Ahl, J. and Goldberger, C. (in Press) Safety and Tolerability of Edivoxetine as Adjunctive Treatment to Selective Seroto-nin Reuptake Inhibitor Antidepressants for Patients with Major Depressive Disorder. *Drugs in Context*.

[11] Ball, S., Atkinson, S., Sparks, J., Bangs, M., Goldberger, C. and Dubé, S. (2015) Long-term, Open-label, Safety Study of Edivoxetine 12 to 18 mg Once Daily as Adjunctive Treatment for Patients with Major Depressive Disorder Who Are Par-tial Responders to Selective Serotonin Reuptake Inhibitor Treatment. *Journal of Clinical Psychopharmacology* (in Press).

[12] Malhotra, A.K., Myrphym Jr., G.M. and Kennedy, J.L. (2004) Pharmacogenetics of Psychotropic Drug Response. *American Journal ofPsychiatry*, **161**, 780-796. http://dx.doi.org/10.1176/appi.ajp.161.5.780

[13] Geller, S.E., Koch, A., Pellettier, B. and Carnes, M. (2011) Inclusion, Analysis, and Reporting of Sex and Race/Eth-nicity in Clinical Trials: Have We Made Progress? *Journal of Women's Health*, **20**, 315-320. http://dx.doi.org/10.1089/jwh.2010.2469

[14] Montgomery, S.A. and Åsberg, M. (1979) A New Depression Scale Designed to be Sensitive to Change. *The British Journal of Psychiatry*, **134**, 382-389. http://dx.doi.org/10.1192/bjp.134.4.382

[15] Williams, J.B., Kobak, K.A., Bech, P., Engelhardt, N., Evans, K., Lipsitz, J., *et al.* (2008) The GRID-HAMD: Standar-dization of the Hamilton Depression Rating Scale. *International Clinical Psychopharmacology*, **23**, 120-129. http://dx.doi.org/10.1097/YIC.0b013e3282f948f5

[16] Chandler, G.M., Iosifescu, D.V., Pollack, M.H., Targum, S.D. and Fava, M. (2010) Research: Validation of the Mas-sachusetts General Hospital Antidepressant Treatment History Questionnaire (ATRQ). *CNS Neuroscience and Thera-peutics*, **16**, 322-325. http://dx.doi.org/10.1111/j.1755-5949.2009.00102.x

[17] Posner, K., Brown, G.K., Stanley, B., Brent, D.A., Yershova, K.V., Oquendo, M.A., *et al.* (2011) The Columbia-Sui-cide Severity Rating Scale: Initial Validity and Internal Consistency Findings from Three Multisite Studies with Ado-lescents and Adults. *The American Journal of Psychiatry*, **168**, 1266-1277. http://dx.doi.org/10.1176/appi.ajp.2011.10111704

[18] McGahuey, C.A., Gelenberg, A.J., Laukes, C.A., Moreno, F.A., Delgado, P.L., McKnight, K.M., *et al.* (2000) The Arizona Sexual Experience Scale (ASEX): Reliability and Validity. *Journal of Sex and Marital Therapy*, **26**, 25-40. http://dx.doi.org/10.1080/009262300278623

[19] Fava, M., Iosifescu, D.V., Pedrelli, P. and Baer, L. (2009) Reliability and Validity of the Massachusetts General Hos-pital Cognitive and Physical Functioning Questionnaire. *Psychotherapy and Psychosomatics*, **78**, 91-97. http://dx.doi.org/10.1159/000201934

[20] Hirata, Y., Goto, T., Takita, Y., Trzepacz, P.T., Allen, A.J., Ichikawa, H. and Takahashi, M. (2014) Long-Term Safety and Tolerability of Atomoxetine in Japanese Adults with Attention Deficit Hyperactivity Disorder. *Asia-Pacific Psy-chiatry*, **6**, 292-301. http://dx.doi.org/10.1111/appy.12119

[21] Adler, L.A., Spencer, T.J., Williams, D.W., Moore, R.J. and Michelson, D. (2008) Long-Term, Open-Label Safety and Efficacy of Atomoxetine in Adults with ADHD: Final Report of a 4-Year Study. *Journal of Attention Disorders*, **12**, 248-253. http://dx.doi.org/10.1177/1087054708316250

[22] Adler, L.A., Spencer, T., Brown, T.E., Holdnack, J., Saylor, K., Schuh, K., *et al.* (2009) Once-Daily Atomoxetine for Adult Attention-Deficit/Hyperactivity Disorder: A 6-Month, Double-Blind Trial. *Journal of Clinical Psychopharma-cology*, **29**, 44-50.

[23] Young, J.L., Sarkis, E., Qiao, M. and Wietecha, L. (2011) Once-Daily Treatment with Atomoxetine in Adults with At-tention-Deficit/Hyperactivity Disorder in Adults: A 24-Week, Randomized, Double-Blind, Placebo-Controlled Trial. *Clinical Neuropharmacology*, **34**, 51-60.

11

The Norwegian 22 July 2011 Terror Acts and Mass Murder: Insanity, Evilness or Both?

Henning Værøy*

Department for Research and Development, Division of Mental Health Services, Akershus University Hospital, Lørenskog, Norway
Email: Heve@ahus.no

Abstract

This review presents unique information rarely seen in a description of a politically extreme right wing terrorist. During the trial following the terror acts in Norway on July 22nd 2011, the author, a forensic psychiatrist was at the time engaged by a national Norwegian newspaper to comment on the court proceedings. The author has later thoroughly gone through all available background material such as the terrorist's childhood, relationship to his mother, childhood psychological evaluation, the interviews made by the forensic psychiatrists and information from the police documents. This information is shared in the review. The author also discusses how it was possible for two pairs of court appointed experienced forensic psychiatrists to arrive at completely different conclusions. One pair concluded with insanity due to Paranoid Schizophrenia and the second pair found no signs of psychotic disorder at all and concluded with Narcissistic Personality Disorder. The court found the terrorist capable to stand trial and sentenced him to 21 years in preventive detention with 10 years to be served before the possibility to apply for an appeal.

Keywords

Terrorism, Insanity, Forensic Diagnosis, Mental Disorders, Personality

1. The 22 July Terror Acts: Background and Consequences

Norway was struck by an outrageous act of terrorism on 22 July 2011. First, the centre of Oslo, including government buildings, was hit by a car bomb, and later a terrorist executed young members of the labour party's youth organisation at an island camp outside Oslo. Within 189 minutes [1], 77 persons lost their lives. Several survived, but had been marked for life.

---

*MD, Dr. in Medical Sciences (Ph.D.), Specialist in Psychiatry.

The court engaged two forensic psychiatrists (FP-1) who, after examining the murderer, concluded that he was suffering from insanity due to paranoid schizophrenia as defined by the *World Health Organization International Classification of Diseases Version* 10 (ICD 10) criteria [2].

Norway is familiar to a certain extent with events involving dangerous psychiatric patients and inadequate hospital security measures. In the past, there have been cases in which psychiatric healthcare treatment programs have not managed to treat and follow up the most dangerous psychiatric patients adequately. The collaboration between psychiatry and the legal system has, in some cases, failed badly in protecting the general population from such severely ill patients. A growing distrust in psychiatric health care is emerging in Norway, and after the insanity conclusion was presented by FP-1 in the Anders Behring Breivik [ABB] case, this frustration and distrust were further encouraged. A public debate on psychiatry's actual role in forensic settings and current practice has followed. During the debate, the court decided to appoint two additional forensic psychiatrists [FP-2] who concluded that the murderer had no signs of insanity or psychosis, but was a political extremist suffering from narcissistic personality disorder [NPD] and traits of antisocial personality disorder [APD]. A recent paper reported on how these issues were handled by the court in the verdict [3].

2. The Terrorist Anders Behring Breivik

2.1. Childhood

In 1981, ABB's mother [4] applied for childcare assistance for her two children, but especially for her son, who was about 2 years old. After separating from her husband in 1980, she was exhausted having to raise the two children as a single parent. The boy was described as very challenging, and a resource family where the children lived during weekends was offered. Later, for a period during 1983 and 1984, the mother once more asked for assistance because she felt that her now 4-year-old son was hyperactive, passive and clingy [5]. The family of three was admitted to the family department of a children's psychiatric hospital for about three weeks, at the end of which a psychologist recommended that custody of the 4-year-old boy should be taken away from his mother. It was argued that the boy was in need of a foster home because he had become contact avoiding, anxious and passive, but with evident restlessness. The child had also developed strategies for getting out of difficult situations, e.g. what was described as a self-imposed avoidant smile [5]. The psychologist also reported that the boy had difficulties with expressing himself emotionally, and that he was passive when playing with others. Despite maintaining some elements of pleasure and joy, he had an almost total lack of spontaneity [5].

During court proceedings in the spring of 1983, the father asked the court to grant him custody of the children. This was based on advice he had received from the family department of the children's psychiatric hospital who stated that unchanged, continued care provided by the mother would most likely increase the boy's risk of developing "serious psychopathology" [6]. In contrast to this, the local public childcare employees basically found nothing wrong with the mother and her two infants. The father lost his case and no longer pursued his claims.

From the forensic report written by FP-2 [7], it is known that ABB visited his father in the south of France for three weeks every summer for some years. He was under crossfire from his parents, being constantly reminded by his mother that his father was an avaricious "criminal" and by his father that his mother was "the crazy one". The report [7] also mentions that the mother had several boyfriends during ABB's upbringing. Two of these became stable father figures, from whom ABB sought support.

Some of the detailed information about the relationship between mother and son in 1983 was initially presented during the 2012 court proceedings. Later, the court prevented publication of this information in the media on the grounds of the mother's right to privacy. What is known from the present author's personal notes from the proceedings is that a psychologist found reason to suspect that the mother transferred her sexual frustrations onto the boy.

ABB also confirmed that he once bought a cake and a dildo as a birthday gift for his mother after her relationship with one of her lovers had ended. Unconfirmed information from ABB's contact with a foster home states that ABB had been encouraged by his mother to touch the foster father's penis in order to observe how it reacted. According to the foster parents, this emerged after a statement from his sister claiming that she had been encouraged to do the same by her father.

2.2. The Mother and Son Relationship

In a recently published book [8], the author chose to publish some previously censored information. In brief,

ABB's mother had been admitted into psychiatric care several times due to problems related to emotional instability and later paranoid delusions and hallucinations. She originally wanted an abortion when she became pregnant with ABB, but failed to submit an application before the legal limit. During the pregnancy, she felt that the unborn child was a difficult foetus due to its general activity, especially its kicking. The latter was perceived as being something the foetus almost did on purpose. She stopped breastfeeding him after 10 months because she could not bear his aggressive sucking which she perceived and consequently described as something destructive. According to the mother, as ABB grew up he became more and more demanding. Other terms used by her were that her son was "hyperactive and clingy".

When ABB was 2 years old, she expressed her fears of what he might do, especially to his sister. The children's psychiatric hospital wrote that they considered her incapable of meeting her son's needs for clarity and structure. The 2-year-old's response to his mother's ambivalence was described as being a devious smile and sometimes laughter. She explained that when she slapped him he always responded by saying that "It didn't hurt, it didn't hurt". Also, the staff at the kindergarten observed that ABB did not cry. Nor did he show other signs of pain when expected, e.g. after a fall. The mother expressed that she wanted "to peel him off me" and that she had a death wish in his regard.

How much the 2 - 3 years old perceived of his mother's thoughts and ideas is impossible to know. After being captured following the terror acts ABB said that "it would have been better if my father and his new wife had won the custody case", referring to the court's ruling when he was around 4 years old. He also made statements like "My mother is not intellectually capable…", "Women don't understand the concept of honour" and "90% of them are emotionally unstable". Likewise, "Fathers should automatically be granted custody of children because those who control the cradle control the world".

The children's psychiatric hospital also wrote that ABB was a victim of his mother's aggressive paranoid projections and fear of sexual intimacy with men in general. Furthermore, as part of the communication between mother and child observed, the hospital described how they lived in a physical symbiosis—as if mother and son were united in one body. "After they were left on their own, Anders for some time slept in his mother's bed with close body contact" [8]. There is no concrete evidence of an incestuous relationship between mother and son, but the hospital refers to an episode in which the mother, in a somewhat "rejectful" manner, allegedly told her son to go and have sexual activity with a person outside the family. In this regard, the link between sexual abuse and the potential development of a pathological personality has been established and described [9].

ABB's mother visited her son in prison before she died in 2013. He was not allowed to attend her funeral.

2.3. Adolescence

The contact between father and son ended in 1995 when ABB was around 15 - 16 years old. In the same period, he was caught twice spraying and tagging trains in Oslo. The police closed the cases and no charges were made.

A police file from 1994 states that ABB did not admit any guilt but agreed to assist in removing the graffiti.

The childcare authorities also opened an investigation, but it was closed shortly after and filed as "nothing further to pursue". School reports [7] state that a teacher described ABB as a person who defended himself intensively and somewhat out of proportion, when, for example, he was late for class. The same teacher associated ABB's behaviour with the reactions of someone living with an almost irrational and constant fear.

ABB performed reasonably well at school. During the court proceedings, friends from school described ABB as an intelligent and physically stronger man than his classmates. He was also the one who helped those who were being bullied [10]. In ABB's mind, looking good was equal to looking strong. At one point, he started weight training and enhanced his progress by using steroids [11].

ABB went to high school from 1995 to 1998 but did not graduate. According to a friend interviewed by FP-2 [7], ABB left high school to start his own business. He had told his friend that he wanted to change other peoples' impression of him and that he wanted to be different from the average student. ABB had also explained that to achieve this, economic success was a major criterion. ABB had a reputation as a person not to start an argument with, but his friend knew of no situations where ABB had actually been violent.

ABB became politically active on the right wing during the high school period and he used to speak about multiculturalism and incompatibility between the Islamic world and Christianity. ABB considered Islam a political ideology and not a religion [7].

ABB claims to have been mentally sane during adolescence, but friends questioned some of his reactions and behaviour. There is no information available to shed light on his psychiatric health during adolescence.

Having heard all witnesses in court, the overall impression is that ABB interacted with only very few close friends during adolescence and that he was happy to be on his own, sometimes for what some people would describe as long periods, without being more specific. However, there is also evidence that he shared apartments with friends for some periods.

There is no known history of stable girlfriends or partners. In court, some of ABB's friends disclosed their thoughts about how ABB could have lied about intimate relations to try to build an image of being the ladies' preferred choice. There are also unconfirmed rumours about sporadic contact with transsexuals.

2.4. Adulthood

At the beginning of his twenties, ABB underwent cosmetic surgery on his mandible, nose and forehead. According to witnesses in court, the results gave him satisfaction [12]. One friend told FP-2 [7] that ABB, at the age of around 25 - 26 years, used anabolic steroids and that he was interested in body building. The same friend mentioned that ABB was more aggressive in that period and that he occasionally smoked cannabis.

During the court proceedings, friends and colleagues explained that ABB had had several businesses, some profitable and others not. Common to most of his business was that they were short-lived and were associated with problems following Norwegian laws and regulations. Among his most notorious activities was a company providing falsified certificates and diplomas. This company was shut down in 2006, after which ABB lived on his savings. To make his savings last longer, he reduced his expenses by moving back to his old room at his mother's apartment.

Friends were asked in court about when ABB decided to move back in with his mother. One of them explained [7] that friends had recommended to ABB's mother not to let him move back in with her, arguing that it was the opposite of doing him a favour. ABB's argument at the time was that after having worked a lot he needed time off to do what he wanted. To ABB, this was not an illegitimate claim but in general no different from other peoples' reasons for taking extended leave. ABB had shared some reflections regarding his childhood alone with his mother who had not managed to take proper care of him during his upbringing, referring especially to the lack of guidance. He had also explained to his friend that children in general needed a stricter upbringing that he had [7].

Of special interest during the court proceedings was the question about the existence of an organisation called the Knights Templar (KT), an ultra-right wing criminal organisation with around 7 founding members. The police had found no proof of its existence but ABB kept insisting that KT was an organisation of which he was a founding member. Also of interest was the question of when ABB started to write his manifesto published just hours before the terror acts and when he started to plan and prepare for the terror acts. The truth may never be known. Still, there is enough evidence to conclude that since 2006 ABB had already made extensive preparations of which precautions to avoid being caught were an important part. As for psychiatric health issues, there is no information about any disorders or problems except for his mother's concerns that he stayed in and played World of Warcraft for days on end.

2.5. Political Activity and Hobbies

ABB joined the ultra-right wing party's Fremskrittspartiet [Fp] youth organisation [FpU] in 1997. There, he expressed strong opinions about immigration, but he was never considered to be a potential terrorist or a mass murderer. ABB later complained critically that the Fp had become too liberal and too busy with being accepted as politically correct in recent years. It is also known that he joined a shooting club in Oslo, which enabled him to acquire weapons legally. ABB had no official military training. All he knew about weapons was based on information from the internet, from his experience at the shooting club, and from firing guns in isolated places out in the wild. During the court proceedings, ABB explained how he prepared for the terror attacks, e.g. by renting an isolated farm, registering as a farmer in order to buy large amounts of nitrogen-based fertilizer, and how he used specific computer-based instruction programs for firearm practice and training on precision aiming. After his arrest, he cynically claimed that these latter mentioned computer programs had been most useful later, during the assassination of the summer camp participants at Utøya.

3. Diagnostic Approach

Guidance for the forensic psychiatric examination is given by the court. The examination by the appointed psychiatrists is based on psychiatric interviews and use of diagnostic criteria and psychometric tools like SCID II. In this case the four appointed individual psychiatrists, although operating in pairs should make separate interviews and arrive at independent conclusions. FP-1 made 13 observations [36 hours] together referring to safety measures as the main reason for why the observations were not made independently. Their approach was publicly criticized by colleagues in open court. The second pair of appointed forensic psychiatrists made their observations separately. The report made by FP-1 offers the psychiatrists' statements and conclusions. It offers very little to quote from the interviews with the terrorist compared to the report from FP-2. Since one purpose with this paper was to present a more detailed picture of ABB, direct information from the interviews are crucial; which is why the report from FP-2 was chosen as main source.

3.1. The Forensic Evaluations

The police's interviews and interrogations of the perpetrator: The forensic psychiatrists' interpretations.

From the FP-2 forensic psychiatrists' report several interviews were made with the terrorist. From these, parts of the dialogue have been transcribed and added to the forensic report. Selected sequences have been translated and are presented below.

From a section of an interview:

The forensic psychiatrist (*FP*-2): "I want to inform you that we have not read the first psychiatric report".

The terrorist (*ABB*): "I am quite impressed that you have been able to control yourself in this regard. My impression is that every psychiatrist in Norway has made their comments, because it must be very tempting to do so in view of the fact that this is such an important case, so—it is impressive indeed".

Talking about the report made by FP-1 [4], *ABB said*: "My impression was that they specifically selected those sources that describe me in the most negative way. Their work was to a large extent based on the technique of "*cut and paste*". My impression, based on reading their report, is that they already at an early stage decided upon what should be the outcome and conclusion. Then they built their case supporting that decision. That is my impression after reading it…"

One of the psychiatrists in FP-2 [7] describes a sequence during an interview with ABB. Parts of this are quoted below.

FP-2: "The media claimed that you presented yourself differently in court when I was present…"

ABB: "I did not think about that at all. I was myself in every way. If you had known me, then you could have foreseen that my presence at the court proceedings would have a great resemblance to a performance. Whatever I say is just a formality. My audience is a small group of persons, a few thousand in Europe, but there may be more. I am aware that this represents a reality which is too strange for most people. But it is a show… I play my part. So, if I say that I expect to receive the war cross with three swords, then, of course I know that I never will get it. And, when I say that I expect to be released immediately, I know that this is not realistic. I am just carrying through what I had planned for a long time".

The terrorist's statements on how he is on a mission to save Norway and Europe from islamisation and how he considers the Marxist Norwegian government as being responsible for ongoing islamisation in Norway is the background for the following.

FP-2: "But why not just be yourself?"

ABB: "In a way I am myself because I present a completely different view on the world, a view which has not been expressed since World War II. This view is of course known in Japan and South Korea. Much of the ideology I represent is normal in Japan and South Korea. It is all about culture and related politics, but to people living in a Marxist society, my ideology seems as strange as it possibly can be".

FP-2: "We will not go into this further, but what you claim to be a Marxist society is in fact a social democracy, or at least most people see it this way, don't they?"

ABB: "I can of course say it is a social democracy. I can distinguish between the two. However, when I say culturally Marxist, what I mean is social democracy as an ideology in which the primary aspects derive from Marxism, like equal rights for both genders… This kind of rhetoric is in many ways a kind of management and ruling technique I may apply, depending on the situation. For those on the left wing this technique is known and used when they stigmatize people as living by a doctrine in which reality is essentially evil. Moreover, we use it on those on the left wing…"

"Are you aware of the 7 questions I asked the other two psychiatrists?"

FP-2: "No, but you may pose them".

ABB: "It is impossible, in such a huge and important case like 22 July, not to become emotionally over-whelmed by the facts. Except for a few minor events, it is the first terrorist attack of such dimensions. The psychiatric society has no experience with politically motivated violence. Not including politically motivated violent persons as a topic in plans for psychiatric studies results in the major problem that psychiatrists don't know how militant nationalists think, how militant Islamists think, or for that matter, how militant Marxists think. This thinking represents an isolated world which I believe only a minority of psychiatrists, if any at all, are familiar with. It is an unknown and strange world and there are no experts in this field. You are not taught about it in school either. I don't know if you have had the opportunity to study it more profoundly, perhaps you can enlighten me?"

FP-2: "No, not in this field. We follow what happens with the same interest as we would do in any other circumstances. It is not a specific part of our profession. We have a mandate to relate to, where the questions regarding insanity or not, level of consciousness and level of mental impairment are the essentials".

ABB says later that: "It is important that you don't underestimate the knowledge about the mentality of especially Al Qaeda or other Islamic militants. These militants have been sources of inspiration for both me and those few individuals I have associated with".

FP-2's interpretation of DVD (*sound only*) *interview of the terrorist made at Utøya on the afternoon and evening of 22 July* 2011.

In their approach to the 22 July interview, FP-2 [7] chose to display large sequences from what the terrorist *de facto* said after having been apprehended at Utøya. Furthermore, they included the description of additional sounds recorded and their interpretation of what they heard.

The first interview by the police was performed in a house at Utøya immediately after apprehension and continued the same evening and the following night. In the background one could hear the noise from the helicopters transporting the wounded off the island. After having listened to the recordings, FP-2 described [7] that they were left with a somewhat strange and peculiar impression. They noted that at a time when 69 dead persons were still on the island and the nation was paralyzed, ABB was sitting down managing to conduct an almost jovial and sociable conversation. He was friendly and polite answering questions, paying close attention not to compromise third parties. He gave the impression of being somewhat agitated. In some sequences, ABB talked about his political point of view in a larger context in which he also played a role. His explanations were rich in detail and also included some details about his preparations for the terror acts. At a certain point, a situation occurred in which the police expressed a strong desire for information about potential fellow terrorists capable of new strikes. ABB on his side focused more on his demands to have access to a computer to offer to collaborate.

He confirmed that he was responsible for the bombing in Oslo and for the killings at Utøya, but showed no signs of emotion in that regard. ABB's statements about fearing for his own life were understandable in view of the fact that during the apprehension, the police were very close to firing shots directly at him, but did not.

3.2. The Remaining Police Interviews Evaluated by FP-2 [7]

FP-2 was appointed after FP-1 had finished their report [4]. The police's interrogations of ABB continued after the report from FP-1 [4]. FP-2 therefore had more interviews to evaluate than FP-1. Regarding the interviews that were evaluated by both teams of psychiatrists, instead of presenting a summary of their interpretations as FP-1 did [4], FP-2 [7] chose to display exact sequences from the police's interrogations.

FP-2 describes ABB's politeness, his initial agitation followed by a calmer period, as did their colleagues [7]. FP-2 underline that they never observed any signs of sadness or signs of regrets during the interviews made available [7]. ABB is described as being cooperative and giving detailed information as long as it did not involve others negatively. In this case, others are those persons who ABB called mentors and fellow founding members of Knights Templar.

FP-2 state that ABB's explanations may in part be judged as being unnecessarily detailed, and furthermore, that he was easily caught by momentary digressions, but also that he was equally easy to get back on track [7].

During some of the interviews FP-2 noticed that ABB, when presenting his global political view and why his terror acts were necessary, had constructed a high and grandiose role for himself. Another observation made was that each time ABB tried to negotiate, he appeared self conscious and demanding.

FP-2 describe [7] how in the interviews made during the police's reconstruction, ABB explained in detail and without any signs of emotional engagement what he did on Utøya. These descriptions are more or less identical to FP-1's version [4]. On the other hand, FP-2's comments [7] based on the same background material give little, if any support to FP-1's conclusion [4] of "moderate associative disturbances".

3.3. Personality Disorders

In their report, FP-2 [7] state that the terrorist displays symptoms of NPD. This condition is classified in ICD 10 [2] as among those in category F 60.8. FP-2 also felt that the symptoms found when examining the terrorist justified a diagnosis of F 60.2 Dissocial personality disorder. In their diagnostic evaluation, FP-2 uses DSM-IV [13] SCID II in the context of the ICD 10 diagnosis. This is not without problems and will be discussed later. FP-1 [4] made no mention of personality disorders in their report.

To fulfil the ICD 10 criteria [2] for specific personality disorders, a number of general criteria must first be met. **Table 1** lists the ICD 10 criteria for personality disorders.

ICD 10 does not specifically define the characteristics of NPD; it is classified as belonging to the category F 60.8 "Other specific personality disorders". The following criteria must be met for the diagnosis F 60.8 [NPD]: "A personality disorder that fits none of the specific rubrics F 60.0 - F 60.7".

DSM-IV-TR (301.81)—The Diagnostic and Statistical Manual of Mental Disorders fourth edition-Text Revised, DSM-IV-TR, defines NPD as shown in **Table 2** and classifies it among the dramatic and emotional subtypes (Cluster B).

FP-2 adopted the DSM-IV diagnostic criteria [13] and in the following text taken from their report, symptoms from the examination of the terrorist have been tested against the various criteria for classification of the DSM-IV axis II disorders:

Avoidant personality disorder—ABB gives the impression of being unafraid, engaged and secure in social situations and he is self-confident, but FP-2 found that ABB is vulnerable to criticism and that he is easily offended. In recent years, he had had very few intimate relationships and has a defensive approach regarding intimate relations. According to FP-2, these evaluations rule out avoidant personality disorder.

Dependant personality disorder—The fact that ABB has managed to take care of himself despite living at his mother's house for longer periods, his self-proclaimed one-man terror cell, being the leader of an anti-Islamic organisation, and finally his planning and execution of the terror acts without involving others, does not support a diagnosis of dependent personality disorder.

Obsessive personality disorder—ABB focuses on details, structures, and how to organize his life. This makes him capable of living a life in which he carries through his intentions. His perfectionism may also reach a point at which it becomes a challenge to complete what he initially planned. Still, this did not influence his business, leisure activities, writing, planning, bomb construction, or other activities. His choice of way of life enabled him to focus on different topics at the same time at the cost of spare time for interaction with friends. ABB prefers to do things himself. He has been careful with spending money and he is rigid and perhaps also stubborn, but he is

Table 1. ICD 10 criteria for personality disorders F 60.

G1	Evidence that the individual's characteristic and enduring patterns of inner experience and behaviour deviate markedly as a whole from the culturally expected and accepted range (or "norm"). Such deviation must be manifest in more than one of the following areas: 1—Cognition (*i.e.* ways of perceiving and interpreting things, people and events; forming attitudes and images of self and others); 2—Affectivity (range, intensity and appropriateness of emotional arousal and response); 3—Control over impulses and need gratification; 4—Relating to others and manner of handling interpersonal situations.
G2	The deviation must manifest itself pervasively as behaviour that is inflexible, maladaptive, or otherwise dysfunctional across a broad range of personal and social situations (*i.e.* not being limited to one specific "triggering" stimulus or situation).
G3	There is personal distress, or adverse impact on the social environment, or both, clearly attributable to the behaviour referred to under G2.
G4	There must be evidence that the deviation is stable and of long duration, having its onset in late childhood or adolescence.
G5	The deviation cannot be explained as a manifestation or consequence of other adult mental disorders, although episodic or chronic conditions from sections F 0 to F 7 of this classification may co-exist, or be superimposed on it.
G6	Organic brain disease, injury, or dysfunction must be excluded as possible cause of the deviation (if such organic causation is demonstrable, use category F 07).

Table 2. DSM-IV-TR criteria for Narcissistic Personality Disorder.

A pervasive pattern of grandiosity (in fantasy or behaviour), need for admiration, and lack of empathy, beginning by early adulthood and present in a variety of contexts, as indicated by five (or more) of the following:

1. Has a grandiose sense of self-importance (e.g., exaggerates achievements and talents, expects to be recognized as superior without commensurate achievements).

2. Is preoccupied with fantasies of unlimited success, power, brilliance, beauty, or ideal love.

3. Believes that he or she is "special" and unique and can only be understood by, or should associate with, other special or high-status people (or institutions).

4. Requires excessive admiration.

5. Has a sense of entitlement, *i.e.* unreasonable expectations of especially favourable treatment or automatic compliance with his or her expectations.

6. Is interpersonally exploitative, *i.e.* takes advantage of others to achieve his or her own ends.

7. Lacks empathy: is unwilling to recognize or identify with the feelings and needs of others.

8. Is often envious of others or believes others are envious of him or her.

9. Shows arrogant, haughty behaviour or attitudes.

It is also a requirement of DSM-IV that a diagnosis of any specific personality disorder also satisfies a set of general personality disorder criteria.

not a collector of items. Some traits of obsessive personality disorder may be present and may consequently influence the total score on the Obsessive Personality Disorder Scale, but FP-2 found no support for this diagnosis.

Paranoid personality disorder—FP-2 concluded that there was no reason to suspect paranoid psychosis based on what they had learned and observed. Regarding his friends, ABB revealed no irrational thinking about their loyalty. FP-2 also concluded that ABB's caution and reluctance in sharing information about his terror plans with others seems realistic and should not in this case be considered as irrational. Other elements like the fact that he often perceives peoples' comments as threatening and offensive may give an SCID II score close to the threshold on this item. FP-2 found that ABB had a score of 3 for 2 of the 7 SCID II items for paranoid personality disorder.

Schizotypal personality disorder—is a condition closely related to psychotic disorders. FP-2 found it necessary to thoroughly examine ABB's behaviour in this regard since FP-1 had concluded that he was suffering from F 20.0 paranoid schizophrenia. ABB's behaviour may in some cases be classified as sufficient for sub-threshold scores, e.g. he had had thoughts about having observed surveillance cars with special antennas outside the farm he rented. On returning to the same farm, he had once found an open door and concluded that it had been opened by others. ABB has never displayed any signs of having had strange perceptions or thoughts about magic and there were no signs of superstition or transference of thoughts. FP-2 noted that ABB has a tendency not to let up when discussing his political views, but otherwise not. FP-2 concluded that everything concerning ABB's political ideas and expression should be considered as being part of belonging to a politically extreme subculture.

Schizoid personality disorder—FP-2 found nothing that would suggest that ABB suffers from schizoid personality disorder.

Histrionic personality disorder—FP-2 found nothing that would suggest that ABB suffers from histrionic personality disorder despite the fact that he seems to greatly enjoy other peoples' attention. The latter is rather a narcissistic trait.

Narcissistic personality disorder—ABB read the first forensic psychiatric report and was most likely influenced by it. He concluded that he is narcissistic, although within a range of behaviour that he considers normal. Having reviewed all information made available to them, FP-2 found that ABB has the following narcissistic traits:

1) ABB displays a grandiose ideation regarding his own importance, even if he sometimes tries to moderate this. The grandiosity is especially evident in his manifesto and in describing his role in Knights Templar. The criterion was met.

2) ABB had had ideas about his own success and power many years before the terror acts. This became evident during the psychiatrists' interviews with him and can also be found when reading the manifesto. The desire

for fame seems to be a strong motivation for ABB in general. The criterion was met.

3) ABB enjoys talking about how he finds it especially motivating to socialize with intelligent persons with a similar high status. He underlines his lack of interest in those who, in his eyes, are of less importance. The criterion was met.

4) ABB is convinced that what he has done is for others to admire, thereby confirming a strong need for admiration. This becomes evident when he is allowed to talk about his political ideology and his terror acts. The criterion was met.

5) The terror acts of 22 July 2011 show that ABB considers he has the right to overrule society's rules and regulations. His reluctance to listen to and discuss other peoples' views may, in retrospect, be associated with his former business activities where he, at times, operated outside the law. The criterion was met.

6) FP-2 found that ABB had made a conscious and strategic choice when he decided to move back to his mother's apartment and remain there for as long as he did. Despite his statements of having had to pay a certain rent, the element of exploitation is recognizable, as is the convenience. The criterion was not fully met.

7) In his own view, ABB is an empathic person. As reference for his ability to recognize and relate to other persons' loss he used his foreseen and accepted loss of family after having performing the terror acts. There were no signs of empathy, remorse or any other emotional signs indicating distress in his statements after the terror acts. This became evident during the reconstructions made on the island of Utøya and later in court. Not showing empathy he explained is due to his ability to de-emotionalize himself. The criterion was met.

8) None of the psychiatrists found signs of envy. ABB has accepted that his friends have made careers, some having well paid jobs. Commenting on his own unsuccessful career, ABB said that he chose to pursue a certain path being well aware of the consequences. The criterion was not met.

9) ABB is clearly arrogant in his behaviour. His arrogance shows itself in many ways e.g., he always insists on being the one with the correct answer. He claims to have read a lot and has no problems with demanding recognition for his hours of reading. To him, his efforts are at least on the level of a university degree. ABB has shown that when other persons' opinions don't fit into his world of ideas, he sets all contradictions aside. The criterion was met.

FP-2 found that 7 of the 9 DSM-IV criteria for SCID II Narcissistic Personality Disorder were met, whereas 5 would have been sufficient for the ICD 10 diagnosis F 60.8 Other specific personality disorders, narcissistic. Furthermore, FP-2 found no symptoms confirming emotional instability. On the contrary, ABB seemed remarkably stable without any emotional aberrations. In this regard, there is unconfirmed information saying that ABB is quite unstable emotionally outside the court room or under observation.

FP-2 also concluded that ABB fulfilled the criteria for the diagnosis of APD. They chose to apply the DSM term antisocial instead of the ICD term dissocial, although these 2 diagnostic systems, to some degree, differ regarding the classification of antisocial behaviour. Based on SCID II for Antisocial Personality Disorder, FP-2 argued that since ABB had no behaviour indicating disturbances before the age of 13 years, the DSM-IV diagnostic criteria were not met. Applying the ICD 10 criteria, they found that the diagnosis F 60.2 Dissocial Personality Disorder was met.

3.4. The Combination of DSM-IV and ICD 10 for Personality Disorders

FP-2 [7] do not explain why they chose to test ABB's personality characteristics against the DSM-IV SCID II criteria and at the same time refer to an ICD 10 diagnosis. It most likely derives from the fact that the criteria for ICD 10 F 60.2 Dissocial Personality Disorder have never been translated into Norwegian. In addition, there is a tradition of using DSM-IV SCID II to confirm suspected, less specific ICD 10 diagnoses, e.g. those clustered under F 60.8 as "Other specific personality disorders". The rationale for FP-2's choice [7] could also be the assumption that the 2 diagnostic systems overlap and that minor differences are irrelevant. In the past, several papers have highlighted the incompatibility issue between the DSM and the ICD diagnostic systems. One study [14] found that when comparing the DSM-III-R to the ICD 10, 60% of the variance in the personality disorder diagnosis represented variance not attributable to the patients. Furthermore, it has also been reported that research results from different studies employing different instruments are not comparable [14]. Another study [15] found that only 29% of the subjects received the same primary diagnosis in each of the 2 systems, an observation perhaps related to the fact that the ICD 10 has a lower diagnostic threshold than the DSM-IV. A study [16] concluded that the sources of disagreement between the latest versions of the 2 systems could be traced to differences in the conceptualization of some of the personality disorders, and differences between the criteria and the diagnostic thresholds. Other papers have also criticized the use of DSM- or ICD-based clinical interviews for the assessment of personality disorders [17]-[19]. In a study on DSM-IV [13] and ICD 10 [2] diagnosis, the least concordant pair of personality disorders was antisocial [DSM-IV] and dissocial [ICD 10] [2]. In view of this and because psychiatric diagnosis are descriptive and have no hard endpoints, the strength of the diagnosis F 60.8 remains a matter for discussion.

3.5. Paranoid Schizophrenia

Paranoid schizophrenia has a central role in this paper since FP-1 concluded that ABB suffers from this according to ICD 10. **Table 3** presents the ICD 10 criteria for schizophrenia and the DSM-IV criteria have been added in order to make comparisons. The paranoid type features delusions or auditory hallucinations. Symptoms like thought disorder, disorganized behaviour or affective flattening are not present in this subtype of schizophrenia. Delusions are persecutory and can be of grandiose nature. Finally jealousy, religiosity, and somatisation may also be present. The APA DSM-V psychosis work group has recommended eliminating the subtypes of schizophrenia contained in the DSM-IV ("Paranoid Type", "Disorganized Type", "Catatonic Type", "Undifferentiated Type", and "Residual Type") and subsuming all of these subcategories under one diagnosis, "Schizophrenia".

3.6. Severe Psychopathology or Classification of Abnormal Behaviour

There are several hypotheses that explain the link between severe psychopathology and personality disorder, none being mutually exclusive [20]. As for schizophrenia, we have learned that patients with this disorder lack emotional and hedonic capacity and are prone to experience negative affect. Furthermore, those who develop schizophrenia have abnormal premorbid personalities [20].

Studying the impact of specific personality traits on symptomatology, disability and outcomes in schizophrenia, it was found that higher extraversion was associated with fewer positive and negative symptoms and less subjective distress. Higher neuroticism was associated with more positive symptoms, more severe delusions and greater distress, whereas psychoticism had no effect on symptomatology [21]. A general profile of high psychoticism, low agreeableness, low conscientiousness and low openness has been shown to represent stable personality characteristics over time, suggesting that they are not due to acute state effects [22]. Based on research, of which selected findings have been referred to above, personality traits seem strongly related to the most common mental illnesses. However, how these traits more specifically relate to psychopathology is less clear.

In the report by FP-1 on ABB [4], there were no indications as to the rationale behind their choice of interpretation of the behaviour observed. Nor was there any discussion regarding whether their classification of

Table 3. ICD 10 and DSM-IV diagnostic criteria for schizophrenia.

Characteristic symptoms	
ICD 10	DSM-IV
At least one of	
Thought echo, thought insertion/withdrawal/broadcast Passivity, delusional perception Third person auditory hallucination, running commentary Persistent bizarre delusions	Bizarre delusions Third person auditory hallucinations Running commentary
Or two or more of	
Persistent hallucinations Thought disorder Catatonic behaviour Negative symptoms Significant behaviour change	Delusions Hallucinations Disorganized speech Grossly disorganized behaviour Negative symptoms
Duration	
More than 1 month	1 month of characteristic symptoms With 6 months of social/occupational dysfunction

symptoms should be considered within the frames of personality disorders or psychopathology. FP-1 thought ABB had grandiose delusions regarding his own role in an extremist universe. He was considered delusional, having bizarre and paranoid qualities that went beyond conspiracy notions about an Islamist take-over of Europe [3].

4. Discussion

4.1. Childhood and Developmental Issues—Lack of Identity

Growing up with a mentally unstable mother as the only caregiver may have influenced the development of ABB's identity. A psychologist recommending foster care for ABB as a 3 - 4 years old child described the child's lack of ability to play and to interact socially. There were obvious psychosocial problems in the family and the father took the mother to court with a custody claim. After the father left, the mother had several lovers and ABB became attached to some. Repeated loss of potential father figures may therefore also have influenced ABB's development as a child.

Following the various testimonies given during the court proceedings, the impression which remains is that ABB's lack of identity gradually surfaced as he grew up. Although a bit blurred around the edges, a picture in which ABB had tried to find a place to fit in since adolescence, both socially and professionally, became much clearer. Seeking a fortune without any parental guidance or mentorship, ABB dropped out of high school, presumably because he felt he could do better without formal education. ABB has a history of having started several businesses, sometimes operating outside the law. At one point, he joined a right wing political organization and tried to make himself a political career, but failed to do so. He also failed to establish relationships on which he could build his own family. He joined the freemasons but rarely participated in meetings. ABB adopted extreme political views beyond the established conservative branches in Norwegian society, thereby excluding himself from the company of potential ideological companions. He ended up as an eccentric, almost bankrupt, moving back in with his mother where he stayed in his room playing computer games for hours and days at the time.

4.2. The Creation of an Identity

The idea of Knights Templar may have been something he picked up reading the history of the masonry. Certainly, some of the terms he later used in his manifesto bear some resemblance to the terms used to describe orders and ranks among the freemasons.

Regardless of whether a terror organisation named Knights Templar exists or not, ABB's belief in such an organisation, even on a fantasy level, underlines his need for something to refer and relate to. Previous research on terrorists has concluded that a common denominator seems to be the need for group identification in order to strengthen one's personal identity and at the same time to reduce one's own and one's group's responsibility [23].

There are many ways to interpret ABB's use of steroids and other performance enhancing substances. Likewise, the cosmetic surgery performed on his nose. One way to consider it is in the context of building and creating an identity as an adult.

4.3. Performance Enhancing Substances

Between 25 April and 15 June 2011, ABB used methandrostenalone 40 mg [4 × 10 mg tablets] daily. From 15 June to 22 July, he used 50 mg stanozolol daily. For 2 - 3 days before 22 July he used a mixture of ephedrine, caffeine and aspirin [Ekastac]. Blood samples taken on 23 July 01:37 and at 01:51 showed the following blood levels: efedrine 0.2 mmol/L, coffeine 19.3 mmol/L, cotinine 1.3 mmol/L. Efedrine and metabolites of stanozolol were found in urine samples. Clinical examination at the time of the blood sampling revealed nothing remarkable except for psychological stress [7]. Due to allergies, ABB had also taken an antihistamine called loratadine for approximately 2 weeks before the terror attacks. Based on the results from blood and urine analysis, there were no indications that ABB was under strong influence of drugs on 22 July.

4.4. The Terrorist's Behaviour—Interviews—Court Room Appearances

During the court proceedings, ABB openly admitted that he had adapted his statements in accordance with

FP-1's conclusion [4]. Thus, FP-2 had different conditions under which to conduct their investigations and evaluations. ABB did not consider himself to be a psychiatric patient and he used every opportunity to repeat his monologue about his political views and aims, emphasizing that his fight was for Norway and Europe aiming to save us all from islamisation. Every morning, at the start of the trial when entering the courtroom, ABB consequently raised his right arm in a salute not unlike the German Nazi salute. When he spoke, ABB made it clear that his aim was to spread his message to as many people as possible. He tried several times but once it became evident what he was going to talk about, he was stopped by the presiding judge. ABB frequently spoke to his lawyers and passed them written notes. He sometimes smiled to those present in the courtroom, and during the testimonies from the survivors and other victims, ABB sometimes looked right at them. He had made it clear that he had no choice regarding what he had done and had no regrets.

Following questions from the victims' lawyers and sometimes from the prosecutors, ABB at times had problems with giving precise answers and he was especially vulnerable regarding his use of historical facts to support his political views.

As the days went by, ABB got more and more used to appearing in court. At the beginning, he answered difficult questions with "I don't remember" and "I don't know", but at a later stage, changed the subject and talked about his "mission". ABB got visibly upset and emotional only once, when he cried during the presentation of a montage of some of his propaganda photos accompanied by music. Once he was asked if he felt anything when witnessing people crying during their appearance in court. He answered that he had to lock everything out in order to avoid emotional reactions. Other times he answered aggressively, especially following questions from the prosecution. With few exceptions, ABB seemed unaffected by what was presented during the long trial.

4.5. The Risk of Under-Interpretation and Over-Interpretation—Differential Diagnosis

Browsing the literature it is hard to find studies on subgroups of assassins. A publication from 1982 [24] refers to a study of presidential assassins in the United States where 4 types of murderers with different personality characteristics are identified. Some are driven by personal interest; some are anxious and dysphoric and in need of acceptance and recognition. Others are emotionless psychopaths and some are suffering from mental disorders [24]. As for classification of ABB, accepting the court's decision and thereby ruling out serious mental disorders like schizophrenia is one important step. Perhaps an excessive focus on mental illness has made it difficult to accept an individual's right to make free and coherent choices even if it means breaking the law. This right is recognized in modern societies as being closely linked to the ability of assuming the responsibility for one's actions accepting the verdict. Regardless of personality, total devotion to a cause or fanaticism may be the motive behind terror acts like those seen in Norway on 22 July 2011. We may provide psychological models for understanding, but we must avoid always looking to psychiatry in our desperate need for an explanation for something we dislike or don't understand.

4.6. Being Prepared to Die in a Terror Act versus Suicide—Different Motivation?

According to Joiner [25], there are two elements which must be present in order for suicidal behaviour to occur: The desire for suicide may have two components: thwarted belongingness and perceived burdensomeness. The first is a sense of social alienation or a failure to form social bonds, while perceived burdensomeness is the sense that one is a burden on persons in their lives. Together, these two elements create the motivational force for the suicidal behaviour. Gunn et al. [26] conclude after having studied 261 suicide notes from 1091 consecutive suicides that Joiner's theory of suicide may apply to only a small percentage of those leaving suicide notes. Joiner [25] used suicide notes to provide supportive evidence for the theory.

In the past, several events have been frequently found to precede suicidal behaviour, i.e. loss events, disrupted interpersonal relationships, job problems and financial difficulties, and events related to physical health [27]. Whether or not the impact of less negative events should be considered as value-neutral or even as positive, remains inconclusive.

Brym and Araj [28] question the assumption that suicide bombers are motivated by an unusually high prevalence of depression and suicidal tendencies as advocated by Merari et al. [29] [30]. The authors conclude that there is reason to question the value of a psychological approach to the study of suicide bombers. They base their points of view on interviews with immediate family members and close friends of Palestinian suicide bombers. They underline the importance of focusing on the political and social roots of the suicide bomber phenomenon.

There is no information about ABB leaving a suicide note. He may have had brief depressive episodes earlier in his life, but there is no information to support that he was severely depressed at the time of performing the terror acts. ABB explained in court that the night before the terror acts, he spent the night at his mother's. After breakfast he started his preparations. He drove the van with the bomb to the government building area. A few meters before he reached the final destination, he made a brief stop reflecting on having reached the point of no return. What seemed to be the motivation was allegedly his political conviction that he was the only person capable of performing the necessary terror acts. ABB later explained in court that when he was about to ignite the fuse which would initiate the sequence leading to explosion, he noticed that volatile gas was leaking from the 950 kg fertilizer bomb material. This scared him since the risk of an immediate explosion after lighting the fuse. Despite this, he convinced himself to go through with ignition.

When apprehended on the island of Utøya, ABB later explained in court that he chose to lay down his weapons when he was addressed by the armed special forces and this despite earlier claiming that he did not expect to survive. Once arrested, he was afraid that the police would torture and kill him. ABB later explained that during his reflections and thoughts about his imminent death, he felt sorry for his family and friends.

5. Author's Comments

Looking back at what we know about the life of ABB, there are factors contributing to difficulties for ABB to create an identity as an independent individual with sufficient self-esteem. Such factors are e.g. being raised by a mentally ill mother, where borders regarding physical contact and sexuality are unclear, thereby causing sexual ambivalence and identity problems. Likewise, living with a mother who constantly devaluates his father may contribute to identity problems. Especially when the mother several times introduced new men to whom ABB got attached before she broke up the relationship. ABB at some point took a role as his mother's caretaker and as an adult he once said to one of his friends that it would have been better if he had been raised by his father, referring to his life with a mother who most likely had been overprotective. As an adult he tried to establish something for himself and made drastic decisions regarding his own future e.g. abandoning school, starting enterprises based on criminal activity like selling false identity papers. All just to fail and move back to his mother's apartment, avoiding contact with successful friends and playing World of Warcraft for days at the time. His attempts to become someone in politics also failed as he lacked the necessary ability to compromise and was regarded as too extreme in his views. His lack of girlfriends despite bragging about their existence to friends who knew better, must also have undermined his self-esteem. Consequently, there is reason to assume that there was a lack of identity in ABB; a lack for which he had to compensate.

ABB explained in court that he understood that his actions were atrocious but underlined their necessity. He also stated during the court proceedings that the future will prove him right and that his actions would later be understood. He also expressed that he saw himself as the one who had to choose between lesser evils and that he was the only one capable of making such a choice at the time. Despite being contradicted by the victims' lawyers, he maintained that he was an empathic person. Such statements have signs of both a self-heroic view and a need for admiration.

During his testimony and explanations ABB was interrupted several times by the judge when he deliberately used his given time to talk about his future political and violent aims. Regardless of the judge's repeated corrections, ABB continued his critical political propaganda. This lack of respect for the court was confirmed by his statement where he clearly expressed that he did not acknowledge the court since it was appointed by the dominant party in the Norwegian government at the time. Persons from the public present in the court room reacted in different ways to what the terrorist said, one time a shoe was thrown, barely missing the terrorist's head. This made him smile back at them.

At some point, ABB created his imaginary kingdom where he was the saviour, thereby maintaining his self-deception of being successful. Could ABB's rage be ascribed, at least in part, to the fact that our society failed to recognize his narcissistic needs?

In court, we learned that ABB had submitted newspaper articles but they were refused, thereby supporting his notion that no one would listen. ABB has confirmed that in his view our society in general is dominated by the left wing; the politicians and the media using all means, including corruption if necessary, to suppress the voices of right wing dissidents. Identifying strongly with the latter group, ABB may have felt like a desperate victim. It is also tempting to speculate that ABB, before planning the terror attacks, perceived society as being ungrateful when refusing him credit for what he was trying to convey. Therefore, one way to look at ABB is through the eyes of a desperate and frustrated man without identity, sufficient social and moral ballast, and with a great need of acknowledgement for his ideas. There may be a need to speak up and protest against what is perceived as lack of respect, and thoughts about punishment may be conceived. All depending on the choices available, to some—after diplomacy, only one road is left open: the use of force. There is a strong impression that ABB had a great need to make a difference. In retrospect perhaps also a need for a life commitment—even something worth dying for? The killings make the element of punishment evident, but there is also the element of self-pity. The latter is found in ABB's description of when he, during his execution of the children, first took aim on a victim and then lowered his gun when he saw a terrified young man that reminded him of himself.

Paranoid schizophrenia, antisocial/dissocial personality disorder and NPD were the 3 diagnoses discussed in the two forensic reports. Expert witnesses testifying in court argued strongly against the diagnosis of paranoid schizophrenia, first of all because the ICD 10 general criteria for schizophrenia were not met. But there were also those who argued that ABB had sufficient symptoms to match the requirements for the DSM-IV diagnosis [3]. Eventually, NPD and traits of APD were chosen as the final diagnosis. Little attention was paid to these classifications since they had no relevance to the court's decision on whether or not ABB might be insane and unaccountable for his actions. Likewise, it had no relevance for his competence to stand trial.

In any classification and categorization of more or less identical signs there will always be diagnostic overlap in the hands of health professionals. The use of specific categorical criteria may yield minor differences. For signs to become symptoms, a choice has to be made. Mental health professionals differ regarding which signs they eventually classify as symptoms.

Diagnostic systems may vary a great deal, up to sevenfold—in their rates of diagnosing schizophrenia [31]. The currently used diagnostic procedures are associated with a number of assumptions [32] [33] and there are notable problems linked to facts, like different disorders existing within the schizophrenia construct. The dimensional nature of a construct makes it difficult to relate to categorical definitions within the same construct [33].

A study applying a modified and expanded version of the Manual for the Assessment of Schizophrenia [MAS] [34] [35] on 660 psychotic patients introduced the term "general schizophrenia factor". This refers to shared factors within the various diagnostic systems based on common symptoms like delusions, formal thought disturbances, hallucinations, and some types of negative symptoms [33]. A study by Landmark *et al.* [34] emphasizes the fact that schizophrenia-related variables show continuous distribution which in turn makes cut-offs between schizophrenic and non-schizophrenic psychosis arbitrary. Skeptics [33] have expressed that: "A dimensional construct is consistent with the interpretation that traditional diagnostic systems are the result of both drawing artificial boundaries on a dimensional construct and emphasizing [or de-emphasizing] different phenomenological and clinical aspects of the construct".

A comparison between the degrees of relationship following application of criteria-based diagnosis—specifically for schizotypal, borderline, avoidant and obsessive-compulsive personality disorders, demonstrated [36] that the choice of assessment methodology may have influenced the clinicians' ratings with consequences for the consistency and intercorrelation measures. Still it was found that these 4 personality disorder subtypes were more interrelated with each other than with the remaining personality diagnoses [36]. A study following patients with borderline personality disorder (BPD) concluded that among those with persistent BPD there is more comorbidity with other personality disorders than in those in whom the BPD had remitted [37].

NPD is not a separate personality disorder in ICD 10, but it is recognized as a specific entity by the DSM diagnostic system. Critics have suggested that pathological narcissism should be described as a range of personality pathology common to several personality disorders, alternatively as a severity dimension, ranging from normal assertiveness to pathological narcissism [38] [39]. As for the validity of the DSM-IV construct, a study has suggested that NPD taxonomic structure might not be a spurious outcome due to the raters' biased expectations, but that, as a whole, it can be defended to maintain NPD as a separate diagnostic category in the DSM nomenclature [40]. With reference to the diagnoses given by the 2 pairs of forensic psychiatrists in the ABB case; *i.e.* paranoid schizophrenia and NPD, many have searched for a plausible explanation behind the different conclusions, including internal weaknesses in the two diagnostic systems used. The diagnosis of paranoid schizophrenia was based on the ICD 10 diagnostic system [2], whereas NPD was based on the DSM-IV [13].

Studying the literature and making the assumption that a diagnosis of schizophrenia in ABB was based on observation of brief prodromal signs that disappeared later, one study caught my attention [41]. Studying the symptoms in 29 patients with prodromal schizophrenia, 48% qualified for one or more current axis I diagnoses, including cannabis dependence, major depressive disorder and alcohol dependence. Interestingly, 48% of the prodromal patients also qualified for an axis II disorder, most commonly schizotypal, followed by BPD. Of special interest was that among the 48% prodromal schizophrenics with concurrent axis II diagnoses, none had NPD, 17% had BPD and 7% had APD [41]. A study of 461 patients with personality disorder investigated how impulsive and aggressive traits related to individual Cluster B personality disorders [42]. It was found that the most frequently diagnosed personality disorder (16.1%) was NPD and that emotional components of aggression such as anger and irritability were prominent features. Interestingly, this is in contrast to what was found in patients with APD in whom instrumental aggression [i.e. physical aggressiveness] is prominent. Consequently, and in accordance with the findings presented [43], patients with NPD were described as quick tempered and in favor of activities without strict rules and regulations. The narcissistic patients were likely to lose control and become aggressive when their irritation increased because of low frustration tolerance [43]. Of interest was also the observation that patients with passive-aggressive personality disorder were similar to those with NPD regarding the propensity to lose their temper [43]. However, in contrast to patients with NPD, the passive-aggressive patients had a hostile and malevolent view of other people [41]. From the descriptions of ABB found in the forensic reports, it is evident that many of the signs observed would fit the description of specific narcissistic personality traits.

Comorbidity between Schizophrenia and Personality Disorders

Literature on comorbidity between psychiatric disorders and personality disorders and especially the more chronic symptom disorders reveal that specific personality disorders are often found [44]. In a recent study on comorbid ICD 10 personality traits in schizophrenia, 65.1% of patients with schizophrenia had a comorbid personality disorder, compared to 19% of the healthy general population. This high comorbidity rate will have a significant impact on the clinical and cognitive characteristics of schizophrenia [45], a conclusion in line with results from earlier studies emphasizing that co-occurrence of independent psychiatric disorders affects phenomenology, course and treatment [46]. According to studies using standardized research instruments [DSM-III], at least 50% of subjects with a personality disorder have two or more co-existing personality disorders [47]-[50].

The research done on Cluster B personality disorders and schizophrenia has mainly focused on comorbid APD and BPD. One study found that only antisocial personality disorder is significantly associated with premeditated aggression in schizophrenia, whereas the other disorders in Cluster B are not [51].

In the case of ABB, some of the signs reported and interpreted as symptoms of paranoid schizophrenia by FP-1 might overlap with symptoms associated with BPD. In fact, the latter diagnosis was one of those also discussed by FP-2. Looking at the comorbidity between schizophrenia and BPD, a study found that about 18% of 142 individuals with diagnosed schizophrenia had comorbid BPD [52]. The patients with both diagnoses showed less improvement in psychiatric symptoms under treatment, particularly for hostility and suspiciousness, but also for global functioning. They were also re-hospitalized more often than the schizophrenia patients without BPD. Co-occurrence of schizophrenia and BPD is therefore not infrequent, and BPD has a significant negative longitudinal impact on the course and outcome in schizophrenia patients [52].

Accordingly, assuming that ABB indeed is suffering from schizophrenia, a comorbid personality disorder would most likely lower his level of functioning and attenuate the intensity of his hostility and suspiciousness. With few exceptions, evidence of such attenuation was clearly not apparent in court. A few times his responses had an aggressive tone. His facial expression, with just a subtle smile, rarely changed, except when he cried during the documentation of his self-made propaganda video. When he responded to comments on his lack of empathy he claimed that he had to protect himself from his own feelings to maintain emotional control.

ABB refused to acknowledge what he considered imposed symptoms of paranoid schizophrenia. Thus, only the investigator's interpretations of signs observed and historical descriptions remained. Even though there were several months between the 2 observations, the fact that such completely different diagnostic conclusions were reached has unsettled many colleagues. Moving from descriptions and observations of phenomena to signs and eventually symptoms is a process subject to many different influences, of which experience and personal choice of the investigators are perhaps the major fasctors. No inter-rater estimates were incorporated into the two reports on the mental health of ABB presented during the court proceedings.

The court's decision of ABB being mentally sane is based on the principle of giving the defendant the benefit of the doubt. The two forensic psychiatric reports were contradictive in their conclusions and essential for the court to answer was the question of whether there was an imminent risk that ABB could commit new atrocities in case he were set free. ABB said several times in court that he had not finished his work, referring to his terror acts. The court was left with no option but to rule against him due to the established imminent threat. In Norway the court has to decide between a time limited and a time non-limited sentence. The non-limited sentences are two; a sentence to psychiatric treatment for the mentally insane and preventive detention for those found mentally sane. In this case on August 24th 2012, ABB was sentenced to 21 years of preventive detention with a minimum of 10 years to be served before he would be entitled to appeal the court's decision. If he after 10 years demands to have his case reopened, the court must once more answer the question of whether there is an imminent risk for new atrocities or not. If yes, the court will have to prolong the sentence.

References

[1]   Stormark, K. (2011) Da terroren rammet Norge. 189 minutter som rystet verden. Kagge Forlag, Oslo.

[2]   World Health Organisation (1992) ICD 10 Classifications of Mental and Behavioural Disorder: Clinical Descriptions and Diagnostic Guidelines. World Health Organisation, Geneva.

[3]   Melle, I. (2013) The Breivik Case and What Psychiatrists Can Learn from It. *World Psychiatry*, **12**, 16-21. http://dx.doi.org/10.1002/wps.20002

[4]   (2011) First Forensic Psychiatric Report. https://sites.google.com/site/breivikarkiv/dokumenter/anders-behring-breivik-rettspsykiatrisk-erklaering-2011-11-29

[5]   Mergård, M. (2012) Voldsom, lunefull og full av uventede innfall. Newspaper Article Aftenposten 14.06. http://www.aftenposten.no/nyheter/iriks/22juli/--Voldsom_-lunefull-og-full-av-uventede-innfall-6850270.html

[6]   Vikås, M., Brenna, J.G., Nygaard, F. and Hopperstad, M. (2011) Psykolog i 1983: Ideelt sett burde han vært i et stabilt fosterhjem. Newspaper Article VG nett 23.12. http://www.vg.no/nyheter/innenriks/terrorangrepet-22-juli-anders-behring-breivik/psykolog-i-1983-ideelt-sett-burde-han-vaert-i-et-stabilt-fosterhjem/a/10024865/

[7]   (2012) Second Forensic Psychiatric Report. http://www.nrk.no/norge/hadde-treningskamerat-fra-midtosten-1.7724579

[8]   Borchgrevink, A.S. (2012) En norsk tragedie (A Norwegian Tragedy). Gyldendal, Oslo.

[9]   Karterud, S., Wilberg, T. and Urnes, Ø. (2010) Personlighetspsykiatri (Personality in Psychiatry). Gyldendal, Oslo, 63.

[10]   Skille, Ø.B. and Bålsrød, K. (2011) En av treningskameratene på ungdomsskolen var jo fra Midtøsten. Interview, National Norwegian Broadcasting 23.07.2011. https://sites.google.com/site/breivikarkiv/dokumenter/anders-behring-breivik-rettspsykiatrisk-erklaering-2012-04-10

[11]   Meland, A. (2011) Dette mislyktes Anders Behring Breivik med. Dagbladet (Norwegian Newspaper), 04.09., 6. www.Dagbladet.no

[12]   Dagbladet (Norwegian Newspaper) (2011) Skrøt av egen briljans, utseende, kjærester og penger. http://www.dagbladet.no/2011/07/27/nyheter/utoya/massedrap/innenriks/17459033/

[13]   American Psychiatric Association (2000) Diagnostic and Statistical Manual of Mental Disorders. 4th Edition, Text Rev., Arlington.

[14]   Bronisch, T. and Mombour, W. (1994) Comparison of a Diagnostic Checklist with a Structured Interview for the Assessment of DSM-III-R and ICD 10 Personality Disorders. *Psychopathology*, **27**, 312-320. http://dx.doi.org/10.1159/000284889

[15]   Sara, G., Raven, P. and Mann, A. (1996) A Comparison of DSM-III-R and ICD 10 Personality Disorder Criteria in an Out-Patients Population. *Psychological Medicine*, **26**, 151-160. http://dx.doi.org/10.1017/S0033291700033791

[16]   Starcevic, V., Bogojevic, G. and Kelin, K. (1997) Diagnostic Agreement between the DSM-IV and ICD 10 DCR Personality Disorders. *Psychopathology*, **30**, 328-334. http://dx.doi.org/10.1159/000285078

[17]   Ottosen, H., Ekselius, L., Grann, M. and Kullgren, G. (2002) Cross-System Concordance of Personality Disorder Diagnosis of DSM-IV and Diagnostic Criteria for Research of ICD 10. *Journal of Personality Disorders*, **16**, 283-292. http://dx.doi.org/10.1521/pedi.16.3.283.22537

[18]   Beltran, R.O., Silove, D. and Llewellyn, G.M. (2009) Comparison of ICD 10 Diagnostic Guidelines and Research Criteria for Enduring Personality Change after Catastrophic Experiences. *Psychopathology*, **42**, 113-118. http://dx.doi.org/10.1159/000204761

[19]   Frances, A.J. and Widiger, T. (2012) Psychiatric Diagnosis: Lessons from the DSM-IV Past and Cautions for the DSM-5 Future. *Annual Review of Clinical Psychology*, **8**, 109-130.

http://dx.doi.org/10.1146/annurev-clinpsy-032511-143102

[20] Andersen, A.M. and Bienvenu, O.J. (2011) Personality and Psychopathology. *International Review of Psychiatry*, **23**, 234-247. http://dx.doi.org/10.3109/09540261.2011.588692

[21] Lysaker, P.H. and Davis, L.W. (2004) Social Function in Schizophrenia and Schizoaffective Disorder: Associations with Personality, Symptoms and Neurocognition. *Health and Quality of Life Outcomes*, **2**, 15.

[22] Kentros, M., Smith, T.E., Hull, J., McKee, M., Terkelsen, K. and Capalbo, C. (1997) Stability of Personality Traits in Schizophrenia and Schizoaffective Disorder: A Pilot Project. *Journal of Nervous and Mental Disease*, **185**, 549-555. http://dx.doi.org/10.1097/00005053-199709000-00003

[23] Stauber, E. (2001) Ethnopolitical and Other Group Violence: Origins and Prevention. In: Chirot, D. and Seligman, M.E.P., Eds., *Ethnopolitical Warfare: Causes, Consequences, and Possible Solutions*, American Psychological Association, Washington DC, 290-304.

[24] Clarke, J.W. (1982) American Assassins: The Darker Side of Politics. Princeton University Press, Princeton.

[25] Joiner Jr., T.E. (2005) Why People Die by Suicide. Harvard University Press, Cambridge.

[26] Gunn III, J.F., Lester, D., Haines, J. and Williams, C.L. (2012) Thwarted Belongingness and Perceived Burdensomeness in Suicide Notes. *Crisis*, **33**, 178-181. http://dx.doi.org/10.1027/0227-5910/a000123

[27] Yen, S., Pagano, M.E., Shea, M.T., Grilo, C.M., Gunderson, J.G., Skodol, A.E., McGlashan, T.H., Sanisow, C.A., Bender, D.S. and Zanarini, M.C. (2005) Recent Life Events Preceding Suicide Attempts in a Personality Disorder Sample: Findings from the Collaborative Longitudinal Personality Disorder Study. *Journal of Consulting and Clinical Psychology*, **73**, 99-105. http://dx.doi.org/10.1037/0022-006X.73.1.99

[28] Brym, R.J. and Araj, B. (2012) Are Suicide Bombers Suicidal? *Studies in Conflict & Terrorism*, **35**, 432-443. http://dx.doi.org/10.1080/1057610X.2012.675550

[29] Merari, A., Diamant, I., Bibi, A., Broshi, Y. and Zakin, G. (2010) Personality Characteristics of "Self Martyrs"/"Suicide Bombers" and Organizers of Suicide Attacks. *Terrorism and Political Violence*, **22**, 87-101. http://dx.doi.org/10.1080/09546550903409312

[30] Merari, A. (2010) Driven to Death. Oxford University Press, Oxford.

[31] Endicott, J., Nee, J., Fleiss, J.L., Cohn, J., Williams, J.B.W. and Simon, R. (1982) Diagnostic Criteria for Schizophrenia. Reliabilities and Agreement between Systems. *JAMA Psychiatry*, **39**, 884-889. http://dx.doi.org/10.1001/archpsyc.1982.04290080006002

[32] Berner, P., Gabriel, E., Katsching, H., Kieffer, W., Koehler, K., Lenz, G., Nutzinger, D., Schanda, H. and Simhandl, V. (1992) Diagnostic Criteria for Functional Psychosis. Cambridge University Press, Cambridge. http://dx.doi.org/10.1017/CBO9780511663208

[33] Peralta, V. and Cuesta, M.J. (2005) The Underlying Structure of Diagnostic Systems of Schizophrenia: A Comprehensive Polydiagnostic Approach. *Schizophrenia Research*, **79**, 217-229. http://dx.doi.org/10.1016/j.schres.2005.05.003

[34] Landmark, J. (1982) A Manual for the Assessment of Schizophrenia. *Acta Psychiatrica Scandinavica*, **65**, 1-85.

[35] Peralta, V. and Cuesta, M.J. (1992) A Polydiagnostic Approach to Self-Perceived Cognitive Disorders in Schizophrenia. *Psychopathology*, **25**, 232-238. http://dx.doi.org/10.1159/000284778

[36] Grilo, C.M., McGlashan, T.H., Morey, L.C., Gunderson, J.G., Skodol, A.E., Tracie, S.M., Sanislow, C.A., *et al.* (2001) Internal Consistency, Intercriterion Overlap and Diagnostic Efficiency of Criteria Sets for DSM-IV Schizotypal, Borderline, Avoidant and Obsessive-Compulsive Personality Disorders. *Acta Psychiatrica Scandinavica*, **104**, 264-272. http://dx.doi.org/10.1034/j.1600-0447.2001.00436.x

[37] Links, P.S., Heslegrave, R. and van Reekum, R. (1998) Prospective Follow-Up Study of Borderline Personality Disorder: Prognosis, Prediction of Outcome and Axis II Comorbidity. *Canadian Journal of Psychiatry*, **43**, 265-270.

[38] Emmons, R.A. (1987) Narcissism: Theory and Measurement. *Journal of Personality and Social Psychology*, **52**, 11-17. http://dx.doi.org/10.1037/0022-3514.52.1.11

[39] Morey, L.C. and Jones, J.K. (1998) Empirical Studies on the Construct Validity of Narcissistic Personality Disorder. In: Roningham, E., Ed., *Disorder of Narcissism: Diagnostic, Clinical and Empirical Implications*, American Psychiatric Press, Washington DC, 351-373.

[40] Fossati, A., Beauchaine, T.P., Grazioli, F., Carretta, I., Cortinovis, F. and Maffei, C. (2005) A Latent Structure of Diagnostic and Statistical Manual of Mental Disorders, Fourth Edition, Narcissistic Personality Disorder Criteria. *Comprehensive Psychiatry*, **46**, 361-367. http://dx.doi.org/10.1016/j.comppsych.2004.11.006

[41] Rosen, J.L., Miller, T.J., D'Andrea, J.T., McGlashan, T.H. and Woods, S.W. (2006) Comorbid Diagnoses in Patients Meeting Criteria for the Schizophrenia Prodrome. *Schizophrenia Research*, **85**, 124-131. http://dx.doi.org/10.1016/j.schres.2006.03.034

[42] Fossati, A., Barratt, E.S., Borroni, S., Villa, D., Grazioli, F. and Maffei, C. (2007) Impulsivity, Aggressiveness, and DSM-IV Personality Disorders. *Psychiatry Research*, **149**, 157-167. http://dx.doi.org/10.1016/j.psychres.2006.03.011

[43] Baumeister, R.F., Bushman, B.J. and Campbell, W.K. (2000) Self-Esteem, Narcissism and Aggression: Does Violence Result from Low Self-Esteem or from Threatened Egoism? *Current Directions in Psychological Science*, **9**, 26-29. http://dx.doi.org/10.1111/1467-8721.00053

[44] Alnaes, R. and Torgersen, S. (1988) The Relationship between DSM-III Symptom Disorders (Axis I) and Personality Disorders (Axis II) in an Outpatients Population. *Acta Psychiatrica Scandinavica*, **78**, 485-492. http://dx.doi.org/10.1111/j.1600-0447.1988.tb06371.x

[45] Moore, E.A., Green, M.J. and Carr, V.J. (2012) Comorbid Personality Traits in Schizophrenia: Prevalence and Clinical Characteristics. *Journal of Psychiatric Research*, **46**, 353-359. http://dx.doi.org/10.1016/j.jpsychires.2011.11.012

[46] Tyrer, P., Gunderson, J., Lyons, M. and Tohen, M. (1997) Extent of Comorbidity between Mental State and Personality Disorders. *Journal of Personality Disorders*, **11**, 242-259. http://dx.doi.org/10.1521/pedi.1997.11.3.242

[47] Pfohl, B., Coryell, W., Zimmerman, M. and Stangl, D. (2006) DSM-III Personality Disorders: Diagnostic Overlap and Internal Consistency of Individual DSM-III Criteria. *Comprehensive Psychiatry*, **27**, 21-34. http://dx.doi.org/10.1016/0010-440X(86)90066-0

[48] Loranger, A.W., Susman, V.L., Oldham, J.M. and Russakoff, M. (1987) The Personality Disorder Examination: A Preliminary Report. *Journal of Personality Disorders*, **1**, 1-13. http://dx.doi.org/10.1521/pedi.1987.1.1.1

[49] Oldham, J.M., Skodol, A.E., Kellman, H.D., Hyler, S.E., Rosnick, L. and Davies, M. (1992) Diagnosis of DSM III R Personality Disorders by Two Structured Interviews: Patterns of Comorbidity. *American Journal of Psychiatry*, **149**, 213-220.

[50] Cold, J. (2013) The Co-Morbidity of Personality Disorder and Lifetime Clinical Syndromes in Dangerous Offenders. *The Journal of Forensic Psychiatry and Psychology*, **14**, 341-366.

[51] Bo, S., Forth, A., Kongerslev, M., Haahr, U.H., Pedersen, L. and Simonsen, E. (2013) Subtypes of Aggression in Patients with Schizophrenia: The Role of Personality Disorders. *Criminal Behaviour and Mental Health*, **23**, 124-137. http://dx.doi.org/10.1002/cbm.1858

[52] Bahorik, A.L. and Eack, S.M. (2010) Examining the Course and Outcome of Individuals Diagnosed with Schizophrenia and Comorbid Borderline Personality Disorder. *Schizophrenia Research*, **124**, 29-35. http://dx.doi.org/10.1016/j.schres.2010.09.005

12

Effects of Religious vs. Conventional Cognitive-Behavioral Therapy on Inflammatory Markers and Stress Hormones in Major Depression and Chronic Medical Illness: A Randomized Clinical Trial

Lee S. Berk[1,2,3], Denise L. Bellinger[2], Harold G. Koenig[3,4,5,6*], Noha Daher[1,7], Michelle J. Pearce[3,4,8], Clive J. Robins[4,9], Bruce Nelson[10], Sally F. Shaw[10], Harvey Jay Cohen[3,5], Michael B. King[11]

[1]Allied Health Studies, School of Allied Health Professions, Loma Linda University, Loma Linda, USA
[2]Department of Pathology and Human Anatomy, School of Medicine, Loma Linda University, Loma Linda, USA
[3]Center for Spirituality, Theology and Health, Duke University, Durham, USA
[4]Department of Psychiatry and Behavioral Sciences, Duke University Medical Center, Durham, USA
[5]Department of Medicine, Duke University Medical Center, Durham, USA
[6]Department of Medicine, King Abdulaziz University, Jeddah, Saudi Arabia
[7]Epidemiology, Biostatistics, and Population Medicine, School of Public Health, Loma Linda University, Loma Linda, USA
[8]School of Medicine, University of Maryland, Baltimore, USA
[9]Department of Psychology and Neuroscience, Duke University Medical Center, Durham, USA
[10]Department of Research, Glendale Adventist Medical Center, Glendale, USA
[11]Division of Psychiatry, Faculty of Brain Sciences, University College, London, UK
Email: *Harold.Koenig@duke.edu

Abstract

Background: Depressive disorder is often accompanied by physiological changes that may adversely affect the course of medical illness, including an increase in pro-inflammatory cytokines. Methods: We examine the effects of religious cognitive behavioral therapy (RCBT) vs. conventional CBT (CCBT) on pro-/anti-inflammatory indicators and stress hormones in 132 individuals with major depressive disorder (MDD) and chronic medical illness who were recruited into a multi-site randomized clinical trial. Biomarkers (C-reactive protein and pro-inflammatory cytokines TNF-α,

---

IL-1β, IFN-γ, IL-6, IL-12-p70), anti-inflammatory cytokines (IL1ra, IL-4, IL-10), and stress hormones (urinary cortisol, epinephrine, norepinephrine) were assessed at baseline, 12 weeks, and 24 weeks. Differential effects of baseline religiosity on treatment response were also examined, along with effects of religiosity on changes in biomarkers over time independent of treatment group. Biomarker levels were log transformed where possible to normalize distributions. Mixed models were used to examine trajectories of change. Results: CRP increased and IL-4, IL-10, and epinephrine decreased over time, mostly in the opposite direction expected (except epinephrine). No significant difference between RCBT and CCBT was found on average trajectory of change in any biomarkers. Religiosity interacted with treatment group in effects on IL-6, such that CCBT was more effective than RCBT in lowering IL-6 in those with low religiosity whereas RCBT appeared to be more effective than CCBT in those with high religiosity. Higher baseline religiosity also tended to predict an increase in pro-inflammatory cytokines INF-γ and IL-12 (p70) and urinary cortisol over time. Conclusions: RCBT and CCBT had similar effects on stress biomarkers. CCBT was more effective in reducing IL-6 levels in those with low religiosity, whereas RCBT tended to be more effective in those with high religiosity. Unexpectedly, higher baseline religiosity was associated with an increase in several stress biomarkers.

Keywords

Cognitive Behavioral Therapy, Religion, Depression, Inflammation, Immune Function, Stress Hormones

---

1. Introduction

Depressive disorder is often accompanied by physiological changes that may adversely affect the course of medical illness, including an increase in pro-inflammatory cytokines such as IL-6, IL-12, IFN-γ, IL-1, and TNF-α [1]-[3], a reduction in anti-inflammatory cytokines such as IL-4 and IL-10 [4] [5], and an increase in stress hormones [6]. Such physiological changes may increase risk of infection [7], vulnerability to and course of malignancy [8] [9], and may lead to inflammatory disorders [10]. The association between depressive disorder and changes in immune and endocrine function is a complex one, though, and this relationship has been argued to be bi-directional in effect [11]. Severe depression may influence levels of inflammation and stress hormones, as inflammation and altered stress hormones can lead to sickness behaviors that resemble depression or lead to depression [4].

The abnormal changes in immunity, inflammation, and stress hormone levels associated with depression have been shown in clinical trials to return back towards normal with a variety of treatments, including antidepressant drug therapy [3] [12] [13], electroconvulsive therapy (TNF-α) [2], and especially, a wide range of psychological interventions [14]-[17].

Religious involvement is widespread in the United States (US) population [18] [19], and religion is often used to cope with psychological stress [20] and medical illness in particular [21]. Religiosity has been reported to prevent the development of depression, increase the speed of depression remission, and may help persons to cope with depression in the setting of chronic medical illness [22]-[24]. Religious involvement has also been associated with lower levels of pro-inflammatory markers such as C-reactive protein (CRP) and IL-6 [25]-[27], higher levels of anti-inflammatory markers such as IL-1ra [28], and lower levels of stress hormones such as cortisol and norepinephrine [29]-[34] in cross-sectional studies. Spiritual interventions have also been shown to alter pro-/anti-inflammatory cytokine levels [35] [36], decrease cortisol [36]-[38], and lower specific catecholamines such as epinephrine and norepinephrine [39] [40].

In a recent clinical trial, we found little difference in outcome between religious cognitive behavioral therapy (RCBT) and conventional CBT (CCBT) in the treatment of major depressive disorder (MDD) in patients with chronic medical illness. In a secondary analysis, there was evidence that outcomes were better for more religious people who received RCBT (possibly due to better treatment adherence) [41]. Thus, we decided to compare the effects of RCBT vs. CCBT on changes in immune/inflammatory biomarker and stress hormone levels during treatment in this same cohort.

Hypotheses

The present analysis examines the effects of religious vs. conventional CBT (RCBT vs. CCBT) on stress biomarkers (inflammation and stress hormones) over 24 weeks during the course of a randomized clinical trial focused on treating persons with MDD and chronic medical illness who were at least somewhat religious or spiritual. We hypothesized that:

1) RCBT will be more effective than CCBT in a) reducing pro-inflammatory cytokines; b) increasing anti-inflammatory cytokines; and c) reducing stress hormones (12-hour urinary cortisol, epinephrine, and norepinephrine);

2) RCBT will be more effective in lowering pro-inflammatory cytokines and stress hormones and increasing anti-inflammatory cytokines in those who are more religious; and

3) Baseline religiosity will predict a decrease in pro-inflammatory cytokines and stress hormones and an increase in anti-inflammatory cytokines over time independent of treatment group.

2. Methods

The methodology involved in the randomized clinical trial has been described in detail elsewhere [41], although we summarize important aspects here. We recruited persons aged 18 to 85 into a multi-site randomized clinical trial (Durham County, North Carolina, and Los Angeles County, California). Potential participants were screened over the telephone, and if they passed this initial screen, were invited to come to the hospital for further screening after signing an informed consent form. Inclusion criteria were 1) one or more chronic medical illnesses present for 6 months or longer; 2) a DSM-IV diagnosis of major depressive disorder made by a structured psychiatric interview, the MINI Neuropsychiatric Interview [42], which follows DSM-IV criteria; 3) mild to moderately severe depressive symptoms (10 to 40 on the 21-item Beck Depression Inventory [BDI-II, which ranges from 0 to 63]) [43]; and 4) religion or spirituality at least somewhat important, assessed by the question "How important is religion/spirituality in your daily life?" ("somewhat important" or more was required). Exclusion criteria were 1) having significant cognitive impairment based on the brief Mini-Mental Stated Exam [44]; 2) having received psychotherapy within the past two months; 3) having a diagnosis of psychotic disorder, substance abuse, or posttraumatic stress disorder (PTSD) on the MINI within the past year; 4) having any history of bipolar disorder (MINI); 5) any active suicidal thoughts (MINI); and 6) having a diagnosis of human immunodeficiency virus/acquired immunodeficiency syndrome (HIV/AIDS), autoimmune diseases, endocrine disorders, a prognosis of less than 6 months, or taking immunosuppressant drugs, given the immune analyzes planned for this report. Those who fulfilled inclusion criteria and had no exclusion criteria then completed a baseline evaluation and were randomized to treatment group by an external group. Interviewers underwent extensive training to ensure that they remained blind to treatment group throughout the study. Duke University Medical Center and Glendale Adventist Medical Center institutional review boards approved the study.

2.1. Interventions

Eight master's level cognitive behavioral therapists conducted the therapy (four delivering CCBT and four delivering RCBT). The intervention consisted of ten 50-minute sessions administered over 12 weeks delivered remotely by telephone (94%); the remaining sessions were conducted by Skype (5%) or online using instant messaging (1%). Remote delivery of therapy was chosen to reduce the effort necessary for those with chronic medical illness to participate.

Conventional CBT was a manual-based intervention following CBT for depression as described by Aaron Beck, focused on altering dysfunctional cognitions and reducing depression-inducing behaviors [45]. If religious issues were brought up during the therapy, the therapist gently redirected the client to more secular ways of approaching the issue.

Religiously integrated CBT was also a manual-based intervention developed specifically for this study. Five version of RCBT were developed so that they would match the religion of the client. First, a Christian version of the CCBT manual was developed [46], and then adapted for Buddhist, Hindu, Muslim, and Jewish clients. University faculty from Jewish, Muslim, Hindu, and Buddhist religious traditions with experience integrating religious beliefs into CBT guided the development of the manuals and workbooks [47]. The faculty also helped to supervise therapists when a client from a particular faith background was enrolled into the study.

There was considerable overlap between the two forms of CBT. Both integrated "spiritual" content into therapy, focusing on forgiveness, gratefulness, altruistic behaviors, and engagement in social activities. Mindfulness meditation was included in CCBT to match the meditative practices that were part of the RCBT intervention. In fact, the only difference between CCBT and RCBT interventions was that RCBT attempted to integrate the client's religious beliefs into the therapy and use them to motivate changes in dysfunctional cognitions and behaviors.

2.2. Measures

Biomarkers. The methods for assessing indicators of inflammation and measures of stress hormones have been described in full elsewhere [34]. In summary, serum inflammatory markers (TNF-α, IFN-γ, IL-1β, IL-4, IL-6, IL-10, IL-12 p70) were measured using Millipore's multiplexed high sensitivity cytokine magnetic bead-based immunoassay kits (Milliplex cat #HSTCMAG-28SK, EMD Millipore, Billerica, MA). IL-1ra was run using the Milliplex Human Cytokine kit (Hcytomag-60K). Intra- and inter-assay coefficients of variation (CV) were <6% and <20% for all cytokines, respectively. All samples were run in duplicate along with duplicate standards that were used to generate a standard curve, and samples were repeated if the CV between the duplicates was greater than 15%.

Serum CRP was measured using enzyme-linked immunosorbent assay (ELISA) kits from Assaypro, St Charles, MO), which have a minimal detection of ~0.25 ng/ml and an intra- and inter-assay CV of 5.0% and 7.1%, respectively. Cortisol concentrations were measured in 12-h overnight urine samples using ELISA kits (Enzo Life Sciences International Inc., Plymouth Meeting, PA) that had a lower limit of detection of 333 pg/ml, and intra-and inter-assay CV of 10.5% and 13.4%, respectively. Cortisol levels were normalized for urine volume using creatinine levels determined by parametric kits that employed the Jaffe reaction (R & D Systems, Minneapolis, MN; minimal detection of 0.01 mg/dL and intra- and inter-assay CV of 3.5% and 4.0%, respectively). All samples were run in duplicate along with duplicate standards that were used to generate a standard curve. If the coefficient of variance between the duplicates was greater than 15%, the assay was repeated for that sample.

Twelve-hour urinary catecholamines (epinephrine and norepinephrine) were determined by high performance liquid chromatography with coulochem detection (HPLC-CD). They were analyzed using EZChrom Elite Software (Scientific Software Inc. Pleasanton, CA). Concentrations were determined based on standards of known concentrations (200 ng/ml) of norepinephrine, epinephrine, and dopamine and expressed as μg/g creatinine to normalize for urine volume.

Religiosity. Standard single item measures of self-rated religiosity, organizational religious activity (attendance at services), and private religious activity (frequency of prayer, meditation, and scripture study) were administered [48], along with multi-item measures of intrinsic religiosity [49] and daily spiritual experiences [50]. To increase the power of the analysis for the primary hypotheses, religious variables were combined into an overall 29-item religiosity measure by summing self-rated religiosity, public and private religious activity, daily spiritual experiences, and intrinsic religiosity (range 44 - 153); alpha for the scale was 0.95.

Demographics and physical health. Demographic characteristics assessed were age and education (continuous in years), gender, race, and marital status. The 12-item Duke Activity Status Index (DASI) [51] was used to measure physical functioning across domains for physical and instrumental activities of daily living (range 12 - 36, with higher scores indicating better function). Medical co-morbidity was assessed using the Charlson Comorbidity Index, which provides a count of and severity ratings for ICD-10 medical illnesses [52]. Severity of overall medical illness was determined using the Cumulative Illness Rating Scale [53].

2.3. Statistical Analysis

Descriptive statistics were used to compare the two treatment groups at baseline (**Table 1**). Given concern over their outlier status, biomarker values more than three standard deviations (97.8% of the normal distribution) above the median value were omitted from analyses. This was done for approximately 3% of values and involved 42 participants assessed over the three time points. Since none of the biomarkers were normally distributed, they were log transformed to normalize their values; because log transformations did not normalize IL-12-p70 and IL-4, analyses were performed on original values.

Table 1. Baseline characteristics of treatment groups.

	CCBT	RCBT
	(n = 67)	(n = 65)
Demographics		
Gender, female (%, N)[1]	65.7 (44)	72.3 (47)
Age, years (mean, SD)	52.5 (13.7)	50.7 (13.3)
Race, white Caucasian (%, N)	58.2 (39)	47.7 (31)
Education, years (mean, SD)	15.2 (3.2)	15.0 (3.5)
Marital status, married (%, N)	41.8 (28)	36.9 (24)
Center, Duke (%, N)	47.8 (32)	46.2 (30)
Religious characteristics		
Affiliation (%, N)		
Christian	92.5 (62)	83.1 (54)
Buddhist	4.5 (3)	6.2 (4)
Jewish	1.5 (1)	6.2 (4)
Muslim	0 (0)	1.5 (1)
Hindu	1.5 (1)	3.1 (2)
Importance, very (%, N)	44.8 (30)	49.2 (32)
Attendance, ≥weekly (%, N)	41.8 (28)	43.1 (28)
Prayer, daily or more (%, N)	38.8 (26)	35.4 (23)
Intrinsic religiosity (mean, SD)	34.5 (8.3)	35.2 (8.4)
Spiritual experiences (mean, SD)	57.5 (16.1)	57.7 (15.9)
Overall baseline religiosity (mean, SD)	102.6 (25.6)	103.3 (25.2)
Depression		
Beck Depression Scale (mean, SD)	25.8 (9.2)	24.8 (7.6)
Depression onset, <12 months (%, N)	70.2 (47)	73.9 (48)
Physical illness severity		
Co-morbidity score (mean, SD)	2.7 (2.4)	2.1 (2.0)
Physical functioning (mean, SD)	29.1 (5.6)	28.7 (5.9)
Illness severity (mean, SD)	6.5 (4.7)	7.1 (5.7)

[1]Column % (N); CCBT = conventional CBT; RCBT = religious CBT. Table adapted from Koenig *et al.* (2015) [41].

In bivariate analyses, mean levels of biomarkers were compared between treatment groups at baseline, 12-week follow-up, and 24-week follow-up using the Student's t-test (**Table 2**). Growth curve modeling using random intercept and slope (mixed effect regression models) examined the effect of the treatment (RCBT vs. CCBT) on trajectory of change of individual inflammatory markers and stress hormones from baseline to 24-week follow-up (**Table 3**). This method allowed for participants with data for at least one time point to be included in the analysis and the retention of participants with missing data. The model included the fixed effects of group, time, and group by time interaction. The primary analysis was an intention-to-treat (ITT) analysis that included all randomized participants; analyses were repeated using a per-protocol (PP) method that included

Table 2. Means (SD) of inflammatory markers and stress hormones at baseline, 12 weeks and 24 weeks by treatment group.

PRO-INFLAMMATORY	CCBT	RCBT	Difference	p[2]
CRP (mg/L)	Mean (SD)[1]	Mean (SD)	Mean (95% CI)	
Intention-to-treat analysis				
Baseline (63 vs. 64)[3]	6.52 (6.64)	5.92 (6.52)	0.61 (−1.70 to 2.92)	0.649
12-week (46 vs. 42)	5.44 (6.67)	7.88 (10.72)	−2.45 (−6.29 to 1.39)	0.287
24-week (30 vs. 24)	8.03 (10.75)	8.09 (6.87)	−0.06 (−4.91 to 4.78)	0.422
Per-protocol analysis				
Baseline (43 vs. 46)	6.64 (6.72)	6.10 (6.40)	0.54 (−2.23 to 3.30)	0.624
12-week (43 vs. 39)	5.34 (6.67)	7.70 (10.6)	−2.36 (−6.32 to 1.60)	0.665
24-week (28 vs. 22)	8.11 (11.03)	8.16 (6.94)	−0.05 (−5.20 to 5.10)	0.410
TNF-α (pg/ml)				
Intention-to-treat analysis				
Baseline (63 vs. 61)	6.92 (3.07)	7.05 (3.76)	−0.13 (−1.35 to 1.09)	0.842
12-week (44 vs. 42)	6.81 (2.20)	6.39 (2.46)	0.42 (−0.58 to 1.41)	0.286
24-week (29 vs. 27)	6.46 (2.18)	6.94 (5.01)	−0.48 (−2.60 to 1.65)	0.847
Per-protocol analysis				
Baseline (45 vs. 43)	6.73 (2.31)	6.27 (2.33)	0.46 (−0.52 to 1.44)	0.313
12-week (41 vs. 38)	6.88 (2.24)	6.30 (2.55)	0.58 (−0.49 to 1.66)	0.172
24-week (27 vs. 24)	6.56 (2.23)	6.85 (5.27)	−0.29 (−2.65 to 2.07)	0.613
IL-1β (pg/ml)				
Intention-to-treat analysis				
Baseline (62 vs. 62)	1.28 (1.07)	1.71 (1.89)	−0.43 (−0.98 to 0.12)	0.570
12-week (44 vs. 43)	1.31 (1.11)	1.25 (1.14)	0.06 (−0.42 to 0.54)	0.245
24-week (29 vs. 27)	1.41 (1.93)	1.17 (1.21)	0.25 (−0.61 to 1.10)	0.302
Per-protocol analysis				
Baseline (44 vs. 44)	1.11 (0.91)	1.46 (1.44)	−0.34 (−0.85 to 0.17)	0.728
12-week (40 vs. 39)	1.28 (1.14)	1.30 (1.18)	−0.03 (−0.54 to 0.49)	0.360
24-week (27 vs. 24)	1.42 (2.00)	1.19 (1.28)	0.23 (−0.71 to 1.17)	0.318
IFN-γ (pg/ml)				
Intention-to-treat analysis				
Baseline (64 vs. 62)	9.91 (8.12)	9.41 (9.11)	0.50 (−2.54 to 3.54)	0.434
12-week (44 vs. 42)	9.27 (7.65)	9.22 (8.40)	0.05 (−3.39 to 3.49)	0.381
24-week (29 vs. 27)	7.90 (5.46)	7.07 (5.58)	0.84 (−2.12 to 3.80)	0.241
Per-protocol analysis				
Baseline (45 vs. 44)	8.45 (6.76)	9.04 (9.01)	−0.59 (−3.94 to 2.76)	0.694
12-week (41 vs. 38)	8.94 (6.78)	9.57 (8.74)	−0.63 (−4.12 to 2.87)	0.421
24-week (27 vs. 24)	8.28 (5.46)	7.34 (5.81)	0.95 (−2.23 to 4.12)	0.209

Continued

IL-6 (pg/ml)				
Intention-to-treat analysis				
Baseline (64 vs. 62)	2.84 (2.57)	2.56 (2.49)	0.28 (−0.61 to 1.17)	0.900
12-week (45 vs. 41)	2.40 (1.78)	2.13 (1.45)	0.27 (−0.43 to 0.97)	0.997
24-week (29 vs. 26)	2.03 (2.06)	2.00 (1.87)	0.03 (−1.04 to 1.10)	0.413
Per-protocol analysis				
Baseline (45 vs. 44)	2.23 (2.06)	2.19 (2.20)	0.04 (−0.85 to 0.94)	0.820
12-week (42 vs. 37)	2.36 (1.79)	2.12 (1.49)	0.24 (−0.50 to 0.99)	0.978
24-week (27 vs. 23)	2.05 (2.12)	1.96 (1.99)	0.09 (−1.09 to 1.26)	0.505
IL-12 p70 (pg/ml)				
Intention-to-treat analysis				
Baseline (64 vs. 62)	2.99 (2.28)	2.95 (3.85)	0.04 (−1.08 to 1.16)	0.946
12-week (43 vs. 41)	2.54 (1.96)	2.24 (1.52)	0.30 (−0.47 to 1.06)	0.439
24-week (29 vs. 27)	1.99 (1.30)	1.85 (1.33)	0.14 (−0.56 to 0.85)	0.682
Per-protocol analysis				
Baseline (45 vs. 44)	2.50 (1.98)	2.46 (2.20)	0.04 (−0.84 to 0.92)	0.928
12-week (40 vs. 37)	2.45 (1.83)	2.31 (1.55)	0.14 (−0.63 to 0.91)	0.719
24-week (27 vs. 24)	2.03 (1.32)	1.81 (1.41)	0.22 (−0.54 to 0.99)	0.563
ANTI-INFLAMMATORY				
IL-1ra (pg/ml)				
Intention-to-treat analysis				
Baseline (64 vs. 63)	33.78 (70.89)	39.10 (71.71)	−5.32 (−30.36 to 19.73)	0.630
12-week (46 vs. 41)	25.65 (40.57)	21.43 (35.93)	4.22 (−12.20 to 20.65)	0.098
24-week (30 vs. 24)	23.43 (27.18)	47.52 (76.74)	−24.09 (−57.77 to 9.58)	0.474
Per-protocol analysis				
Baseline (46 vs. 46)	23.62 (38.27)	48.42 (81.50)	−24.80 (−51.32 to 1.72)	0.974
12-week (43 vs. 38)	26.52 (41.75)	22.21 (37.22)	4.30 (−13.29 to 21.89)	0.09
24-week (28 vs. 22)	24.63 (27.74)	51.16 (79.27)	−26.53 (−26.53 to 62.96)	0.440
IL-4 (pg/ml)				
Intention-to-treat analysis				
Baseline (63 vs. 58)	12.72 (12.72)	12.33 (11.89)	0.38 (−4.06 to 4.83)	0.865
12-week (43 vs. 43)	9.95 (8.46)	11.07 (11.25)	−1.12 (−5.39 to 3.15)	0.605
24-week (28 vs. 27)	6.77 (6.46)	7.15 (10.42)	−0.39 (−5.12 to 4.35)	0.870
Per-protocol analysis				
Baseline (45 vs. 43)	11.47 (10.34)	11.51 (11.92)	−0.04 (−4.76 to 4.68)	0.986
12-week (40 vs. 39)	9.53 (8.42)	11.75 (11.55)	−2.22 (−6.74 to 2.30)	0.437
24-week (26 vs. 24)	6.73 (6.67)	7.84 (10.86)	−1.10 (−6.31 to 4.11)	0.671

Continued

IL-10 (pg/ml)				
Intention-to-treat analysis				
Baseline (63 vs. 59)	9.43 (8.85)	9.09 (12.56)	0.34 (−3.59 to 4.26)	0.101
12-week (43 vs. 42)	8.05 (9.13)	5.74 (8.10)	2.31 (−1.41 to 6.04)	0.016
24-week (28 vs. 27)	6.23 (5.34)	4.91 (8.62)	1.32 (−2.59 to 5.24)	0.012
Per-protocol analysis				
Baseline (45 vs. 43)	8.71 (8.73)	7.70 (11.18)	1.01 (−3.23 to 5.25)	0.209
12-week (40 vs. 38)	8.12 (9.42)	6.13 (8.41)	1.99 (−2.05 to 6.03)	0.038
24-week (26 vs. 24)	6.16 (5.49)	5.29 (9.09)	0.87 (−3.47 to 5.22)	0.023
STRESS HORMONES				
Cortisol (mg/L creatinine)				
Intention-to-treat analysis				
Baseline (62 vs. 62)	35.50 (19.56)	32.70 (17.45)	2.80 (−3.79 to 9.39)	0.379
12 weeks (46 vs. 42)	31.15 (19.63)	30.56 (18.42)	0.59 (−7.50 to 8.68)	0.937
24 weeks (28 vs. 27)	23.19 (9.09)	28.60 (27.36)	−5.41 (−16.70 to 5.88)	0.959
Per-protocol analysis				
Baseline (43 vs. 46)	35.90 (20.62)	31.43 (17.07)	4.47 (−3.49 to 12.42)	0.293
12 weeks (44 vs. 38)	30.41 (19.07)	31.24 (18.87)	−0.83 (−9.19 to 7.54)	0.821
24 weeks (26 vs. 23)	23.99 (8.94)	30.66 (29.16)	−6.67 (−19.68 to 6.35)	0.986
Epinephrine (mg/L creatinine)				
Intention-to-treat analysis				
Baseline (62 vs. 63)	12.22 (20.95)	10.29 (17.57)	1.93 (−4.89 to 8.75)	0.576
12 weeks (44 vs. 43)	5.73 (5.55)	5.28 (4.22)	0.45 (−1.65 to 2.56)	0.779
24 weeks (30 vs. 27)	5.55 (4.49)	3.67 (3.15)	1.88 (−0.20 to 3.96)	0.067
Per-protocol analysis				
Baseline (46 vs. 46)	12.58 (22.24)	10.86 (19.92)	1.72 (−7.03 to 10.46)	0.87
12 weeks (42 vs. 39)	5.75 (5.66)	5.13 (4.06)	0.63 (−1.55 to 2.79)	0.273
24 weeks (28 vs. 23)	5.35 (4.23)	3.90 (3.17)	1.45 (−0.69 to 3.60)	0.098
Norepinephrine (mg/L creatinine)				
Intention-to-treat analysis				
Baseline (61 vs. 62)	52.20 (42.08)	50.08 (28.79)	2.12 (−10.79 to 15.03)	0.85
12 weeks (46 vs. 41)	60.85 (44.05)	52.01 (35.07)	8.83 (−8.28 to 25.95)	0.748
24 weeks (30 vs. 27)	52.04 (35.50)	43.87 (34.52)	8.17 (−10.46 to 26.80)	0.198
Per-protocol analysis				
Baseline (44 vs. 45)	56.44 (47.59)	53.29 (31.47)	3.15 (−13.93 to 20.23)	0.715
12 weeks (44 vs. 37)	61.49 (44.64)	51.31 (32.35)	10.18 (−7.36 to 27.73)	0.76
24 weeks (28 vs. 23)	53.93 (35.94)	45.11 (35.42)	8.81 (−11.38 to 29.01)	0.197

CCBT = Conventional cognitive-behavioral therapy; RCBT = religious CBT; SD = standard deviation, CI = confidence intervals; CRP = C-reactive protein (acute phase protein), TNF-α = tumor necrosis factor-α, IL = interleukin, IFN = interferon. [1]Means and SD (standard deviations) are for original data (not log transformed); [2]p values are for analyses using log transformed data, except for IL-4 and IL-12; [3]N (sample size) for CCBT vs. RCBT; mean values, SD, and mean differences are for raw data.

Table 3. Effect of RCBT vs. CCBT on trajectory of change in inflammatory biomarkers and stress hormones from baseline to 24 weeks.

	B	SE	t value	p
PRO-INFLAMMATORY				
Log CRP (mg/L)				
Intent-to-treat (ITT) *analysis*				
Time	0.07	0.04	1.82	0.071
Main effect of group	0.10	0.13	0.77	0.441
Group × time interaction	−0.07	0.06	−1.17	0.242
Per-protocol (PP) analysis				
Time	0.09	0.04	2.03	0.044
Main effect of group	0.13	0.15	0.87	0.385
Group × time interaction	−0.09	0.06	−1.51	0.135
Log TNF-α (pg/ml)				
Intent-to-treat analysis				
Time	−0.01	0.01	−1.40	0.163
Main effect of group	0.01	0.04	0.30	0.767
Group × time interaction	0.00	0.01	−0.02	0.98
Per-protocol analysis				
Time	0.00	0.01	−0.41	0.681
Main effect of group	0.05	0.04	1.18	0.242
Group × time interaction	−0.01	0.01	0.60	0.549
Log IL-1β (pg/ml)				
Intent-to-treat analysis				
Time	−0.03	0.03	−1.06	0.293
Main effect of group	0.04	0.14	0.30	0.765
Group × time interaction	0.04	0.04	0.81	0.417
Per-protocol analysis				
Time	−0.03	0.03	−0.77	0.442
Main effect of group	0.03	0.17	0.16	0.874
Group × time interaction	0.03	0.05	0.69	0.492
Log IFN-γ (pg/ml)				
Intent-to-treat analysis				
Time	−0.02	0.02	−1.19	0.237
Main effect of group	0.05	0.10	0.45	0.654
Group × time interaction	0.02	0.03	0.81	0.417
Per-protocol analysis				
Time	−0.02	0.02	−0.67	0.501
Main effect of group	0.02	0.13	0.16	0.876
Group × time interaction	0.02	0.03	0.71	0.478

Continued

Log IL-6 (pg/ml)				
Intent-to-treat analysis				
Time	0.01	0.04	0.13	0.897
Main effect of group	0.04	0.12	0.34	0.738
Group × time interaction	−0.03	0.06	−0.46	0.645
Per-protocol analysis				
Time	0.03	0.04	0.62	0.533
Main effect of group	0.00	0.15	−0.01	0.990
Group × time interaction	−0.02	0.06	−0.36	0.716
IL-12 p70 (pg/ml)				
Intent-to-treat analysis				
Time	−0.18	0.08	−2.16	0.033
Main effect of group	−0.09	0.57	−0.17	0.869
Group × time interaction	0.06	0.12	0.52	0.602
Per-protocol analysis				
Time	−0.17	0.09	−1.90	0.059
Main effect of group	−0.13	0.46	−0.29	0.774
Group × time interaction	0.07	0.12	0.55	0.587
ANTI-INFLAMMATORY				
Log IL-1ra (pg/ml)				
Intent-to-treat analysis				
Time	−0.04	0.05	−0.78	0.436
Main effect of group	0.06	0.19	0.33	0.741
Group × time interaction	0.05	0.07	0.78	0.436
Per-protocol analysis				
Time	−0.05	0.06	−0.89	0.377
Main effect of group	−0.02	0.23	−0.08	0.935
Group × time interaction	0.07	0.08	0.91	0.364
IL-4 (pg/ml)				
Intent-to-treat analysis				
Time	−2.31	0.71	−3.28	0.001
Main effect of group	−0.18	2.53	−0.07	0.945
Group × time interaction	0.49	0.99	0.49	0.625
Per-protocol analysis				
Time	−1.45	0.64	−2.27	0.025
Main effect of group	−0.03	2.62	−0.01	0.99
Group × time interaction	−0.32	0.89	−0.36	0.719

Continued

Log IL-10 (pg/ml)				
Intent-to-treat analysis				
Time	−0.12	0.04	−2.87	0.005
Main effect of group	0.11	0.16	0.66	0.514
Group × time interaction	0.13	0.06	2.11	0.037
Per-protocol analysis				
Time	−0.11	0.05	−2.33	0.021
Main effect of group	0.09	0.19	0.47	0.642
Group × time interaction	0.12	0.06	1.93	0.056
STRESS HORMONES				
Log Cortisol (mg/L creatinine)				
Intent-to-treat analysis				
Time	−0.03	0.02	−1.34	0.181
Main effect of group	0.08	0.07	1.18	0.241
Group × time interaction	−0.04	0.03	−1.17	0.245
Per-protocol analysis				
Time	−0.01	0.03	−0.53	0.598
Main effect of group	0.11	0.08	1.36	0.175
Group × time interaction	−0.05	0.04	−1.38	0.170
Log Epinephrine (mg/L creatinine)				
Intent-to-treat analysis				
Time	−0.24	0.05	−4.86	<0.0001
Main effect of group	−0.19	0.13	−1.43	0.156
Group × time interaction	0.13	0.07	1.88	0.063
Per-protocol analysis				
Time	−0.25	0.05	−4.51	<0.0001
Main effect of group	−0.15	0.15	−0.98	0.328
Group × time interaction	0.11	0.08	1.52	0.130
Log Norepinephrine (mg/L creatinine)				
Intent-to-treat analysis				
Time	−0.04	0.03	−1.29	0.200
Main effect of group	−0.06	0.08	−0.76	0.447
Group × time interaction	0.05	0.04	1.15	0.253
Per-protocol analysis				
Time	−0.04	0.03	−1.34	0.184
Main effect of group	−0.07	0.09	−0.78	0.438
Group × time interaction	0.05	0.04	1.04	0.301

RCBT = religious CBT; CCBT = Conventional cognitive-behavioral therapy; CRP = C-reactive protein (acute phase protein), TNF-α = tumor necrosis factor-α, IL = interleukin, IFN = interferon. B = unstandardized coefficient for "time" indicates change in biomarker during the course of therapy (independent of group); the "main effect of group" represents the average difference between treatment groups (RCBT = 1, CCBT = 0); and for the "group × time interaction" indicates whether the two groups changed at the same rate; B's are from mixed effects growth curve models; SE = standard error; p = significance level; N = 121 - 127 for ITT analyses and 88 - 92 for PP analyses; log-transformed data used, except for IL-4 and IL-12.

Understanding Psychiatry

only those who received at least 5 of the 10 treatment sessions (to determine changes in biomarkers in those who received at least half of the treatment).

To examine the differential effect that baseline religiosity had on the effectiveness of RCBT vs. CCBT, we entered the summed measure of baseline religiosity and its interaction with treatment group into the mixed models above (**Table 4**). If the interaction was statistically significant or nearly so (p < 0.10), we dichotomized the summed religiosity variable at the mid-point into low and high religiosity categories and repeated the analysis (group, time, group by time interaction) in each category. To examine the effect of baseline religiosity on the trajectory of change in biomarkers regardless of treatment group, we entered baseline religiosity into the mixed model, along with group, time, and group by time interaction (**Table 5**). Statistical analyses were performed using SAS (version 9.3; SAS Institute Inc., Cary, North Carolina). The significance level was set at p=0.05 for all endpoints without correction for multiple comparisons given the exploratory nature of these analyses.

3. Results

As reported in the parent study [41], a total of 450 potential participants were screened between June 2011 and June 2013, of whom 187 were assessed by in-person screening and 132 were randomized to treatment group. Three clients who did not fulfill inclusion/exclusion criteria were mistakenly randomized in the trial, but were included to keep randomization intact. The characteristics of the sample are described in **Table 1**. Participants scored an average of 25.3 ± 8.5 on the BDI, which indicates moderate depression severity (but well above the cutoff of 10 for depression on the scale). There were no significant differences between treatment groups on any of the characteristics in **Table 1**. As reported elsewhere, mean level of depressive symptoms in both groups decreased progressively during the course of treatment (from 25.3 ± 8.5 at baseline to 11.8 ± 9.4 at 12-week and 11.8 ± 11.2 at 24-week), with no difference between RCBT and CCBT [41]. Median levels of *baseline* CRP, pro-inflammatory cytokines, and stress hormones tended to be higher in this sample compared to those in a community sample of non-depressed persons enrolled in the Midlife in the United States Study (MIDUS) [34].

Based on the existing research suggesting a relationship between stress biomarkers and depression, we expected that a change (*i.e.*, decrease) in depression severity during the course of treatment would be correlated with a decrease in pro-inflammatory biomarkers, an increase in anti-inflammatory cytokines, and a reduction in urinary stress hormones. However, decrease in severity of depressive symptoms was not significantly correlated with changes in pro-inflammatory proteins or cytokines (CRP, $r = -0.03$, $p = 0.810$; TNF-α, $r = -0.03$, $p = 0.745$; IL-1β, $R = 0.02$, $p = 0.887$; IFN-γ, $r = 0.08$, $p = 0.440$; IL-6, $r = 0.07$, $p = 0.507$; IL-12, $r = -0.05$, $p = 0.675$), changes in anti-inflammatory cytokines (IL-1ra, $r = -0.00$, $p = 0.984$; IL-4, $r = -0.00$, $p = 0.984$; IL-10, $r = 0.04$, $p = 0.736$), or changes in urinary stress hormones (cortisol, $r = 0.08$, $p = 0.469$; epinephrine, $r = -0.01$, $p = 0.953$; norepinephrine, $r = -0.05$, $p = 0.651$). This is despite the fact that depressive symptoms decreased in the overall trial population by an average of 13.9 points on the BDI-II, with changes ranging from a decrease of 38 points to an increase of 29 points. Similarly, there was a wide range of change in biomarkers during the study.

3.1. Effect of RCBT vs. CCBT on Biomarkers

In the ITT analysis that addressed our primary hypothesis, no difference was found between RCBT and CCBT in their effects on stress biomarkers in any comparison at baseline, 12 weeks, or 24 weeks, except for the anti-inflammatory cytokine IL-10, where a greater reduction was seen with RCBT at both 12 and 24 weeks (**Table 2**, **Figure 1**). The PP analysis among clients who had received at least 5 of the 10 treatment sessions also indicated no differences except for IL-10, supporting the findings from the ITT analysis.

Several pro-inflammatory, anti-inflammatory, and stress hormone indicators changed significantly over time in the mixed effects growth curve models (in both expected and unexpected directions) (**Table 3**). The ITT analysis indicated that the stress hormone epinephrine decreased significantly over time in the expected direction (time B $= -0.24$, SE [standard error] $= 0.05$, t $= -4.86$, p < 0.0001) (**Figure 2**). However, contrary to expectations the anti-inflammatory cytokines IL-4 and IL-10 also decreased over time (IL-4 time B $= -2.31$, SE $= 0.71$, t $= -3.28$, p $= 0.001$; IL-10 time B $= -0.12$, SE $= 0.04$, t $= -2.87$, p $= 0.005$). Also, pro-inflammatory acute phase protein CRP increased over time, an effect which in the PP analysis became significant (time B $= 0.09$, SE $= 0.04$, t $= 2.03$, p $= 0.044$) (**Figure 3**).

However, there was no significant difference in average treatment effects (*i.e.*, main effect of group) between RCBT and CCBT on any biomarker, including IL-10, in either ITT or PP analyses.

Table 4. Interaction between baseline religiosity and treatment group on trajectory of change in inflammatory markers and stress hormones.

	B	SE	t value	p
PRO-INFLAMMATORY				
Log CRP (mg/L)				
Intent-to-treat analysis (ITT)	0.00	0.00	−0.19	0.853
Per-protocol analysis (PP)	0.00	0.00	−0.28	0.779
Log TNF-α (pg/ml)				
ITT	0.00	0.00	−0.30	0.763
PP	0.00	0.00	−0.41	0.683
Log IL-1β (pg/ml)				
ITT	0.00	0.00	−0.92	0.360
PP	−0.01	−0.01	−1.08	0.282
Log IFN-γ (pg/ml)				
ITT	0.00	0.00	−0.49	0.628
PP	0.00	0.00	−0.71	0.478
Log IL-6 (pg/ml)				
ITT	−0.01	0.00	−1.98	0.050
PP	−0.01	0.00	−2.66	0.009
IL-12 p70 (pg/ml)				
ITT	−0.02	0.02	−0.95	0.345
PP	−0.01	0.02	−0.36	0.721
ANTI-INFLAMMATORY				
Log IL-1ra (pg/ml)				
ITT	−0.01	0.01	−1.94	0.055
PP	−0.02	0.01	−2.14	0.034
IL-4 (pg/ml)				
ITT	−0.12	0.08	−1.57	0.118
PP	−0.12	0.08	−1.45	0.149
Log IL-10 (pg/ml)				
ITT	−0.01	0.01	−1.54	0.126
PP	−0.01	0.01	−1.21	0.228
STRESS HORMONES				
Log Cortisol (mg/L creatinine)				
ITT	0.00	0.00	−1.45	0.148
PP	0.00	0.00	−1.15	0.250
Log Epinephrine (mg/L creatinine)				
ITT	0.00	0.00	−0.70	0.486
PP	0.00	0.00	0.29	0.776
Log Norepinephrine (mg/L creatinine)				
ITT	0.00	0.00	−0.05	0.963
PP	0.00	0.00	0.41	0.682

CRP = C-reactive protein, TNF-α = tumor necrosis factor-α, IL = interleukin, IFN = interferon; B = unstandardized coefficient for the religiosity by group interaction term in the mixed effects growth curve model; SE = standard error; p = significance level; N = 121 - 127 for ITT analyses and 88 - 92 for PP analyses; log transformed data used, except for IL-4 and IL-12.

Table 5. Effect of baseline religiosity on trajectory of change in inflammatory markers and stress hormones independent of treatment group.

	B	SE	t value	p
PRO-INFLAMMATORY				
Log CRP (mg/L)				
Intent-to-treat analysis (ITT)	0.001	0.002	0.66	0.511
Per-protocol analysis (PP)	0.001	0.002	0.47	0.642
Log TNF-α (pg/ml)				
ITT	0.000	0.001	0.18	0.857
PP	0.000	0.001	0.78	0.438
Log IL-1β (pg/ml)				
ITT	0.001	0.002	0.59	0.556
PP	0.001	0.003	0.37	0.713
Log IFN-γ (pg/ml)				
ITT	0.004	0.002	2.42	0.017
PP	0.005	0.002	2.28	0.024
Log IL-6 (pg/ml)				
ITT	0.001	0.002	0.35	0.725
PP	0.000	0.002	0.23	0.820
IL-12 p70 (pg/ml)				
ITT	0.021	0.011	1.96	0.052
PP	0.007	0.008	0.90	0.369
ANTI-INFLAMMATORY				
Log IL-1ra (pg/ml)				
ITT	0.003	0.003	1.15	0.252
PP	0.002	0.004	0.62	0.539
IL-4 (pg/ml)				
ITT	0.027	0.040	0.67	0.502
PP	0.017	0.042	0.39	0.694
Log IL-10 (pg/ml)				
ITT	0.001	0.003	0.54	0.593
PP	0.000	0.003	−0.13	0.899
STRESS HORMONES				
Log Cortisol (mg/L creatinine)				
ITT	0.001	0.001	1.83	0.069
PP	0.002	0.001	1.77	0.079
Log Epinephrine (mg/L creatinine)				
ITT	0.000	0.001	0.24	0.808
PP	0.001	0.000	0.69	0.490
Log Norepinephrine (mg/L creatinine)				
ITT	0.000	0.001	0.15	0.880
PP	0.000	0.001	−0.11	0.914

CRP = C-reactive protein, TNF-α = tumor necrosis factor-α, IL = interleukin, IFN = interferon; B = unstandardized coefficient for the baseline religiosity term in the mixed effects growth curve model; SE = standard error; p = significance level; N = 121 - 127 for ITT and 88 - 92 for PP analyses; log transformed data used in analyses, except for IL-4 and IL-12.

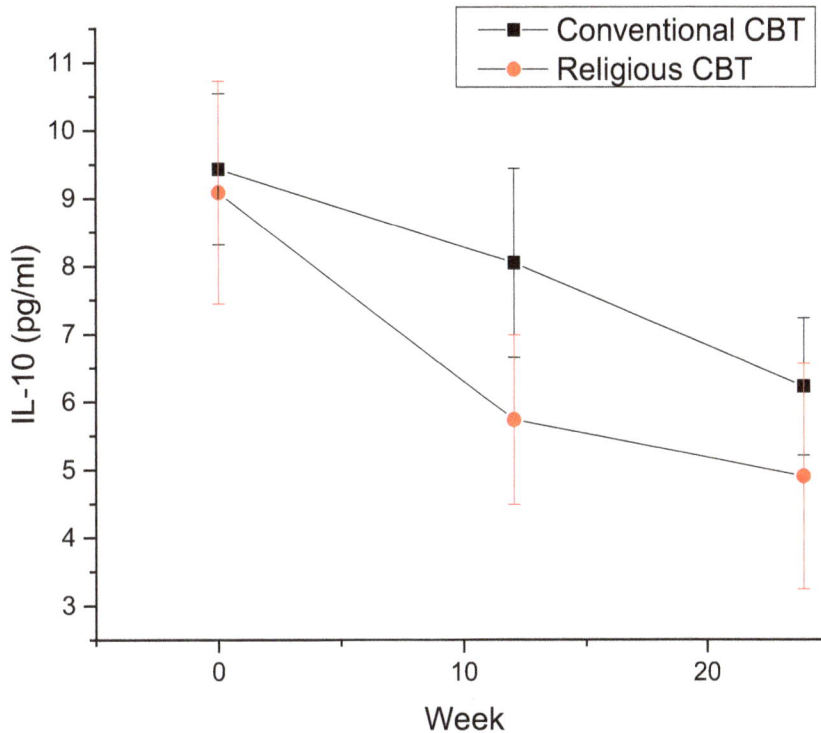

Figure 1. Effects of RCBT vs. CCBT on average level of anti-inflammatory cytokine interleukin 10 (IL-10) (±standard error). Mixed model intent-to-treat analysis (log transformed): time B = −0.12, p = 0.005; main effect of group B = 0.11 (where RCBT = 1), p = 0.514; group × time interaction B = 0.13, p = 0.037.

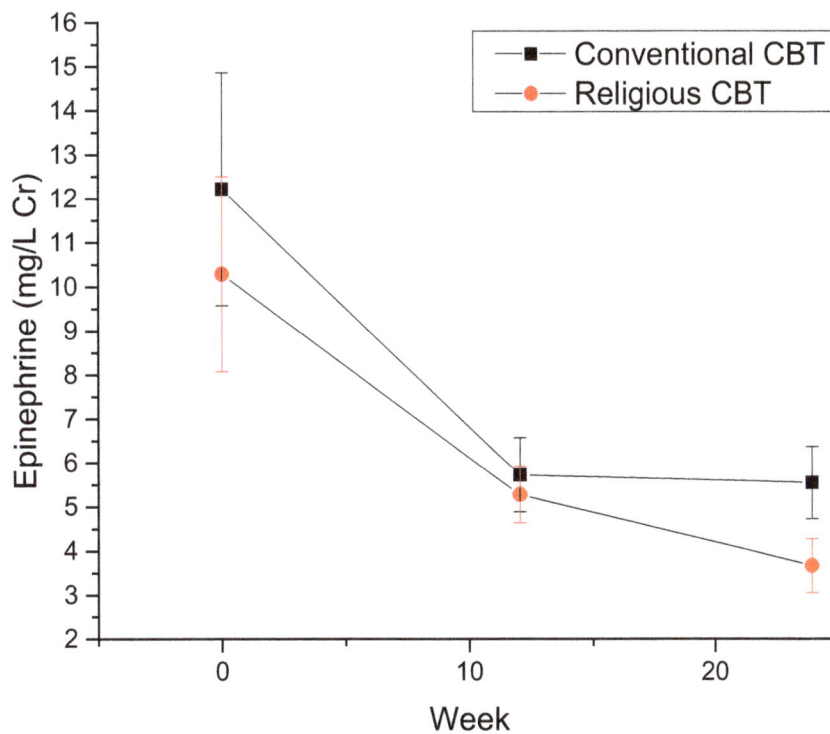

Figure 2. Effects of RCBT vs. CCBT on average level of urine epinephrine (±standard error). Mixed model intent-to-treat analysis (log transformed): time B = −0.24, p < 0.0001; main effect of group B = −0.19, p = 0.156; group × time interaction B = 0.13, p = 0.063.

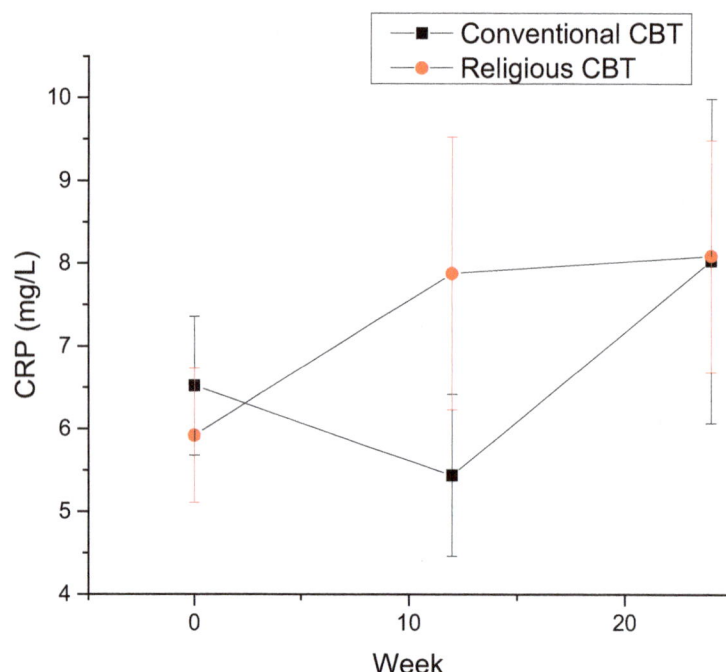

Figure 3. Effects of RCBT vs. CCBT on average level of C-reactive protein (CRP) (±standard error). Mixed model intent-to-treat analysis (log transformed): time B=0.07, p = 0.071; main effect of group B = 0.10, p = 0.441; group × time interaction B = −0.07, p = 0.242.

3.2. Differential Effects of Religiosity

With regard to the impact of RCBT vs. CCBT in those with higher and low religiosity scores, no significant effect was seen on any pro-inflammatory, anti-inflammatory, or stress hormone outcome examined in the ITT analysis, except for IL6 (**Table 4**). For IL-6, the interaction between overall religiosity and treatment group in the mixed effect growth curve model was significant in both ITT and PP analyses (B = −0.007, SE = 0.003, t = −1.98, p = 0.050, and B = −0.011, SE = 0.004, t = −2.66, p = 0.009, respectively). The ITT analysis in the low religiosity group indicated that CCBT was more effective than RCBT in lowering IL-6 levels (main effect B = 0.38, SE = 0.15, t = 2.52, p = 0.014, n = 62); this was replicated in the PP analysis (main effect B = 0.48, SE = 0.18, t = 2.62, p = 0.011, n = 44). In those with high religiosity, RCBT was no more effective than CCBT in the ITT analysis (main effect B = −0.28, SE = 0.19, t = −1.44, p = 0.155, n = 64), but was more effective in the PP analysis (main effect B = −0.47, SE = 0.24, t = 2.00, p = 0.050, n = 45) (**Figure 4**).

3.3. Effect of Baseline Religiosity on Biomarkers

When overall religiosity was entered into the mixed effects growth curve models, effects were observed on changes in several biomarkers over time independent of treatment group (**Table 5**). The effects, however, were not as hypothesized. Results from the ITT analysis indicated that greater religiosity at baseline predicted an increase in pro-inflammatory cytokines IFN-γ (B = 0.004, SE = 0.002, t = 2.42, p = 0.017) and IL-12-p70 (B = 0.021, SE = 0.011, t = 1.96, p = 0.052), and tended to predict an increase in urinary cortisol (B = 0.001, SE = 0.001, t = 1.83, p = 0.069). Religiosity had no significant effect on any other biomarker.

4. Discussion

To our knowledge, this is the first study to compare the effects of religiously-integrated CBT compared to conventional CBT on changes in a wide range of pro-inflammatory, anti-inflammatory, and stress hormone biomarkers in persons with major depressive disorder and chronic medical illness who were at least somewhat religious or spiritual. Despite the finding that a number of these biomarkers changed during the course of therapy, neither RCBT nor CCBT were effective in reducing pro-inflammatory cytokines. The only exception in this re-

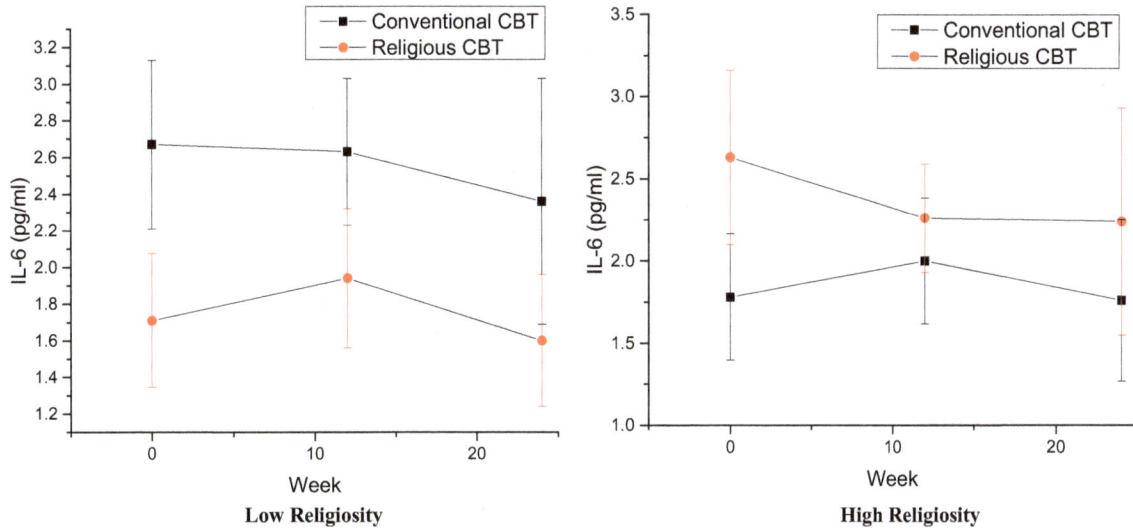

Figure 4. Effects of RCBT vs. CCBT on the average level (original values) of pro-inflammatory cytokine interleukin-6 (IL-6) (±standard error) in those with low and high religiosity. Low religiosity: mixed model per-protocol analysis (log transformed): time B = 0.09, p = 0.084; main effect of group B = 0.48, p = 0.011; group × time interaction B = −0.13, p = 0.063 (n = 44); high religiosity: mixed model per-protocol analysis (log transformed): time B = −0.03, p = 0.719; main effect of group B = −0.47, p = 0.050; group × time interaction B=0.08, p = 0.446 (n = 45).

gard emerged from the moderator analysis. In the low religiosity group, CCBT was significantly more effective in reducing the pro-inflammatory cytokine IL-6, whereas in the high religiosity group, RCBT was more effective in reducing IL-6 in the per protocol analysis. Baseline religiosity, however, predicted an increase in pro-inflammatory cytokines IFN-γ and IL-12-p70 and tended to do likewise with urinary cortisol (which is usually associated with greater depression [54] [55]).

4.1. Interpretation

The only findings in this study that supported our hypotheses were the reduction in urinary epinephrine over time as MDD was treated and the interaction of religiosity with treatment type for the marker IL-6. The former is consistent with prior research indicating higher levels of stress hormones in those with MDD and a decline in those hormones in response to treatment [56]. The latter is consistent with our original report that CCBT tended to be more effective than RCBT in the treatment of MDD in those who were less religious, whereas RCBT tended to be more effective in those who were more religious [41].

Why, however, was RCBT in general not more effective than CCBT in reducing pro-inflammatory cytokines, increasing anti-inflammatory cytokines, and reducing stress hormones, biomarkers known to be associated with MDD? One finding that may have influenced these results was that change in depressive symptoms was not associated with change in any of the inflammatory markers or stress hormones measured here, despite a sharp mean drop in BDI-II scores over the time of the trial. Had there not been such a decrease in symptoms, we might have attributed the failure to detect differences in treatment effect to the mild to moderate level of depression at baseline (ranging from 10 to 42). This lack of an association between change in depression with treatment and change in biomarkers remains an unexplained finding. If changes in biomarker levels during the study were not related to changes in depression, then the treatments for depression examined here may not have had much of an effect on changes in biomarkers either. Several biomarkers (four of twelve) did change during the study, although the change was in expected (one) and unexpected directions (three). There was no way, however, to determine whether those changes were due to a treatment effect, regression to the mean, or a chance finding, given the inconsistent pattern of change and lack of a no-treatment control group.

Failure to find a difference in biomarker change between RCBT and CCBT may also have been due to the similarity of the interventions. Both therapies addressed dysfunctional cognitions and behaviors and did so in broadly spiritual ways (focusing on meaning and purpose, forgiveness, gratitude, altruism, social connections, etc.), with the only difference being the religious nature of motivations for change. Given that studies comparing two types of psychotherapy often do not report significant differences [57], and given the many similarities in the two treatment approaches examined here, perhaps failure to find a difference in clinical or physiological outcomes is not too surprising.

The positive correlation between baseline religiosity and an increase in pro-inflammatory markers was also a curious and unexpected finding given prior research. Could religious people have become more physiologically stressed by the treatment even though their depressive symptoms lessened? Might the religious element of RCBT have stressed certain individuals with its reference to religious issues, even though the CBT elements helped? Neither of these explanations are likely since the effect was present in both RCBT and CCBT groups (*i.e.*, was independent of treatment group). A "healthy" physiological response may also differ depending on the condition. The goal of treatment is to produce an optimal balance in pro- and anti-inflammatory responses, and this could involve an increase in certain inflammatory biomarkers such as IFN-γ that can actually decrease in response to stress [58].

4.2. Limitations

A number of limitations in the present study may have influenced our findings. First, our sample consisted of persons with chronic medical illnesses who were taking a wide range of medications that could influence levels of inflammatory markers and stress hormones. Although we did our best to exclude individuals with obvious inflammatory disorders and those taking drugs that suppress the immune system or affect endocrine functions, individuals with conditions or on medication that could have affected the results of biomarker analyses may have ended up in the sample. This likely added to the variance in our outcomes, making it difficult to identify differences between treatments or associations with depressive symptoms or religiosity. Second, none of the biomarkers were normally distributed, and two of the biomarkers (IL4 and IL-12) could not be normalized with log transformation, factors which may have also influenced our results.

Third, the trial population included some participants whose MDD symptoms were only mild in severity. The findings may have been quite different had only participants with severe major depression been included. Fourth, treatment was delivered remotely by telephone, which may not have the same results as in-person treatment. However, recent evidence on CBT delivered in primary care suggests there is little difference in efficacy and that adherence may be better when therapy is delivered by telephone [59] [60]. Finally, many statistical comparisons were conducted to compare RCBT vs. CCBT on each of the 12 stress biomarkers in the ITT analysis and per-protocol analyses, as well as to test the moderating effects of religiosity and the effects of baseline religiosity on outcomes, increasing the likelihood of a Type 1 error. We chose to use a traditional significance level of 0.05 because of the exploratory nature of these analyses and the relatively small sample (which was not powered to detect changes in biomarker levels). Had we corrected our p-value for multiple comparisons the significance level would have been closer to 0.001.

Nevertheless, the study also has a number of strengths. First, it was a multi-site randomized clinical trial conducted on the East and West coasts of the US that tested reasonable hypotheses based on the existing literature. Second, the interventions were structured and manual-based, administered by experienced therapists, and were administered in a standard dose (ten 50-minute sessions). Third, we diagnosed MDD using a structured psychiatric interview (MINI) and examined changes in depressive symptoms using a standard measure that is widely used in clinical trials of depression in primary care (BDI-II). Fourth, we measured religiosity in a comprehensive manner that is seldom done in studies of this nature. Fifth, we assessed a wide range of stress biomarkers known to be associated with depressive disorder and often found to be responsive to treatment. Finally, our use of mixed effects growth curve models enabled us to make maximum use of the available data.

5. Conclusion

Neither RCBT nor CCBT were consistently effective in reducing pro-inflammatory cytokines, increasing anti-inflammatory cytokines, or reducing stress hormones in this sample of persons with chronic medical illness and major depressive disorder. The only exception was that CCBT had a greater impact on reducing the pro-inflammatory cytokine IL-6 in those with low religiosity, while RCBT seemed to have a greater effect on IL-6 in those with higher religiosity. Religiosity, however, predicted an increase in pro-inflammatory cytokines and the stress hormone cortisol over time independent of treatment group, which was not expected. Whether these findings are due to chance, given the multiple statistical comparisons, or due to the trial design will need to be determined by future research that seeks to replicate these results.

Funding

Funding support provided by the John Templeton Foundation.

References

[1] Howren, M.B., Lamkin, D.M. and Suls, J. (2009) Associations of Depression with C-Reactive Protein, Il-1, and Il-6: A Meta-Analysis. *Psychosomatic Medicine*, **71**, 171-186. http://dx.doi.org/10.1097/PSY.0b013e3181907c1b

[2] Hestad, K.A., Tonseth, S., Stoen, C.D., Ueland, T. and Aukrust, P. (2003) Raised Plasma Levels of Tumor Necrosis Factor Alpha in Patients with Depression: Normalization during Electroconvulsive Therapy. *Journal of Electroconvulsive Therapy*, **19**, 183-188.

[3] Guglu, C., Kara, S.H., Caliyurt, O., Vardar, E. and Abay, E. (2003) Increased Serum Tumor Necrosis Factor-Alpha Levels and Treatment Response in Major Depressive Disorder. *Psychopharmacology*, **170**, 429-433. http://dx.doi.org/10.1007/s00213-003-1566-z

[4] Leonard, B.E. and Myint, A. (2009) The Psychoneuroimmunology of Depression. *Human Psychopharmacology*, **24**, 165-175. http://dx.doi.org/10.1002/hup.1011

[5] Zorrilla, E.P., Luborsky, L., McKay, J.R., Rosenthal, R., Houldin, A., Tx, A., McCorkle, R., Seligman, D.A. and Schmidt, K. (2001) The Relationship of Depression and Stressors to Immunoloigcal Assays: A Meta-Analytic Review. *Brain, Behavior, and Immunity*, **15**, 199-226. http://dx.doi.org/10.1006/brbi.2000.0597

[6] Miller, A.H. (1998) Neuroendocrine and Immune System Interactions in Stress and Depression. *Psychiatric Clinics of North America*, **21**, 443-463. http://dx.doi.org/10.1016/S0193-953X(05)70015-0

[7] Evans, D.L., Ten have, T.R., Douglas, S.D., Gettes, D.R., Morrison, M., Chiappini, M.S., *et al.* (2002) Association of Depression with Viral Load, CD8 T Lymphocytes, and Natural Killer Cells in Women with HIV Infection. *American Journal of Psychiatry*, **159**, 1752-1759. http://dx.doi.org/10.1176/appi.ajp.159.10.1752

[8] Thaker, P.H., Lutgendorf, S.K. and Sood, A.K. (2007) The Neuroendocrine Impact of Chronic Stress on Cancer. *Cell Cycle*, **6**, 430-433. http://dx.doi.org/10.4161/cc.6.4.3829

[9] Lutgendorf, S.K., DeGeest, K., Sung, C.Y., Arevalo, J.M., Penedo, F. and Lucci III, J. (2009) Depression, Social Support, and Beta-Adrenergic Transcription Control in Human Ovarian Cancer. *Brain, Behavior, & Immunity*, **23**, 176-183. http://dx.doi.org/10.1016/j.bbi.2008.04.155

[10] Zautra, A.J., Yocum, D.C., Villanueva, I., Smith, B., Davis, M.C., Attrep, J. and Irwin, M. (2004) Immune Activation and Depression in Women with Rheumatoid Arthritis. *Journal of Rheumatology*, **31**, 457-463.

[11] Irwin, M.R. and Miller, A.H. (2007) Depressive Disorders and Immunity: 20 Years of Progress and Discovery. *Brain, Behavior, and Immunity*, **21**, 374-383. http://dx.doi.org/10.1016/j.bbi.2007.01.010

[12] Hannestad, J., DellaGiola, N. and Bloch, M. (2011) The Effect of Antidepressant Medication Treatment on Serum Levels of Inflammatory Cytokines: A Meta-Analysis. *Neuropsychopharmacology*, **36**, 2452-2459. http://dx.doi.org/10.1038/npp.2011.132

[13] Castanon, N., Leonard, B.E., Neveu, P.J. and Yirmiya, R. (2002) Effects of Antidepressants on Cytokine Production and Actions. *Brain, Behavior, and Immunity*, **16**, 569-574. http://dx.doi.org/10.1016/S0889-1591(02)00008-9

[14] Dahl, J., Ormstad, H., Aas, H.C.D., Malt, U.F., Bendtz, L.T., Sandvik, L., Brundin, L. and Andreassen, O.A. (2014) The Plasma Level of Various Cytokines Are Increased during Ongoing Depression and Are Reduced to Normal Levels after Recovery. *Psychoneuroendocrinology*, **45**, 77-86. http://dx.doi.org/10.1016/j.psyneuen.2014.03.019

[15] van Middendorp, H., Geenen, R., Sorbi, M.J., van Doornen, L.J. and Bijlsma, J.W. (2009) Health and Physiological Effects of an Emotional Disclosure Intervention Adapted for Application at Home: A Randomized Clinical Trial in Rheumatoid Arthritis. *Psychotherapy & Psychosomatics*, **78**, 145-151. http://dx.doi.org/10.1159/000206868

[16] Antoni, M.H., Lechner, S., Diaz, A., Vargas, S., Holley, H., Phillips, K., McGregor, B., Carver, C.S. and Blomberg, B. (2009) Cognitive Behavioral Stress Management Effects on Psychosocial and Physiological Adaptation in Women Undergoing Treatment for Breast Cancer. *Brain, Behavior, and Immunity*, **23**, 580-591. http://dx.doi.org/10.1016/j.bbi.2008.09.005

[17] Roberts, A.D.L., Papadopoulos, A.S., Wessely, S., Chalder, T. and Cleare, A.J. (2009) Salivary Cortisol Output before and after Cognitive Behavioral Therapy for Chronic Fatigue Syndrome. *Journal of Affective Disorders*, **115**, 280-286. http://dx.doi.org/10.1016/j.jad.2008.09.013

[18] Pew Forum (2007) US Religious Landscape Survey. http://religions.pewforum.org/

[19] The Gallup Poll (2009) State of the States: Importance of Religion. http://www.gallup.com/poll/114022/state-states-importance-religion.aspx

[20] Pargament, K. (1997) The Psychology of Religion and Coping. Guilford Press, New York.

[21] Koenig, H.G. (1998) Religious Beliefs and Practices of Hospitalized Medically Ill Older Adults. *International Journal of Geriatric Psychiatry*, **13**, 213-224.
http://dx.doi.org/10.1002/(SICI)1099-1166(199804)13:4<213::AID-GPS755>3.0.CO;2-5

[22] Koenig, H.G., Cohen, H.J., Blazer, D.G., Pieper, C., Meador, K.G., Shelp, F., Goli, V. and DiPasquale, R. (1992) Religious Coping and Depression in Elderly Hospitalized Medically Ill Men. *American Journal of Psychiatry*, **149**, 1693-1700. http://dx.doi.org/10.1176/ajp.149.12.1693

[23] Koenig, H.G. (2007) Religion and Remission of Depression in Medical Inpatients with Heart Failure/Pulmonary Disease. *Journal of Nervous and Mental Disease*, **195**, 389-395.

[24] Koenig, H.G., George, L.K. and Peterson, B.L. (1998) Religiosity and Remission of Depression in Medically Ill Older Patients. *American Journal of Psychiatry*, **155**, 536-542. http://dx.doi.org/10.1176/ajp.155.4.536

[25] Koenig, H.G., Cohen, H.J., George, L.K., Hays, J.C., Larson, D.B. and Blazer, D.G. (1997) Attendance at Religious Services, Interleukin-6, and Other Biological Indicators of Immune Function in Older Adults. *International Journal of Psychiatry in Medicine*, **27**, 233-250. http://dx.doi.org/10.2190/40NF-Q9Y2-0GG7-4WH6

[26] Lutgendorf, S.K., Russell, D., Ullrich, P., Harris, T.B. and Wallace, R. (2004) Religious Participation, Interleukin-6, and Mortality in Older Adults. *Health Psychology*, **23**, 465-475. http://dx.doi.org/10.1037/0278-6133.23.5.465

[27] King, D.E., Mainous III, A.G. and Pearson, W.S. (2002) C-Reactive Protein, Diabetes, and Attendance at Religious Services. *Diabetes Care*, **25**, 1172-1176. http://dx.doi.org/10.2337/diacare.25.7.1172

[28] Bellinger, D.L., Berk, L.S., Koenig, H.G., Daher, N., Pearce, M.J., Robins, C.J., Nelson, B., Shaw, S.F., Cohen, H.J. and King, M.B. (2014) Religious Involvement, Inflammatory Markers and Stress Hormones in Major Depression and Chronic Medical Illness. *Open Journal of Psychiatry*, **4**, 335-352. http://dx.doi.org/10.4236/ojpsych.2014.44040

[29] Dedert, E.A., Studts, J.L., Weissbecker, I., Salmon, P.G., Banis, P.L. and Sephton, S.E. (2004) Private Religious Practice: Protection of Cortisol Rhythms among Women with Fibromyalgia. *International Journal of Psychiatry in Medicine*, **34**, 61-77. http://dx.doi.org/10.2190/2Y72-6H80-BW93-U0T6

[30] Tartaro, J., Luecken, L.J. and Gunn, H.E. (2005) Exploring Heart and Soul: Effects of Religiosity/Spirituality and Gender on Blood Pressure and Cortisol Stress Responses. *Journal of Health Psychology*, **10**, 753-766. http://dx.doi.org/10.1177/1359105305057311

[31] Ironson, G., Soloman, G.F., Balbin, E.G., O'Cleirigh, C., George, A., Kumar, M., *et al.* (2002) The Ironson-Woods Spirituality/Religiousness Index Is Associated with Long Survival, Health Behaviors, Less Distress, and Low Cortisol in People with HIV/AIDS. *Annals of Behavioral Medicine*, **24**, 34-48. http://dx.doi.org/10.1207/S15324796ABM2401_05

[32] Carrico, A.W., Ironson, G., Antoni, M.H., Lechner, S.C., Duran, R.E., Kumar, M., *et al.* (2006) A Path Model of the Effects of Spirituality on Depressive Symptoms and 24-h Urinary-Free Cortisol in HIV-Positive Persons. *Journal of Psychosomatic Research*, **61**, 51-58. http://dx.doi.org/10.1016/j.jpsychores.2006.04.005

[33] Chan, C.L., Ho, R.T., Lee, P.W., Cheng, J.Y., Leung, P.P., Foo, W., *et al.* (2006) A Randomized Controlled Trial of Psychosocial Interventions Using the Psychophysiological Framework for Chinese Breast Cancer Patients. *Journal of Psychosocial Oncology*, **24**, 3-26. http://dx.doi.org/10.1300/J077v24n01_02

[34] Bellinger, D.L., Berk, L.S., Koenig, H.G., Daher, N., Pearce, M.J., Robins, C.J., Nelson, B., Shaw, S.F., Cohen, H.J. and King, M.B. (2014) Religious Involvement, Inflammatory Markers and Stress Hormones in Major Depression and Chronic Medical Illness. *Open Journal of Psychiatry*, **4**, 335-352. http://dx.doi.org/10.4236/ojpsych.2014.44040

[35] Pace, T.W., Negi, L.T., Adame, D.D., Cole, S.P., Sivilli, T.I., Brown, T.D., *et al.* (2009) Effect of Compassion Meditation on Neuroendocrine, Innate Immune and Behavioral Responses to Psychosocial Stress. *Psychoneuroendocrinology*, **34**, 87-98. http://dx.doi.org/10.1016/j.psyneuen.2008.08.011

[36] Witek-Janusek, L., Albuquerque, K., Chroniak, K.R., Chroniak, C., Durazo-Arvizu, R. and Mathews, H.L. (2008) Effect of Mindfulness Based Stress Reduction on Immune Function, Quality of Life and Coping in Women Newly Diagnosed with Early Stage Breast Cancer. *Brain, Behavior, and Immunity*, **22**, 969-981. http://dx.doi.org/10.1016/j.bbi.2008.01.012

[37] Sudsuang, R., Chentanez, V. and Veluvan, K. (1991) Effect of Buddhist Meditation on Serum Cortisol and Total Protein Levels, Blood Pressure, Pulse Rate, Lung Volume and Reaction Time. *Physiology & Behavior*, **50**, 543-548. http://dx.doi.org/10.1016/0031-9384(91)90543-W

[38] Walton, K.G., Fields, J.Z., Levitsky, D.K., Harris, D.A., Pugh, N.D., Schneider, R.H., *et al.* (2004) Lowering Cortisol and CVD Risk in Postmenopausal Women: A Pilot Study Using the Transcendental Meditation Program. *Annals of the New York Academy of Sciences*, **1032**, 211-215. http://dx.doi.org/10.1196/annals.1314.023

[39] Jin, P. (1992) Efficacy of Tai Chi, Brisk Walking, Meditation, and Reading in Reducing Mental and Emotional Stress. *Journal of Psychosomatic Research*, **36**, 361-370. http://dx.doi.org/10.1016/0022-3999(92)90072-A

[40] Curiati, J.A., Bocchi, E., Freire, J.O., Arantes, A.C., Braga, M., Garcia, Y., *et al.* (2005) Meditation Reduces Sympa-

thetic Activation and Improves the Quality of Life in Elderly Patients with Optimally Treated Heart Failure: A Prospective Randomized Study. *Journal of Alternative and Complementary Medicine*, **11**, 465-472. http://dx.doi.org/10.1089/acm.2005.11.465

[41] Koenig, H.G., Pearce, M.J., Nelson, B., Shaw, S.F., Robins, C.J., Daher, N., Cohen, H.J., Berk, L.S., Bellinger, D., Pargament, K.I., Rosmarin, D.H., Vasegh, S., Kristeller, J., Juthani, N., Nies, D. and King, M.B. (2015) Religious vs. Conventional Cognitive-Behavioral Therapy for Major Depression in Persons with Chronic Medical Illness. *Journal of Nervous and Mental Disease*, **203**, 243-251. http://dx.doi.org/10.1097/NMD.0000000000000273

[42] Sheehan, B.V., Lecrubier, Y., Sheehan, K.H., Amorim, P., Janavs, J., Weiller, E., *et al.* (1998) The Mini International Neuropsychiatric Interview (MINI): The Development and Validation of Structured Diagnostic Psychiatric Interview for DSM-IV and ICD-10. *Journal of Clinical Psychiatry*, **59**, 22-33.

[43] Beck, A.T., Ward, C.H., Mendelson, M., Mock, J. and Erbaugh, J. (1961) An Inventory for Measuring Depression. *Archives of General Psychiatry*, **4**, 561-571. http://dx.doi.org/10.1001/archpsyc.1961.01710120031004

[44] Koenig, H.G. (1996) An Abbreviated Mini-Mental State Exam for Medically Ill Elders. *Journal of the American Geriatrics Society*, **44**, 215-216. http://dx.doi.org/10.1111/j.1532-5415.1996.tb02449.x

[45] Beck, A.T., Rush, J., Shaw, B.F. and Emery, G. (1979) Cognitive Therapy of Depression. Guilford Press, New York.

[46] Pearce, M.J., Koenig, H.G., Robins, C.J., Nelson, B., Shaw, S.F., Cohen, H.J. and King, M.B. (2015) Religiously-Integrated Cognitive Behavioral Therapy: A New Method of Treatment for Major Depression in Patients with Chronic Medical Illness. *Psychotherapy*, **52**, 56-66. http://dx.doi.org/10.1037/a0036448

[47] Religious Cognitive Behavioral Therapy Manuals (2014) Duke University Center for Spirituality, Durham, NC. Theology and Health. Manuals and Workbooks at: http://www.spiritualityandhealth.duke.edu/index.php/religious-cbt-study/therapy-manuals

[48] Koenig, H.G., Meador, K.G. and Parkerson, G. (1997) Religion Index for Psychiatric Research. *American Journal of Psychiatry*, **154**, 885-886. http://dx.doi.org/10.1176/ajp.154.6.885b

[49] Hoge, D.R. (1972) A Validated Intrinsic Religious Motivation Scale. *Journal for the Scientific Study of Religion*, **11**, 369-376. http://dx.doi.org/10.2307/1384677

[50] Underwood, L.G. and Teresi, J.A. (2002) The Daily Spiritual Experiences Scale: Development, Theoretical Description, Reliability, Exploratory Factor Analysis, and Preliminary Construct Validity Using Health-Related Data. *Annals of Behavioral Medicine*, **24**, 22-33. http://dx.doi.org/10.1207/S15324796ABM2401_04

[51] Hlatky, M.A., Boineau, R.E., Higginbotham, M.B., Lee, K.L., Mark, D.B., Califf, R.M., Cobb, F.R. and Pryor, D.B. (1989) A Brief Self-Administered Questionnaire to Determine Functional Capacity (The Duke Activity Status Index). *American Journal of Cardiology*, **64**, 651-654. http://dx.doi.org/10.1016/0002-9149(89)90496-7

[52] Charlson, M.E., Pompei, P., Ales, K.L. and Mackenzie, C.R. (1987) A New Method of Classifying Prognostic Comorbidity in Longitudinal Studies: Development and Validation. *Journal of Chronic Disease*, **40**, 373-383. http://dx.doi.org/10.1016/0021-9681(87)90171-8

[53] Linn, B., Linn, M. and Gurel, L. (1968) Cumulative Illness Rating Scale. *Journal of the American Geriatrics Society*, **16**, 622-626. http://dx.doi.org/10.1111/j.1532-5415.1968.tb02103.x

[54] Myint, A.M., Leonard, B.E., Steinbusch, H.W. and Kim, Y.K. (2005) Th1, Th2, and Th3 Cytokine Alterations in Major Depression. *Journal of Affective Disorders*, **88**, 167-173. http://dx.doi.org/10.1016/j.jad.2005.07.008

[55] Dowlati, Y., Herrmann, N., Swardfager, W., Liu, H., Sham, L., Reim, E.K. and Lanctôt, K.L. (2010) A Meta-Analysis of Cytokines in Major Depression. *Biological Psychiatry*, **67**, 446-457. http://dx.doi.org/10.1016/j.biopsych.2009.09.033

[56] Veith, R.C., Lewis, N., Linares, O.A., Barnes, R.F., Raskind, M.A., Villacres, E.C., Murburg, M.M., Ashleigh, E.A., Castillo, S., Peskind, E.R., Pasculay, M. and Halter, J.B. (1994) Sympathetic Nervous System Activity in Major Depression. Basal and Desipramine-Induced Alterations in Plasma Norepinephrine Kinetics. *Archives of General Psychiatry*, **51**, 411-422. http://dx.doi.org/10.1001/archpsyc.1994.03950050071008

[57] Wampold, B.E., Mondin, G.W., Moody, M., Stich, F., Benson, K. and Ahn, H. (1997) A Meta-Analysis of Outcome Studies Comparing Bona Fide Psychotherapies: Empirically, "All Must Have Prizes." *Psychological Bulletin*, **122**, 204-215. http://dx.doi.org/10.1037/0033-2909.122.3.203

[58] Zorrilla, E.P., Luborsky, L., McKay, J.R., Rosenthal, R., Houldin, A., Tax, A., McCorkle, R., Seligman, D.A. and Schmidt, K. (2001) The Relationship of Depression and Stressors to Immunological Assays: A Meta-Analytic Review. *Brain, Behavior, and Immunity*, **15**, 199-226. http://dx.doi.org/10.1006/brbi.2000.0597

[59] Mohr, D.C., Ho, J., Duffecy, J., Reifler, D., Sokol, L., Burns, M.N., *et al.* (2012) Effect of Telephone-Administered vs. Face-to-Face Cognitive Behavioral Therapy on Adherence to Therapy and Depression Outcomes among Primary Care Patients: A Randomized Trial. *Journal of the American Medical Association*, **307**, 2278-2285. http://dx.doi.org/10.1001/jama.2012.5588

[60] Kalapatapu, R.K., Ho, J., Cai, X., Vinogradov, S., Batki, S.L. and Mohr, D.C. (2014) Cognitive-Behavioral Therapy in Depressed Primary Care Patients with Co-Occurring Problematic Alcohol Use: Effect of Telephone-Administered vs. Face-to-Face Treatment—A Secondary Analysis. *Journal of Psychoactive Drugs*, **46**, 85-92. http://dx.doi.org/10.1080/02791072.2013.876521

13

Sex Work, Motivations for Entry, and the Combined Impact of Both on Mental Health: A Case Report of Japanese Female Patients within Therapeutic Relationships

Masayo Uji

Department of Bioethics, Kumamoto University Graduate School of Medical Sciences, Kumamoto, Japan
Email: ujimasayo@hotmail.co.jp

Abstract

The purpose of this study was to explore the motivations for entry into the sex industry. The narratives of four Japanese female psychiatric patients with a past experience of sex work were used for analysis. I identified not only practical factors such as financial difficulties or lack of job skills, but also various psycho-social factors, namely: weak emotional ties with their mothers since infancy, their mothers' tendency to prioritize sons over daughters, unremitting needs for maternal care, fear of rejection and object-seeking behavior, desire to control others, envy and aggressive self-destructive behavior, difficulties in establishing female peer relationships during adolescence, proneness to dependency on male objects through sexual relationships, past histories of crime and delinquency, weak internal motivation, frequent acting out, and addictive behaviors. In this article I discussed whether their mental maladjustment was purely the product of their past experiences as sex workers, or whether in fact both the maladjustment and the motivations for entry were derived from personality characteristics developed since infancy. Although not applicable to every Japanese sex worker, this article presents a preliminary hypothesis regarding the contribution of the above multi-dimensional factors to the motivations for entry, and the following mental maladjustment.

Keywords

Motivation, Sex Industry, Psycho-Social Factors, Maladjustment, Personality Characteristics

1. Introduction

A considerable number of studies have examined the motivations for entry into the sex industry, which for the purpose of this article includes the hostess trade. Disregarding factors that are highly culturally specific, most studies are in broad agreement regarding the motivations for entering or remaining in the sex trade, including financial motivation [1]-[3]; childhood physical or sexual abuse [1] [2] followed by loss of self-worth [4]; disrupted family life [4]; runaway behavior [2]; homelessness and experience of life on the street [4]; views of prostitution as exciting, glamorous, and empowering [2]; emotional support within a companionship [3]; drug abuse [1]-[3]; desire to gain the attention and acceptance of adults [4]; and self-identity as a professional woman [3]. Some research has referred to the differences between runaway girls and filial daughters [3], and between juvenile and adult prostitutes [2]. But it is also appropriate to consider that motivating factors, their number, and the degree to which each contributes to entry into the sex trade vary from individual to individual. Usually these factors do not contribute singly, but rather interact with each other or form part of a chain reaction [4]. Cusick [4] emphasized that "whatever the power of personal experiences that incline a person towards prostitution, this can still only be possible in specific cultural condition". Studies exploring these motivations within the Japanese cultural context are scarce.

From the viewpoint of clinical psychiatry, examining the entry into the sex trade as well as any subsequent negative experiences is important in terms of understanding the way in which personality pathology contributes to the motivation for sex work and to psychological maladjustment after entry. Previous research has reported a high prevalence of mental disorders among sex workers, such as mood disorder [1] [5], anxiety disorder [5], and PTSD [1] [5]; however, it is not clear whether these disorders cause entry into sex work or are its byproducts. In her literature review, Cusick [4] referred to several articles which viewed engagement in prostitution as a result of various pathologies, such as latent homosexuality, oedipal fixation, low intelligence, emotional disturbance, sex confusion, and poor self-image.

This study did not aim to identify a universal pattern concerning entry into the sex industry and any consequent psychological maladjustment. Rather, as a preliminary work targeting a small number of individuals with past experience as sex workers or hostesses who also had mental disorders, it sought to explore the factors related to motivations for sex work and to psychological maladjustment. More specifically, it examined whether maladjustment was the result of engagement with the sex industry or whether it was instead caused by each individual's dispositional personality characteristics, which also contributed to the motivations for entry.

The approach of most previous studies, some of which are referenced above, was to conduct in-depth interviews with women who used to be or who were still sex workers, focusing mainly on their experience related to sex work. The concern with this approach is that by asking direct questions regarding the women's entry into the sex trade, the interviewer is likely to receive a direct answer (e.g., money) that does not touch on underlying motivations. This problem is further compounded if the interview is only a "one-off." As explained in the previous paragraph, this trial study sought to examine personality characteristics that had been shaped by each subject's interpersonal relationships since infancy, both inside and outside the family. As such, multiple conversations over a significant length of time were desirable. Therefore, this study was based on the stories of four women narrated within therapeutic relationships lasting at least one year, with varying therapy frequencies.

In summary, this report focused on patients with mental disorders who had experience as sex workers. The goals of the study were:

1) to identify the psycho-social factors that influenced entry into sex work, and

2) to determine whether the subjects' maladjustment arose from the above factors or it was primarily the byproduct of sex work.

2. Methods

As noted in the introduction, female patients with a past experience of sex work were chosen as the subjects of this study. Their narratives were taken from clinical records between August 1st 2008 and August 31st 2014. I had treated, or was treating them as the consulting psychiatrist or the psychotherapist in a designated consulting room of one of two hospitals in Japan. I selected four patients from whom I had obtained enough information regarding their life history during consultation or psychotherapy for meaningful analysis. I first identified experiences that seemed to be related to entry into the sex industry or hostess trade, regardless of whether the relations were direct or indirect. Next, I determined the psycho-social factors that seemed to have influenced the subjects' maladjustment. Finally, I evaluated whether their mental maladjustment was purely the product of their past experiences as sex workers or hostesses, or whether both the maladjustment and the motivations for entry were derived from personality characteristics developed since infancy. The research protocol was approved by the Ethical Committee of Kumamoto University (Institutional Review Board).

3. Results

The outlines of the four patients' life histories, including their course of entry into sex work, are sketched below.

3.1. Ms. A

Ms. A visited a psychiatric clinic due to increasing irritability and depressive mood during pregnancy, when she was in her late twenties. In particular, since being pregnant she found herself unable to control her aggressive feelings towards her mother, with whom she had not lived for about a decade. She lived with her husband and her daughter, who was still a baby. She frequently became irritated towards her daughter and in calmer moments worried that her actions might contribute to future mental illness in the child. Ms. A was irritated not only when her daughter showed frustration by crying, but also when she sought greater intimacy. A similar dynamic occurred in her relationship with her dog, namely irritation when the dog desired affection. I provided Ms. A with 30 minutes of psychotherapy once or twice a month. She was diagnosed with hysteroid personality [6] [7] in addition to major depressive disorder.

Ms. A had many of the characteristics typically cited by previous studies as indicative of likely entrance into the sex trade: failure to finish high school, runaway episodes, delinquency, financial difficulties, and lack of job skills. The patient also reported her father's bankruptcy, her parents' marital disharmony followed by divorce, and her subjectively perceived maternal indifference and hatred. Academically, since elementary school she had always ranked in the lowest tier performance-wise. Her relationships with her female friends during childhood were unstable, although marked by less conflict than in later years. She was afraid that she was disliked by them, or that her closest friend would prefer a classmate over her. During the higher grades of elementary school, she once engaged in shoplifting and once stole her friend's stationery, which one of her younger sisters reported to her friend. Even when her teacher directly asked her whether she actually stole her friend's stationary, she never confessed her misconduct. Her mother was consistently indifferent about these episodes, and gave her no instructions or guidance. Ms. A occasionally felt that her mother did not love her. She dropped out of senior high school within the first year because she was not interested in studying. She dated a succession of boys, one of whom was violent toward her. The boyfriend once entered her house through the window of her room at night and began acting violently. Her mother came up to her room and opened the door, but quickly left her room as if she had not seen anything. Immediately following this incident, Ms. A accompanied the man home and stayed with him overnight. She became pregnant with him and subsequently terminated the pregnancy. When informed of the pregnancy, her mother recommended physical exercise to cause a miscarriage. Soon after dropping out of senior high school, Ms. A ran away and moved to a female friend's house. The relationship with this woman quickly soured due to mutual harassment, and they broke contact. This pattern is representative of Ms. A's relationships with other women. When she was 16 years old she started prostitution because she did not have money to pay her mobile phone bills. She had earlier taken part-time jobs in pachinko parlors and restaurants, but was unable to continue these for more than one month. The reasons for these short time frames were not fully verbalized in therapy, but there was a vague mention of a lack of trust in colleagues. Ms. A believed she did not possess the skills for any work other than prostitution. She initially sought clients through classified adverts. Because she perceived her first customer to be very kind, and he did not use force during the encounter, she did not regard the idea of sex with strangers as particularly objectionable. This, coupled with the significant financial rewards, kept her in this line of work. After running away she started working in brothels. During her work as a prostitute she once suffered physical violence, and in a separate incident was almost robbed. She gradually came to abhor being touched by unfamiliar men and quit the job. In total, she continued this job for about five years, but changed brothels several times due to unstable interpersonal relationships. She sometimes took unannounced time off, and on other occasions quit without notice, not responding to her managers' phone calls. She behaved as she pleased. Underlying this impulsive, seemingly irrational behavior was likely an inability to communicate a need for emotional support, which she refused to acknowledge but which had been withheld by her mother since her infant years. After leaving prostitution, she started working as a hostess at a bar where she met her current husband. They got married when she was found to be pregnant, although the pregnancy resulted in a miscarriage. After several years she became pregnant again. This time, however, she gave birth to a healthy female daughter. As noted earlier, she found child-rearing overwhelming, which led her to seek early-hour childcare for her daughter before she was a year old. It was difficult for Ms. A to establish mutually reliable companionships with the mothers of other babies, a fact she did not admit to herself. Following her pregnancy she occasionally returned to her mother's house, an expression of the unconscious expectation of maternal care that had always gone unfulfilled due to the mother's indifference. Ms. A was not able to communicate so as to receive her mother's attention. She was not brave enough to show her attachment towards the mother. Overcoming her fear of rejection would have been too difficult. Therefore, all she could do was to hope that her mother would initiate conversation, a hope that remained unrealized. In this situation, instead of feeling emotional pain, she defended against it by devaluing her mother as an incomprehensible person. This pattern reoccurred in her relationship with her female boss, whom she described as a nervous person. She dismissed as of no use the idea of initiating communication with both her mother and boss. Her husband was relatively cooperative. However, she did not feel a sense of reliance on him and did not initiate conversation. At the same time, she felt envy toward him, as she perceived him as having been raised in a favorable family environment. She tried to alleviate her stress by eating chocolate, shopping, and smoking.

She visited my clinic every two or three weeks at the beginning and even now. She occasionally cancels therapy or is late. One of the reasons for this could be because she is not accustomed to keeping promises or being punctual. Furthermore, her verbal ability to describe her emotions and life events is relatively poor due to the lack of communication with her mother since infancy, lack of perceived acceptance by her therapist, and depressive mood. Therefore, of all four women in this study, the information from Ms. A regarding psycho-social factors related to entry into the sex industry and psychological maladjustment is the most limited.

3.2. Ms. M

The second patient, Ms. M, visited my clinic in her early twenties due to depressive mood, binge eating, and anxiety. She lived with her parents and grandparents. When I first met her, she could not talk at much length, and instead her mother gave me information on the circumstances behind the symptoms. For this patient, I conducted 30-minute psychotherapy sessions every two weeks. She was diagnosed with hysteroid personality [6] [7] in addition to eating disorder and major depressive disorder.

She had no memory of emotional ties with her mother during infancy or childhood. As in the case of Ms. A, Ms. M's perceived maternal parenting was indifferent and insensitive. When she was in the fourth grade of elementary school, she temporarily became anorexic, likely an expression of unconscious desire to be cared for by her mother. She had an older brother and a younger sister. The mother was basically slow to notice her daughters' poor health and emotional pain, but showed comparatively more affection towards her son. When becoming adults, although Ms. M and her sister strengthened unity by criticizing their mother behind her back because of her unfair distribution of affection between the son and daughters, the relationship between the sisters was also conflictive over the parents' care.

During elementary school Ms. M was physically assaulted by a male classmate and was touched sexually by a male schoolteacher. Her mother expressed anger with this teacher at home, without ever confronting him, but even as an adult Ms. M had no negative feelings toward him. During junior high school, she was bullied by her female classmates and became isolated from them, but was not able to talk back to the bullies. At some point in the third grade of junior high school, she started going to a cram school to study for the senior high entrance examination. Shortly afterward she stopped attending junior high school. The reason for this unusual decision was that it was too noisy for her to study in the classroom because some students, who had already been admitted to a senior high school based on the recommendation of the junior high school principal, chatted a lot during recess. However, the underlying reason for her dropping out was assumed to be her difficulties in establishing reliable relationships with her classmates. She made her mother drive her to the cram school, reflecting the same attitude she currently adopts in demanding that her mother drive her to the hospital where she receives psychiatric treatment, despite the availability of other measures that would increase her independence. After a short time at the cram school she came to have a romantic relationship with a male teacher, resulting in a competitive relationship with a female friend, and once again isolation from her peer group. Although her academic performance was relatively good, she was not accepted by the senior high school she applied for. She attended another high school, where she focused almost exclusively on her appearance in order to avoid being teased by both old and new classmates as well as to rebuild a new self. She occasionally stayed out at night with her boyfriend, and on other occasions shoplifted, both of which elicited parental reprimands.

After graduating from senior high school, she attended a vocational school to become a hairdresser and began living by herself. However, she was not able to cope with the strict atmosphere of the school, and quit within the first year. She then started working at a night club, a fact her parents did not learn of until she developed psychiatric symptoms a few years later. She worked for three years as a club hostess. Her responsibilities were not limited to entertaining male customers, but also involved engaging in false romantic relationships, including dating, outside the club. She said she was happy to tempt male customers. Also, like her colleagues, she enjoyed buying brand-name bags and wearing gorgeous dresses. Some customers annoyed her because they put pressure on her. One tried to initiate sex, but she expressed her rejection by crying and resisting physically. However, she was instructed by the club manager to focus on extracting as much money from them as possible, an order she subsequently followed without question.

It was not the above stressful events in her hostess job, but rather a romantic breakup with her cohabitant, and subsequently living on her own, that brought about depressive feelings, bulimia, and withdrawal from society. She disclosed these feelings to her younger sister, who also used to live alone. Her sister told their mother to take Ms. M to a psychiatric clinic, which resulted in my consultation. After recovering from her most severe depressive symptoms, she attended an appointment with her therapist wearing very revealing clothes and extravagant accessories.

After commencing psychiatric care, she returned to her parents' home to live. At the practical level, her parents were cooperative, for instance driving her to the hospital, purchasing an exercise machine she wanted in order to lose weight, and buying a puppy as she requested. On the other hand, when her parents did not respond in the way she expected, she perceived it as rejection, which led to bulimia and depressive mood. In contrast to her appropriate acknowledgment of her father's support, she tended to deny her mother's routine care, to devalue her, and to characterize her as a person who was slow to notice things, an image of her mother she had held since childhood. Despite the fluctuation of her bulimic and depressive symptoms, they gradually decreased in frequency and severity, and within three years she decided to enter a junior college for training as a child care specialist. Before entering the college she took driving lessons, during which she came to have romantic feelings towards an instructor, and she sought a date with him several times. Eventually the man agreed and she lived with him every weekend. Her therapist at the time interpreted this romantic involvement as a way to gain emotional stability in the face of her inability to focus on her own issues by supporting herself. The pattern seemed to be a repetition of her junior high school period when she had a relationship with the teacher at the cram school.

3.3. Ms. R

The third patient, Ms. R, visited my clinic in her mid-thirties with depressive and anxious feelings. The life events before her maladjustment were divorce and bankruptcy caused by her husband's debt. She had signed a guarantee form without asking her husband the meaning of the documents. This blithe acquiescence to others' requests was frequently manifested in her interpersonal relationships. We met for 45-minute psychotherapy sessions once a week. She was diagnosed with "as if personality" [8] in addition to major depressive disorder.

Her life history was somewhat unique in the context of contemporary Japanese society. She began living in a shrine with her grandparents when she was three years old, while her parents continued to live with her two-year-old brother. The reasons for her separation from her parents were never made clear. Her strong attachment to her grandparents and intense conflict between her grandmother and mother offered a possible explanation, but were not sufficient to rationally explain the separation.

The grandfather used to take her to an Izakaya (a Japanese-style bar). Ms. R said that his care of her after she used the toilet was a good memory. This struck me as strange for two reasons. First, the grandfather used his bare hand instead of paper to wipe her, an act that seemed to contain a sexual element lost on Ms. R. Second, it seemed in this situation that the grandmother would be the most appropriate person to take on the mothering role. However, it became clear later that throughout Ms. R's life, any person, regardless of gender, could be the second mother, the object she wanted to control to fulfill her emotional needs of dependency. This relationship with significant others is consistent with the object relations described by Winnicott [9], who writes that for an infant in the early phase of life, their father exists as "another mother." When Ms. R was four years old, after her grandfather's death, she started living with her grandmother in a love hotel, where the grandmother was working as a live-in staff member. The grandmother was the second wife of the grandfather, so Ms. R was not a blood relative of this woman. In normal circumstances, the death of a child's only blood relative in their home environment would lead to the child being returned to the parents, but that was not the case in this instance. The grandmother started work at midnight, at which time Ms. R was frequently awake. She tried to alleviate her loneliness by holding a doll. This intolerable loneliness was subjectively experienced again and again later in her life, and was the excuse for many of her attitudes and behaviors, regardless of whether they were morally or legally acceptable. In senior high school, Ms. R was shocked to learn that she had in fact lived with her grandmother in a love hotel, and felt strong shame. However, she planned to keep it a secret between her and her grandmother.

She returned to her parents' house with her grandmother when she was six years old. During elementary school, her school performance was excellent. Therefore her elementary school life was relatively easy compared to high school, despite the existence of a strict female teacher whom she prayed would become sick. In the context of her family life, she experienced intense envy toward her younger brother, who had strong emotional ties to their mother and received much maternal praise for his comparatively better school performance. She always felt emotionally distant from her mother. Ms. R even felt that her mother disliked her, and that she would prefer it if her brother were the only child. This relationship was exacerbated by the mother's conflict with the grandmother, to whom Ms. R felt strong attachment. She worked hard in order to surpass her brother in school performance where she could, which she expected to bring about maternal approval and praise. However, no success in this regard was able to bring her a sense of accomplishment. When she occasionally disclosed a variety of somatic symptoms to her mother, she was simply encouraged to go to school. These somatic symptoms seemed to be disclosed in order to elicit maternal care. However, the mother was not empathetic enough to recognize this underlying emotional motivation.

In junior high school, Ms. R was bullied and socially excluded due to her physical appearance, which she blamed on her mother because she did not provide any guidance on personal grooming. This bullying came to an end when a popular boy in Ms. R's class became her friend.

Ms. R's focus in senior high school was to get the attention of classmates by entertaining them. Underlying this behavior was an intense feeling of envy toward a few more popular female classmates. Ms. R sometimes made up stories about herself and even engaged in self-destructive, risky behavior so that her physical appearance would back up her narratives. She strongly disliked losing the attention of others.

Ms. R had a weak grasp on the concept of personal opinion. For as long as she could remember, she avoided expressing her opinions to others in order to avoid the risk of being disliked due to conflict. However, this behavior pattern produced the opposite results to those she expected, namely, she lost credibility with classmates.

In senior high school, again isolated in her class, Ms. R was comforted by a man who lived in her neighborhood. At the end of her final year of senior high school, her teacher recommended that she attend welfare vocational school because she was the only one in her class who had not decided on her future course. She followed this advice without any careful consideration.

To attend the vocational school, Ms. R had to live separately from her family. This caused unbearable loneliness, so every night she visited her friends or invited them to her apartment. After graduating from the school, she started working at a welfare facility for the elderly. A male coworker who initially visited her at home frequently eventually remained in the house as a cohabitant, an action with which she expressed neither agreement nor disagreement. It should be emphasized here that Ms. R knew when she started living with this man that he was her friend's boyfriend. Although Ms. R expressed neither agreement nor disagreement towards cohabitation, she disclosed to her therapist her envy toward this female friend and was convinced she could make the man choose her instead. Despite her success in winning over her friend's boyfriend, her cohabitation with him was emotionally draining. He frequently went out with his male friends at night, which again brought her intolerable loneliness, and he left the housework to her. She sometimes saw him chatting with female colleagues. For these reasons, she harbored anger towards the boyfriend, jealousy towards her female colleagues, and most of all, the fear that he would forget about her. None of these negative feelings were verbally expressed. Instead, they drove her to actions from which she expected to gain his attention and approval, including going on a diet, visiting hospitals due to the somatic symptoms caused by his absence at night, and changing her hairstyle and fashion. However, it was difficult to gain his attention to a satisfactory degree, and she therefore eventually engaged in sexual relationships with other men, some of whom were his friends. These sexual relationships alleviated her nighttime loneliness. She expected that he would be told of her sexual relationships with other men and believed that this would result in both his jealousy towards the men and an increase in his attention and love towards her.

At some point in the fifth year of their cohabitation, they broke up when the man began dating another woman. Ms. R.'s female colleagues tried to comfort and cheer her up, but she told me that in fact they looked down on her as someone who had been miserably abandoned. Before the breakup she had harbored feelings of superiority toward female colleagues who did not have a boyfriend, and she believed that these colleagues were now enjoying proving her wrong. Despite these negative feelings toward her colleagues, she accepted their attention because she was unable to be alone. She also called on her mother, broke down over the impossibility of giving up her boyfriend, and revealed plans to win him back. However, her mother told her that her planned actions were completely undignified. This admonition disappointed her expectation that her mother would manage Ms. R's difficulties by any means. Following this, Ms. R began to desperately tempt many men in whom she had no genuine interest. Every weekend, she returned to her parents' home with a different man. Behind this behavior was the message to her mother that Ms. R was comparatively more valuable because she could attract many men. If any of these men fell in love with Ms. R, she abruptly rejected them by avoiding them. She believed that she could control any man by having a sexual relationship with him. Her promiscuity came to be known in her neighborhood. She then married a man who treated her very kindly while they dated. He pushed for the marriage; again, she expressed neither agreement nor disagreement.

Several years into the marriage she could no longer deny that her husband carried a huge debt. Now in her early thirties, to help repay this debt she started working as a club hostess at his request. Despite her anger toward her husband, she obeyed his request because her husband also worked at night and her new work therefore alleviated her loneliness. When she was working at the club, she met a male customer known only as the "president," who invited her to become a prostitute. She did just as the "president" required, including dealing with violent customers and having a sexual relationship with the "president" in return for his favor and a privileged position above the other prostitutes. In addition to prostitution, she became addicted to shoplifting and illegal drugs. Lack of sleep led to frequent traffic accidents, for which she did not feel any responsibility; she asked an insurance company representative for help in avoiding having to pay compensation. Furthermore, she was unable to concentrate on her daytime job due to sleepiness, and had an affair with a male colleague who had a wife and children. These issues at her workplace caused her colleagues to develop negative feelings toward her. When she perceived their anger and rejection, she quickly quit the job. She even adopted self-destructive behavior, for instance ingesting a detergent when she felt unable to tolerate the difficulties in her interpersonal relationships. Her income increased, but she hardly spent any money on food and gradually lost weight. Every morning when she returned home, she left her night's earnings on a table in the living room for her husband. Her husband, having been told by a friend that she was working as a prostitute, thought she must be mentally ill and recommended she be hospitalized. She offered to divorce, a means of expressing her rejection of him. In her mind, the only reason she entered the sex industry was external, namely her husband's request that she work at night for money. Similarly, she attributed her anorexia to not having enough money to eat because her husband needed it to pay back his debt. However, this was inconsistent with a fact that emerged in a later therapy session, that she sometimes stole money from the husband's wallet.

Ms. R did divorce her husband, after which she returned to her parents' house and began visiting my clinic. Within a few months after returning to her parents' house, she became bulimic due to anxiety and fear she experienced at night while her parents were asleep, resulting in a 30 kg weight gain. She eventually started working at a welfare facility near the house. As occurred during senior high school and in her twenties, she harbored envy toward a woman who seemed to be blessed with a fortunate home life and who had gained popularity, in particular with male colleagues. Also, her stereotypic interpersonal behaviors always manifested in all relationships in which she detected even a hint of warmth, whether with colleagues or others. She experienced disappointment at failed attempts to elicit praise, care, support, or approval by meeting assumed expectations, expressing false empathy, and giving small gifts. Once, she was made fun of by her female colleagues, probably because she had always tried to give the image of being a model professional. Her colleagues' behaviors caused strong feelings of rejection and resentment. In the past, this type of situation would cause her to quickly enter into sexual relationships with men, but this time she tried to escape from her painful experiences in the real world by watching a movie whose protagonist was a prostitute. However, against her expectations, the prostitute in the story was killed by her mother.

Ms. R's relationship with her mother was the archetype for all others, including those described above. As in childhood, she continued to tell her mother about her somatic symptoms, but this never resulted in expressions of care. Furthermore, she occasionally made her parents drive her to the hospital, which she justified by her bad physical condition. Currently, she gives money to fund her mother's gambling addiction, but her mother's gratitude usually does not last longer than a few seconds. In therapy sessions she has expressed sadness and loneliness, as well as anger and denigration towards the mother. She even told me that she envied her mother, as "she seems to live with fewer constraints." When at a family party she thought she succeeded through various means at socially isolating her mother from the party attendees, her aggression was satisfied and she reported the incident to me with pleasure.

3.4. Ms. S

The fourth patient, Ms. S, was in her early twenties when she first visited me. She perceived as having been tortured by negative interpersonal life events with almost all people with whom she was currently or had previously been in contact, resulting in intense resentment followed by repeated self-destructive acting out, i.e. overdosing and bulimia. She also had many experiences of abandonment. I met with her for 45 minutes of psychotherapy every week. She was diagnosed with borderline personality disorder. During the treatment, she asked me to prescribe many minor tranquilizers, an expectation I could not fulfill.

She lived with her parents and one of two older brothers. This brother was schizophrenic and both parents had to devote themselves to taking care of him, which Ms. S resented. Throughout her life history, she perceived that she was regarded by her parents as less important than her brothers. Ms. S had been sexually exploited repeatedly by an elder brother during her elementary school years. Ms. S felt that she was not allowed to disclose this to others, including her mother, and thought her home life forbade her from romantic involvement outside the household. But she came to have romantic feelings toward boys at school, which resulted in uncomfortable feelings of conflict. After entering her twenties, she told her mother about the past negative sexual experiences with her brother. Behind this disclosure was her envy and aggression towards the elder brother, although these feelings were actually more intense towards his wife. For Ms. S, his happy marriage was impossible to accept, without his consideration of and regret over his past misconduct. Before the brother's marriage, Ms. S's perception of him had not been necessarily negative, rather, she liked him, but after his marriage she was possessed by the idea that the wife was the only women her brother loved, and she was used just as a tool for his sexual desire. She experienced these feelings of aggression and envy not only toward this woman, but toward any who seemed to be happy, including her mother: "My mother was able to get married, but I am not."

As with the three women already discussed, Ms. S could not recall expressing her emotional needs to her mother until pre-adolescence, though since adolescence this has not been the case. At school as a preadolescent, a relationship with a male schoolteacher was very discordant. In addition, Ms. S had difficulties establishing stable relationships with her classmates. She always felt that she was treated badly and insulted by classmates as well as other schoolmates. When she was in the fifth grade of elementary school, her father told her to check on her mother, who was participating in a community meeting that night, because he was afraid that the mother was engaged in an affair. Ms. S currently feels anger toward her father regarding this event because he did not care about her security but was instead focused solely on her mother, toward whom she felt strong envy.

Immediately before graduating from senior high school, Ms. S started having sexual relationships with anonymous men who picked her up on the roadside, and later learned she could earn money by having sex. Her motivations behind this were to show her father that she was able to earn money and have sex with many men. She said that her father occasionally boasted of his numerous past sexual relationships, and when she asked him to buy something he looked down on the fact that she was unable to earn money.

Thus the initial reasons for these behaviors were defiance towards her father, and later, desire for money. However, once she started prostitution, Ms. S's initial needs were further complicated by emotional dependence, *i.e.* to be cared for by the males in these sexual relationships. From these men's perspective, she was something to be bought. Inevitably, her fears of abandonment were realized repeatedly.

At one point she became pregnant due to a sexual relationship with a married man. Her age and economic status meant that abortion was her only viable option. The man refused to pay for the procedure and when pressed, threatened to expose Ms. S's prostitution to her mother. Ms. S expressed her resentment toward the man to her mother, who remonstrated with him, unsuccessfully, under the impression that the baby had been conceived conventionally outside a worker-client relationship.

Continuing her independent work, Ms. S also started a job as a prostitute in an adult entertainment establishment. When she was initially approached by a man recruiting for the business, her reaction was one of fear. But when the man began to back off, her fear of abandonment was stimulated and she agreed to take the job. Her income was approximately ten thousand dollars per month, almost all of which was spent on hairstyle and lavish dresses. At some point, her mother intuited her line of work and scolded her. However, Ms. S ignored her.

Because she was always sensitive to the words of others, she again started to perceive disapproval, rejection, and disrespect in both staff and customers, and she frequently voiced her displeasure. One of the customers once told her she was "crazy." Her maladjustment necessitated frequent workplace changes, with her longest stay in any one establishment being merely three months. However, she was not able to quit prostitution because she did not have any skills she felt confident she could use for other work.

Eventually, however, she was sexually and financially exploited by her manager, and rumors of violence and enforced drug consumption in the work place led her to quit out of fear. She also stopped her work as an independent prostitute. After quitting prostitution, she impulsively entered a few sexual relationships with unrealistic expectations her partners could not fulfill. After having consensual sex a number of times, she expressed rage at having been, in her view, used.

Once she turned twenty years old, she disclosed to her mother her traumatic childhood sexual experience with her brother. Her mother responded: "it cannot be helped, because it has already happened." This seemed to be a microcosm of Ms. S's relationship with her mother: her expectations always being betrayed by her mother's unempathetic attitudes towards her. Her father's response was even worse, as he believed that she must have made up the story. These reactions re-traumatized her 10 years after the initial events.

After repeated breakups with men, she was eager to have peer relationships with women, which had not been possible during her adolescence. However, once these relationships began, she experienced unbearable envy, feelings of rejection, and aggression toward the women. For example, at the vocational rehabilitation center she started attending after launching psychotherapy, she felt envy toward women who had graduated from university or who were popular with male members. Therefore, it was difficult for her to have long-lasting reliable relationships with women. In various social milieus, she was often excluded from women's company. Her unfulfilled needs were transformed into aggression, which her mother was not able to empathize with, which further drove her to abandonment fear and the action of testing and evaluating her mother: for instance, how her mother advised her on difficulties, whether her mother responded to her requests such as to be driven to the hospital, whether her mother gave her pocket money, whether her mother believed her side of any story, and so on. Ms. S frequently became disappointed in her interactions with her mother and would stay in her room with the cat or became angry and shouted at her mother.

4. Discussion

4.1. Factors That Were Common to More Than One Patient

Here, I would like to outline the common factors identified in at least two of the four women.

1) Weak emotional ties with their mothers since infancy

Without exception, the maternal attachment of each woman was weak during the period of infancy and elementary school. Their mothers were comparatively indifferent, insensitive, and inconsiderate towards them, rather than abusive, authoritarian, and didactic.

2) Unremitting need for maternal care, fear of rejection, and object-seeking behaviors

Even after becoming adults, Ms. M, Ms. R., and Ms. S still had an intense expectation to be cared for by their mothers. They attempted to obtain maternal care through appeals for practical assistance, such as requests for hospital lifts or money. Ms. R tried to gain her mother's affection by fueling her mother's addiction. In the case of Ms. A, the emotional needs were suppressed and latent. These women's need to be cared for was not limited to their mothers, but extended to many people, especially male objects whose rejection they always feared.

3) Desire to control others

Ms. R tried to control others through disclosing somatic symptoms, expressing false empathy, and pandering. In the case of Ms. M, symptoms of an eating disorder could be viewed as a strategy for controlling others. Ms. R and Ms. S tried to manipulate others through self-destructive behaviors. All women except Ms. A made their parents drive them to the hospital, although they themselves were able to drive.

4) Envy and aggressive self-destructive behaviors

All patients except Ms. M expressed feelings of envy toward their mothers, female friends, relatives, spouses, and siblings. Ms. A confided in me her envy toward her husband. Furthermore, she expressed occasional hatred toward her baby and dog, specifically with regard to their dependence on her, as they freely sought her affection in a manner that had never been possible for her. In the case of Ms. M, due to narcissistic pride, she seemed to deny her envious feeling towards her siblings in relation to her mother's unfair distribution of affection. Rather than recognizing her own envy, she devalued her mother. Aggressive self-destructive behaviors as retaliation were prominent in the cases of Ms. R and Ms. S. Both disclosed intense feelings of envy towards women who seemed to be happy and who had succeeded in gaining a male's attention or having a stable partner, including, in the case of Ms. S, her mother. Ms. S not only harbored envy toward her mother but also competitive feelings toward her father, who boasted of his sexual experiences, and these feelings drove her to engage in anonymous sexual relationships.

5) Mothers prioritizing sons over daughters

Of the four women, all three who had male siblings believed that their mothers experienced and exhibited more affection for their male siblings than for them. Ms. R further felt that she was an unwanted child and that her mother was fully emotionally satisfied by her son.

6) Difficulties in establishing female peer relationships during adolescence and proneness to dependency on male objects through sexual relationships

Without exception, all four women were unable to establish trustful relationships with female friends and were inclined to sexual relationships with the opposite gender. This pattern formulated in adolescence continued to the present time.

7) Past histories of crime and delinquency

Histories of shoplifting were reported by three patients—Ms. A in childhood, Ms. M in late adolescence, and Ms. R in her early thirties. Furthermore, Ms. R used to be addicted to an illegal drug.

8) Weak internal motivation

Refusal to attend school and dropping out were reported by Ms. A, Ms. M, and Ms. S. Even acknowledging the strict school atmosphere, these women's internal motivation [10] to perform well academically seemed to be comparatively weak. This weak motivation was also seen in their inability to keep a job, and in Ms. A's failure to attend therapy with regularity. In particular, Ms. R's motivation for school and job performance was always external, in that she tried to elicit attention and praise from her mother and other people. The egos of these women were always at risk of intense internal aggressive impulses when their expectations of others went un-realized.

9) Longing for beautiful external appearance

This was identified in the cases of Ms. M and Ms. S, and was caused at least in part by their competitive feelings with other women as well as their attempts to reassert their value.

10) Frequent acting out

Most of the women did not seem to carefully consider their difficulties before making decisions. Rather, they resolved their conflictive situations by acting out, for instance by running away, quitting their jobs, having sexual relationships, binge eating, and overdosing.

11) Addictive behaviors

These occurred in every woman if we regarded binge eating as an addictive behavior. The objects of addiction were varied, including food, consumer goods, illegal drugs, and minor tranquilizers. Ms. R's compulsive devotion in the context of interpersonal relationships, and her shoplifting (also conducted by two other women), can also be seen as addictive behaviors. In addition to this, Ms. R and Ms. S were addicted to sexual relationships with anonymous men.

12) Past negative sexual experiences

Ms. M was sexually abused by a schoolteacher, although she did not necessarily view this as negative. Ms. S's sexual exploitation by a family member was defined as "negative" only after the perpetrator's marriage.

13) Lack of job skills coupled with financial difficulties

Ms. A believed that she lacked any job skills other than those of a sex worker. At first appearance, Ms. R became a prostitute to repay her husband's debt, but other factors, such as intolerable loneliness at night and desire for her husband's praise as well as protest against him, make for more convincing reasons. In her case, the feeling of omnipotence gained by controlling men through sexual relationships was a prominent factor. Ms. S tried to earn a significant amount of money to prove to her father that she could do so, which meant that her motivation regarding income was more psychological than financial. This could be applicable for every woman except Ms. A, in whom purely financial motivations were not improbable.

14) Intra-familial disharmony

Ms. A reported clear marital disharmony between her parents. Ms. R identified conflict between her mother and mother-figure (grandmother).

4.2. Interpretations

Based on the numerous factors identified in the clinical materials above, I would like to present a broad hypothesis regarding the motivations underlying entry into the sex industry and hostess trade. The most prominent factors were these women's weak maternal bonds since infancy, and their intense emotional needs toward significant others, including their mothers. The lack of "experience of omnipotence" [11] within the mother-infant relationship led to Ms. R and Ms. S's inability to give up their omnipotent expectations of significant others. Ms. R always tried to guess others' motivations and wants, desperate to fulfill them and thus gain favors through pseudo-empathetic attitudes and object-satisfying behaviors. These would then convince her that she could control others in the way she desired. When this conviction was betrayed, she immediately turned to acting out by way of promiscuity, self-destructive behavior, or negligence of her job duties. Ms. S's expectations of emotional care were too intense to be realized, resulting in aggressive acting out following feelings of rejection. Ms. A was not able to initiate conversation due to fear of rejection, leading to interpersonal relationships that seemed to replicate that with her mother. These women's inability to express their emotional needs straightforwardly led them to try to temporarily fulfill their needs by coercing practical assistance. Ms. M's anorexia during elementary school could be regarded as an unconscious intention to both test and evaluate her mother through challenging behaviors [12].

In addition to the lack of maternal care within the dyadic relationship with the mother, in the context of triadic family relationships three women perceived they were being neglected by their mothers in comparison with their male siblings. Ms. A was the exception because she did not have a male sibling. Insufficient maternal care and support, as observed in Ms. A and Ms. M, also played a crucial role in the development of conflict with a female sibling. These women's weak emotional ties with their mothers resulted in their failure to incorporate the "ego-supporting mother" [13] and acquire the "capacity to be alone" [13], which in turn caused intense object-seeking tendencies. These women ended up feeling disappointed and rejected by their chosen object of the moment due to this individual's failure to fulfill their emotional needs, and this usually resulted in feelings of aggression toward the objects. This aggression was not initially experienced with the chosen objects, instead having its origin in the archetypical relationship with the mother, toward whom the women felt intense feelings of envy. This envy was re-experienced with various chosen objects: Ms. S had an intense envy of her parents' sexual relationship, Ms. R was envious of her female friends and colleagues, and Ms. A experienced envy of her husband. These frequently aroused feelings of envy could be attributed to a basic lack of satisfaction in the maternal care received. Although Ms. M did not clearly express her envy, this was not necessarily an indication of its absence.

The above factors made it difficult for these women to experience a psychologically healthy adolescence. Blos [14] defined adolescence as the "second individuation process". In this process, an adolescent's ego struggles to repress the incestuous fantasies that increase with genital impulses caused by physical sexual maturation [15], and adolescents disengage themselves from infantile objects (parents) [14]. Keeping distance from their parents and family members usually causes the adolescent's ego to become unstable, resulting in new attachments to various love objects outside of the family whom the adolescents choose as substitutes for their abandoned parents. Despite the passionate and exclusive nature of the attachment on each occasion, each relationship is very fickle and is easily replaced by the next object, which should be distinguished from the adult's stable interpersonal relationships [15]. However, these transient relationships are crucial in order for the adolescent to attain psychological balance. Blos [16] writes that the object choice of early adolescence is the adolescent's friend. The choice is based on the narcissistic nature, as the adolescent chooses and loves anyone without whom they cannot achieve their ideal self-image, which contributes to their narcissistic balance. Despite the girl's bi-sexual object choice during early adolescence compared to the boy's homosexual object choice, the lack of female friends causes emotional crisis for girls, such as despair, depression, and loss of interest [16]. As Japan has become more westernized, communities have become less close-knit, which has driven some individuals to feel isolated [17]. The "circle-based self" is used to alleviate this feeling of isolation through temporary peer circles, usually of the same gender, and has its roots deep in adolescent mentality. Nishizono [17] hypothesizes that in contemporary society, it also functions as a mental support for young adult men, regardless of whether the members' motivations for organizing the circle is constructive or pathological. He added that the need for the "circle-based self" is more intense among women than men, and failure to belong to such a circle results in mental maladjustment. The four women analyzed in this article were not able to benefit from the mental support of a circle due to fear of rejection, envy, and desire to obtain others' attention and approval, all of which arose from a lack of self-esteem.

Addictive behaviors, including binge eating and shoplifting, can be regarded as ways of latching onto a transitional object [18], primarily because these individuals have not incorporated the "ego-supporting mother" [13], and secondarily because they have not been able to establish a mutually reliable relationship with a new significant other due to un-relinquished omnipotent expectations and lack of empathy. Ms. R's anorexia could be considered an expression of aggression towards her husband, who had failed to provide her with care and attention, by provocatively attacking her own body.

These women's casual sexual relationships can be understood in terms of their trying to alleviate feelings of isolation and thereby recover self-esteem. Allowing others to exploit their sexuality seemed to be the quickest way to get these individuals' attention, despite the false nature of this activity. Blos [16] writes that females' delinquent sexual behavior is based on pseudo-sexuality: a manifestation of their defense against the strong regressive pull to the pre-oedipal mother. He also writes that this sexual behavior is a form of revenge against their mother, who they feel rejected them, by showing that they have somebody, an interpretation which could be applicable to Ms. R. For each of the four women in this study, gorgeous dresses were the strategy through which to assert her superior value, primary to her mother, but also to other women. Other anti-social behaviors such as shoplifting could be regarded as a way of gaining their mothers' attention. When they broke down immediately after failed relationships with men, they regressed to depending on their mothers by manipulating them.

Another shared feature among the four women was the lack of sound ego-function, due to failure to incorporate the mother's ego function. Their tolerance for frustration was extremely low, and they tended to lack the ability to find solutions to problems, resulting in refusal to attend or dropping out of school. Ms. R's relatively favorable school performance was motivated by the desire for her mother's praise. Her motivation was always external: her object's transient attitudes toward her determined whether she devoted herself to a job or abandoned it. In the cases of Ms. A and Ms. S, low ego-function resulted in the failure to acquire job skills, and the sex industry seemed to be the easiest way to fulfill emotional and material needs. In addition to the incorporation of the mother's ego function during infancy, Blos [16] discusses the importance of the latency period, when a child becomes able to use a variety of ego activities, "sublimatory, adaptive and defensive in nature", developed through identification with parents. These then bring about the child's "sense of self-esteem derived from achievement and mastery" and "inner resourcefulness". Freud [15] writes that in the latent period, complete dependency on parents during infancy is usually replaced by the introjection of objects, including parents and teachers, which strengthen the child's ego function, giving them a sense of self-esteem. It might be assumed that in the cases of the four women discussed in this article, lack of experience being dependent on their parents during infancy made it difficult to obtain stable and flexible ego-function during the subsequent latency period. They were thus lacking in internal motivation derived from ego-function.

Negative sexual experiences during childhood were reported by two women. Neither of these necessarily perceived the perpetrators negatively at the time, and instead viewed them positively. The weak emotional ties with their mothers appeared to have made them value attention from anyone as emotional comfort. It was probable that these past sexual experiences opened their eyes to the possibility of obtaining attention through sexual contact, which formed a basis for their later entry into the sex industry when they had maladaptive interpersonal relationships.

From here, I would like to discuss the disparities between previous research and my own observations. Past studies have reported that a significant number of prostitutes at some point experience homelessness or street life. However, this was not the case for any of the four women discussed in this article. This might be due to the culture in which they live. In Japan, young people are more dependent on their parents, even in conflictive relationships, which would deter them from runaway behavior and protect them from homelessness and street life. Furthermore, as seen in the case of Ms. A, young people who run away due to conflict with their parents can usually find a friend who will take them in, even if their relationship is not a strong one.

In this research, the primary factors that seemed to have mobilized these women to enter the sex industry or hostess trade were related to their personality pathologies. This might be due to the fact that the four women were clinical patients. If non-clinical women had been evaluated instead, more practical factors such as financial difficulties, low academic performance, lack of job skills, and experience with homelessness may have been identified. One additional difference between the current study and previous articles was that among the four women, none was proud of being a sex worker.

Finally, the second research question of this study should be discussed. In my view, these women's current maladjustment cannot be viewed purely as a byproduct of their experience as sex workers. Rather, entering as well as leaving the sex industry can be seen as stages leading to later maladjustment. Retrospectively viewing their life histories, the primary indicator of later maladjustment appeared to be the lack of stable and warm emotional ties with their mothers in early life. This factor interacted in complicated ways with many other factors, such as sexual trauma, difficulties in cultivating ego function, family dynamics, and failure to complete the "second individuation process" [14] through peer relationship during adolescence. As Blos [16] noted, "in female delinquents the infantile instinctual organization breaks through with the onset of puberty and finds a bodily outlet in genital activity". He defined this as pseudo-sexuality, behind which wass "an unduly deep and lasting attachment to the pre-oedipal mother [16]". He adds that the motivation of young prostitutes is due to their emotional constellation. In my view, this statement cannot be generalized to all sex workers. However, inferring from the four women described above, the motivation for entry into the sex industry or hostess trade is strongly influenced by the pre-oedipal mother, at least in clinical populations.

4.3. Limitations

First, the four women analyzed in this article was not homogenous in terms of age of entry into the sex industry, type of sex industry or hostess trade, social status, or educational background. It is plausible that if we analyze a homogenous group, more common factors will be obtained.

Second, it is probable that I obtain a limited range of information useful for this study because my purpose of interviewing these patients is to treat their mental disorders. However, I believe that in many ways, evaluating countless narratives during psychotherapy in the context of a deep therapeutic relationship can be more valuable than a small number of interviews tailored to investigate a particular research topic. It might be difficult for some patients to disclose their past experiences due to fear of rejection by the therapist. However, this could also be the case outside of therapeutic relationships, including in the context of research interviews.

4.4. Conclusion

Through analysis of limited clinical materials, this study reached the conclusion that entry into the sex industry was intrinsically related to each patient's entire emotional constellation, although in some cases material or practical factors were involved to a minor degree. For certain women, working in the sex industry can be regarded as an attempt to compensate for unmet emotional needs of dependency at the cost of their own sexuality. Entry into the sex industry resulted in additional traumatic experiences because for men these women were simply sexual targets, not the objects of love. In the author's view, the sex industry exploited the vulnerabilities of these women's personalities.

Acknowledgements

The author would like to express deep gratitude to the four patients, as well as to Emeritus Professor of Fukuoka University, Masahisa Nishizono, who supervised her in treating these patients.

Conflict of Interest

There is no conflict of interest to declare.

References

[1] Chudakov, B., Ilan, K., Belmaker, R.H. and Cwikel, J. (2002) The Motivation and Mental Health of Sex Workers. *Journal of Sex and Marital Therapy*, **28**, 305-315. http://dx.doi.org/10.1080/00926230290001439

[2] Cobbina, J.E. and Oselin, S.S. (2011) It's Not Only for the Money: An Analysis of Adolescent versus Adult Entry into

Street Prostitution. *Sociological Inquiry*, **81**, 310-332. http://dx.doi.org/10.1111/j.1475-682X.2011.00375.x

[3] Hwang, S.L. and Bedford, O. (2004) Juveniles' Motivations for Remaining in Prostitution. *Psychology of Women Quarterly*, **28**, 136-146. http://dx.doi.org/10.1111/j.1471-6402.2004.00130.x

[4] Cusick, L. (2002) Youth Prostitution: A Literature Review. *Child Abuse Review*, **11**, 230-251. http://dx.doi.org/10.1002/car.743

[5] Rössler, W., Koch, U., Lauber, C., Hass, A-K., Altwegg, M., Ajdacic-Gross, V. and Landolt, K. (2010) The Mental Health of Female Sex Workers. *Acta Psychiatrica Scandinavica*, **122**, 143-152. http://dx.doi.org/10.1111/j.1600-0447.2009.01533.x

[6] Easser, B.R. and Lesser, S.R. (1965) Hysterical Personality: A Re-Evaluation. *The Psychoanalytic Quarterly*, **34**, 390-405.

[7] Zetzel, E.R. (1968) The So-Called Good Hysterics. *The International Journal of Psychoanalysis*, **49**, 256-260.

[8] Deutsch, H. (1942) Some Forms of Emotional Disturbance and Their Relationship to Schizophrenia. *The Psychiatric Quarterly*, **11**, 301-432.

[9] Winnicott, D.W. (1960) Ego Distortion in Terms of True and False Self. In: Winnicott, D.W., Ed., *The Maturational Processes and the Facilitating Environment: Studies in the Theory of Emotional Development*, Karnac Books, London, 140-152.

[10] Ryan, R.M. and Deci, E.L. (2000) Self-Determination Theory and the Facilitation of Intrinsic Motivation, Social Development, and Well-Being. *American Psychologist*, **55**, 68-78. http://dx.doi.org/10.1037/0003-066X.55.1.68

[11] Winnicott, D.W. (1962) Ego Integration and Child Development. In: Winnicott, D.W., Ed., *The Maturational Processes and the Facilitating Environment: Studies in the Theory of Emotional Development*, Karnac Books, London, 56-63.

[12] Nishizono, M. and Yasuoka, H. (1979) Wrist Cutting Syndrome. *Japanese Journal of Clinical Psychiatry*, **8**, 1309-1315.

[13] Winnicott, D.W. (1958) The Capacity to Be Alone. In: Winnicott, D.W., Ed., *The Maturational Processes and the Facilitating Environment: Studies in the Theory of Emotional Development*, Karnac Books, London, 29-36.

[14] Blos, P. (1967) The Second Individuation Process of Adolescence. *Psychoanalytic Study of Child*, **22**, 162-186.

[15] Freud, A. (1966) Defense Motivated by Fear of the Strength of the Instincts Illustrated by the Phenomena of Puberty. The Ego and the Mechanisms of Defense (Revised Edition). Karnac Books, London, 137-172.

[16] Blos, P. (1962) On Adolescence: A Psychoanalytic Interpretation. The Free Press, a Division of Macmillan Inc, New York.

[17] Nishizono, M. (1999) Pathology of Circle-Based Self and Psychotherapy. *Japanese Journal of Psychotherapy*, **25**, 444-447 (in Japanese).

[18] Winnicott, D.W. (1953) Transitional Object and Transitional Phenomena. *International Journal of Psychoanalysis*, **34**, 89-97.

14

Efficacy of Quality of Life Therapy on Increasing Happiness in Patients with Major Depressive Disorder

Hossein Jenaabadi[1], Bahareh Azizi Nejad[2*], Ghazal Fatehrad[3]

[1]Faculty of Educational Sciences and Psychology, University of Sistan and Baluchestan, Zahedan, Iran
[2]Department of Educational Science, Payame Noor University, Tehran, Iran
[3]Department of Management and Economic, Science and Research Branch, Islamic Azad University, Tehran, Iran
Email: hjenaabadi@ped.usb.ac.ir, *bahareh19@gmail.com

Abstract

Introduction: The present study sought to examine the effectiveness of quality of life therapy on increasing happiness among patients with major depression. **Methods:** The research followed an experimental research design with an experimental and a control group. To this end, among the statistical population of the study that consisted of all individuals with major depression disorder, 30 individuals were randomly selected and placed in two groups (experimental and control). The experimental group individually received an intervention with a trend based on quality of life improvement for 10 sessions. The control group received no such treatment. Beck's Depression Inventory and Oxford Happiness Questionnaire were used in two occasions of pretest and posttest. Data analysis was performed using descriptive statistics and multivariate analysis of covariance. **Results:** The results revealed that quality of life therapy reduced depression and increased happiness among the subjects on the posttest (p < 0.01). **Conclusion:** This research found two important results. First, it was revealed that quality of life therapy had high efficiency in treating depression considered as a resistant disorder to treatment. Second, it was indicated that focus on happiness in the treatment of major depression disorder can significantly help patients recover.

Keywords

Quality of Life Therapy, Happiness, Depression

---

*Corresponding author.

1. Introduction

Major depression is a disorder included of a set of disabling symptoms [1]. From the diagnostic perspective, depression is one of the most widespread diagnoses in mental disorders which encompasses many individuals with different backgrounds in the form of an epidemic [2] [3]. It is predicted that in 2020 the prevalence of this disorder will reach the second global rank diagnosis for each age group as well as each gender, while less than 25% of these patients will have access to effective therapy [4]. According to DSM data, major depression is a disorder recognized with one or several periods of major depression without backgrounds of mania treatment, mixed or hypomania. A period of major depression takes at least two weeks, typically, the person is either depressed or loses her/his interest to most activities. The individual who is diagnosed with major depressive disorder should at least meet four symptoms of a list of symptoms including changes in appetite and weight, changes in sleep and activity, absence of energy, guilt feeling, difficulties in thinking and decision-making, and recurrent death and suicidal thoughts [5].

Major depression is a recurrent disease with a variety of social, economic, physical and mental consequences [6]. It significantly affects quality of life through long term pain, disruption in occupation, in education, and in domestic or interpersonal relationships, or even committing suicide [7]. It is associated with high economic loss because of disability and repeated absence [8]. Considering the disabling effects and great human, economic and social issues associated with this disorder, a variety of approaches have been designed to treat major depression. One of the mostly used therapeutic approaches is the cognitive-behavior approach. However, the problem of this type of treatment is high recurrence of the disorder after apparently successful therapy [9]. One of the suggestions about the lack of effectiveness of this approach is the absence of attention to happiness and quality of life. Nowadays, with the appearance and spread of health psychology and positive psychology, attitudes toward disorders have left the medical framework as well as the single factor model. Researchers believe that it is better to account for the development of mental disorders by defective life styles and low quality of life and therapy should be associated with revision, reformation and change in quality of life and increasing individual capabilities, exploring personal resources and new strengths and providing satisfaction of life and well-being in individuals and societies [10].

There is a consensus among researchers that the construct of quality of life consist of objective factors as well as subjective factors (internal well-being). Objective factors consist of literacy level, income level, working conditions, marital status, security, socioeconomic position, and mental indices on the basis of individuals' assessment and perception of the level of satisfaction as well as happiness etc. [11]. Therefore, an increase in happiness contributes to one of the component of quality of life (subjective component) and increases quality of life. Regarding the influence of happiness on quality of life among individuals and society and to prevent recurrence of depression, Frisch introduced a new approach through modulation of cognitive-behavior approach and positive psychology known as quality of life therapy [12].

The approach of quality of life therapy is one of the innumerable approaches in the positive psychology that supports the approach of life satisfaction to increase human happiness and quality of life. This approach combines Aaron T. Beck's cognitive approach in the clinical area, Csikszentmihalyi's activity theory and Seligman's positive psychology. In addition to those with disorders such as depression, the group targeted by this approach contains normal and healthy individuals, who are going to experience higher levels of well-being, mental health and in general quality of life. In this approach, principles and skills are taught to help patients identify, follow and meet needs, goals and wishes in the important and valuable areas of life. Areas which are presented in this approach include: 1-Physical health, 2-Self-esteem, 3-Goals and values, 4-Job, 5-Money, 6-Game, 7-Learning, 8-Creativity, 9-Helping others, 10-Love, 11-Friends, 12-Children, 13-Relatives, 14-House and neighbors, 15-Society, 16-Wife and 17-Life in general [12].

The quality of life therapy that is mainly focused on providing happiness and life satisfaction through cognitive-behavior change in five main concepts including circumstances, attitudes, standards that we define for ourselves, importance, and other factors influencing satisfaction of life (CASIO). These are five strategies for providing satisfaction in such areas, which enhance quality of life on the basis of providing satisfaction with the distance between what the person wants and what he/she has. This model changes these five contexts and helps patients enhance their satisfaction and happiness. Moreover, this method offers principles to deal with an increase in happiness. These principles consist of positive concepts, attitude, strengths and schemas or beliefs that assist in creating stable and enduring happiness and satisfaction [12].

Research studies on measuring the effectiveness of this approach also generally suggest its high effectiveness. For example, Ghasemi found that quality of life group therapy, combined of the positive psychology and the cognitive-behavior approach, enhances indices of mental health as well as mental well-being [13]. Toghyani *et al.*

also indicated that the quality of life therapy can increase positive affection and decrease negative affection and as a result can enhance male adults' mental health [14]. Padash found that quality of life therapy contributes to happiness of married men and women [15]. Abedi compared this approach to the cognitive-behavior approach among children with obsessive-compulsive disorder and their mothers and concluded that it increased satisfaction of life and quality of life of children and their mothers and also reduced their anxiety symptoms [16].

Considering the relatively low success of the current therapies in treating depression and the lack of attention to increase the level of happiness of individuals with depression and the claim of the quality of life therapy approach on increasing capabilities and happiness, this research sought to investigate the efficiency of this approach on increasing happiness of depressed individuals.

2. Materials and Methods

This was an experimental study with pretest-posttest including a control and an experimental group and Ethics committee approval taken. The population included all inhabitants of Zahedan with major depression disorder referred to one of the consultation centers in Zahedan. To determine the sample among the individuals with depression referred to health centers, 48 individuals were selected among those who showed willingness to participate in the research and their score on the Beck's depression scale was 13 or higher. These individuals were interviewed by a psychotherapist using a structured clinical interview. Of these, 36 individuals were diagnosed with symptoms of major depression, among which 30 individuals were randomly selected and placed in two groups (experimental and control), each including 15 individuals. The inclusion criteria included:

1. As diagnosis was done as per DSM-IV TR, a patient should have depression, meet the DSM-IV TR criteria for depression and show no co morbidity with other I disorders.

This line should be, according to me, as diagnosis was done as per DSM-IV TR.

2. The patient should not receive medication or psychotherapy for his/her current problem.

3. The problem should not be related to drug abuse or medicine use.

4. The problem should not be related to specific physical or neurological diseases.

3. Instruments

3.1. Beck's Depression Inventory-Revised Form

This instrument is a self-report 21-item questionnaire developed to assess symptoms of depression. Each of the items has 4 options which are scored from zero (mental health symptoms) to 3 (acute and deep symptoms of depression). Items indicate four degrees of depression. The total score ranges from zero to 63 and the cut-off point for screening is 13. Its designers considered scores of 10 and higher as mild depression, 20 to 28 as moderate depression, and 29 to 63 as severe depression. The questionnaire was translated into Persian and its validity was checked. Internal consistency for the BDI on Iranian students was reported 87% and its test-retest reliability was 73% [15]. Results of Beck, Steer and Brown indicated that the questionnaire has high internal consistency [17]. Moreover, another research study reported its alpha coefficient which was 91%, the correlation calculated between scores on two halves of the test was 89% and the test-retest coefficient within a week was 94%.

3.2. Oxford Happiness Questionnaire

The scale was developed by Argyle and Lu [18]. It has 29 items. Each of the items has 4 options scored from 0 to 3. Therefore, the maximum total score is 87. The total score ranges from 0 to 87. Both validity and reliability of the questionnaire have been checked in various research studies. For example, Argyle and Lu calculated the reliability of this scale using the Cronbach's alpha on 347 subjects and reported that its alpha was 90% [18]. Alipour and Norbala also conducted the same study on 132 Iranian subjects and obtained its alpha value which was 93% [19]. Many research studies have reported that the validity of this questionnaire is appropriate [20] [21]. Francis *et al.* [22] and Byani [23] reported a significant correlation of 52% and 65%, respectively between the results of this questionnaire and the Beck's depression questionnaire. In addition, Alipour and Norbala confirmed the reliability of the questionnaire using face validity method [19].

3.3. Research Procedure

In this research 30 patients diagnosed with major depression and showed no comorbidity with other I disorders were randomly selected. Selected subjects were randomly divided into two groups (experimental and control (waiting list group)). Afterwards, each group of subjects was asked to attend a briefing session aimed to inform subjects of the purpose of the study and obtain their consent to participate in the research. Additionally, the agreement form was completed by each patient. They were assured that all presentations of therapeutic sessions and results of the inventories will be kept confidential and no other organization or individual will have access to them and results would be presented collectively and anonymously. Considering patients convenience, the treatment sessions were scheduled with regard to their working conditions. Subjects placed in the control group were assured that the same therapy will be conducted on them after performing the research procedure. Participants answered the two mentioned inventories (pretest) in the briefing session. After the briefing session, the participants in the experimental group individually received a treatment based on the quality of life therapy in 10, 45-minute sessions. Each treatment session was conducted in a week. The control group received no such treatment. The control group did the same when the research process was fully completed. The synopsis of the therapy sessions were as follows: *Session* 1 (establishing relationships, describing the major depression disorder and the effect of happiness on the disorder, teaching the quality of life therapy approach to the patients, discussing 16 domains of satisfaction with life, determining the members' problem scope, homework: thinking about how we can improve our quality of life); *Session* 2 (reviewing the previous session homework, discussing self-esteem and its role in increasing happiness and current skills in these areas, homework: using skills in daily life especially applying the technique of BAT); *Session* 3 (reviewing the previous session homework, discussing and reviewing the CASIO model in self-respect, discussing health issues and presenting related skills, homework: using skills in daily life, particularly applying the technique of TAC); *Session* 4 (reviewing the previous session homework, discussing goals and values, discussing the principles of quality of life, explaining the principles and application of these principles to increase satisfaction, homework: using skills in daily life, especially applying the technique of DAP); *Session* 5 (reviewing the previous session homework, discussing friends or relatives and its role in life satisfaction, presenting relevant skills, homework: use of skills in daily life especially the techniques of writing a letter and egg basket); *Session* 6 (reviewing the previous session homework, discussing the role of free time in increasing happiness, presenting related skills, homework: implementing the plan or routine leisure time or recreation hobby); *Session* 7 (reviewing the previous session homework, discussing learning, presenting related skills, homework: use of problem-solving skills in daily life, particularly applying the technique of problem-solving); *Session* 8 (reviewing the previous session homework, providing positive psychology techniques to prevent recurrence, homework: providing three basic principles of happiness: inner richness, quality of time and meaning-seeking); *Session* 9 (reviewing the previous session homework, discussing the principles and the scope and application of the principles in the area of relationships); and *Session* 10 (reviewing the previous session, reviewing all therapy sessions and conclusions).

4. Results

In **Table 1**, the mean and standard deviation of the pretest and posttest on the depression and happiness inventories are demonstrated for both groups.

To test the assumptions of analysis of covariance, Box's M statistic was used. Box's M statistic is 959.4 and F statistics is 52.1. The significance level is 206.6 ($p < 0.05$). Therefore, it is indicated that the assumption of homogeneity of variance matrices-covariance is met. After presenting the assumptions, in order to compare the

Table 1. Mean and standard deviation of the groups on the pretest and posttest.

Steps		Depression			Happiness		
	Group	Mean	SD	Mean	SD	Frequency
Posttest	Experimental	13.21	26.3	36.44	44.2	15
	Control	15.22	35.3	28.47	05.1	15
	Total	33.21	37.3	36.44	09.1	30
Pretest	Experimental	38.11	44.1	20.58	63.1	15
	Control	20.20	70.3	13.48	15.1	15
	Total	43.16	26.5	43.51	12.1	30

groups' mean scores on the posttest, MANCOVA was used. Accordingly, the pre-test scores were controlled as the covariate and then the posttest scores were compared. To compare the posttest scores of the depression and happiness inventories, after controlling the pretest, multivariate analysis of covariance was used. Since the test shows significant differences between the dependent variables, to evaluate the effect of each of the variables, one-way ANCOVA was used. The results are presented in **Table 2**.

As **Table 2** indicates, the difference between these two groups, regarding the level of depression on the posttest, is significant [$p < 0.0001$, f (1, 26) = 30.19]. Additionally, the difference between these two groups, considering the level of happiness on the posttest, is significant [$p < 0.0001$, f (1, 26) = 27.103]. It can be concluded that quality of life therapy reduces depression and increases happiness in individuals with major depression.

5. Discussion and Conclusion

The present study sought to examine the effectiveness of quality of life therapy on increasing happiness among patients with major depression. In this regard, it was revealed that quality of life therapy had high effectiveness in reducing depression and increasing happiness in individuals with major depression. The results are consistent with the results of other research studies confirming the effectiveness of quality of life therapy in reducing mental diseases and increasing happiness. For the example, the results are consistent with the results of Ghasemi who found that quality of life group therapy combined of the positive psychology and the cognitive-behavior approach enhanced indices of mental health and mental well-being [13]. Likewise, Toghyani *et al.* indicated that the quality of life therapy can increase positive affection and decrease negative affection and as a result can enhance male adults' mental health [14]. Moreover, Sin and Lyubomirsky suggested that positive psychotherapies can increase happiness [24]. Finally, the results are in line with Mitchell *et al.*'s study who found that compared to problem-solving-based psychotherapies or using placebo, positive psychotherapies increased happiness much higher [25].

To explain these results, several points should be mentioned. First, this approach has a general or universal view to life and its goals in each phase of the intervention is related to patients' general goals in life, so that patients are able to observe a direct relationship between an intervention or homework and realization of major needs, goals and demands. In addition, assessing and conceptualizing patients' difficulties and capabilities provide a universal viewpoint to life that is based on operating in sixteen areas of daily life with any psychological or physical difficulty, disorder or disability. The other reason for the effectiveness of this approach is the search for efficient goals known as goals and values. In this type of therapy, a part of goals and values, basic skills for controlling life and temperament control skills to prevent immobility in conformity and compatibility and to prevent chronic issues and difficulties, and to control negative emotions and organize their life in search of personal goals in important areas of life are taught to the patients. More importantly, this approach is a logo therapy aiding patients to find the most meaningful things which lead to happiness and health in the present time and in future [19].

Table 2. Results of analysis of covariance to compare the posttest scores of depression and happiness.

Source	Dependent Variable	Sum of Squares	df	Mean Square	F	sig	Chi Eta	Test Power
Pretest D	D	858.362	1	858.362	186.43	0.000	624.0	1
	H	859.2	1	859.2	652.0	427.0	024.0	122.0
Pretest H	D	780.4	1	780.4	569.0	457.0	021.0	112.0
	H	227.113	1	227.113	817.25	0.000	498.0	998.0
Group	D	200.162	1	200.162	304.19	0.000	426.0	988.0
	H	947.452	1	947.452	276.103	0.000	799.0	1
Error	D	458.218	26	402.8				
	H	030.114	26	386.4				
Total	D	58363	30					
	H	8336	30					

D: Depression, H: Happiness.

The main limitation of the current study was this subject that there are other studies in other disorders where quality of life therapy is used, such as Sharp (2002), Lambert (2006); therefore, there was no way to compare the obtained results with other new therapeutic approaches. Moreover, all steps were performed by the researcher, with the possibility of bias in subjects' responses to the inventories. Therefore, a comparison between different therapeutic approaches to treat major depression along with cooperation of therapists and subjects are recommended.

References

[1]   Dozois, D.J. and Dobson, K.S. (2002) Handbook of Assessment and Treatment Planning for Psychological Disorders. Guilford Press, New York.

[2]   Sharp, L.K. and Lipsky, M.S. (2002) Screening for Depression a Cross the Life Span: A Review of Measures for Use in Primary Care Settings. *American Family Physician*, **66**, 1001-1008.

[3]   Lambert, K.G. (2006) Rising Rates of Depression in Today's Society: Consideration of the Roles of Effort Based Rewards and Enhanced Resilience in Day-to-Day Functioning. *Neuroscience & Biobehavioral*, **30**, 497-510. http://dx.doi.org/10.1016/j.neubiorev.2005.09.002

[4]   World Health Organization (2007) What Is Depression? http://www.who.int/mentalhealth/management/depression/definition/en/index.Html

[5]   American Psychiatric Association (2014) Diagnostic and Statistical Manual of Mental Disorders. 4th Edition, American Psychiatric Association, Washington DC.

[6]   Segal, Z.V., Williams, J.M.G. and Teasdale, J.D. (2002) Mindfulness-Based Cognitive Therapy for Depression: A New Approach to Preventing Relapse. Guilford, New York.

[7]   Kaltenthaler, E., Shackley, P., Stevens, K., Beverley, C., Parry, G. and Chilcott, J.A. (2002) A Systematic Review and Economic Evaluation of Computerized Cognitive Behavior Therapy for Depression and Anxiety. Technical Report, Core Research, Alton.

[8]   Spitzer, M. (2009) Thought Suppression as a Cognitive Vulnerability Factor for Depression an FMRI Study. Hanna Lo, Heilbronn.

[9]   Joseph, S. and Lindley, A.P. (2006) Positive Therapy (A Meta Theory for Psychological Practice). Rutledge Press, USA.

[10] Seligman, M.E.P. and Csikszentmihalyi, M. (2010) Positive Psychology: An Introduction. *American Psychologist*, **55**, 5-14. http://dx.doi.org/10.1037/0003-066X.55.1.5

[11] Lambert, M. and Naber, D. (2013) Current Issues in Schizophrenia: Overview of Patients Acceptability, Functioning Capacity and Quality of Life. *CNS Drugs*, **18**, 5-17. http://dx.doi.org/10.2165/00023210-200418002-00002

[12] Frisch, M.B. (2006) Quality of Life Therapy. John Wiley & Sons Press, New Jersey.

[13] Ghasemi, N. (2011) The Effectiveness of Quality of Life Group Therapy on Mental Health. *Journal of Clinical Psychology*, **10**, 23-33.

[14] Toghyani, M., Kalantari, M., Amiri, S. and Molavi, H. (2014) The Effectiveness of Quality of Life Therapy on Subjective Well-Being of Male Adolescents. *Procedia-Social and Behavioral Sciences*, **30**, 1752-1757. http://dx.doi.org/10.1016/j.sbspro.2011.10.338

[15] Padash, Z. (2011) The Effectiveness of Quality of Life Therapy on Happiness. *Journal of Counseling and Family Psychotherapy*, **1**, 115-130.

[16] Abedi, M.R. and Vostanis, P. (2014) Evaluation of Quality of Life Therapy for Parents of Children with Obsessive-Compulsive Disorder in Iran. *European Child & Adolescent Psychiatry*, **19**, 605-613. http://dx.doi.org/10.1007/s00787-010-0098-4

[17] Beak, A.T., Steer, R.A. and Brown, G.K. (1996) An Inventory for Measuring Depression. *JAMA Psychiatry*, **4**, 561-571. http://dx.doi.org/10.1001/archpsyc.1961.01710120031004

[18] Argyle, M. and Lu, L. (1990) The Happiness of Extraverts. *Personality and Individual Differences*, **11**, 1011-1017. http://dx.doi.org/10.1016/0191-8869(90)90128-E

[19] Alipour, N. and Norbala, A. (1999) Validity and Reliability of Oxford Happiness Inventory. *Journal of Thinking and Behavior*, **18**, 55-65.

[20] Hills, P. and Argyle, M. (2011) Happiness, Introversion-Extroversion and Happy Factors. *Personality and Individual Differences*, **30**, 595-608. http://dx.doi.org/10.1016/S0191-8869(00)00058-1

[21] Furnham, A. and Cheng, H. (1999) Personality as a Predictor of Mental Health and Happiness in the East and West. *Personality and Individual Differences*, **27**, 395-403. http://dx.doi.org/10.1016/S0191-8869(98)00250-5

[22] Francis, L.J., Brown, I.B., Lester, D. and Philipchalk, R. (1998) Happiness as Stable Extraversion: A Cross-Cultural Examination of Reliability and Validity of Oxford Happiness Inventory among Students in the U.K., U.S.A., Australia and Canada. *Personality and Individual Differences*, **24**, 167-171.
http://dx.doi.org/10.1016/S0191-8869(97)00170-0

[23] Byani, A. (2006) Validity and Reliability of Happiness-Depression Scale. *Journal of Science and Research in Psychology*, **29**, 73-83.

[24] Sin, N. and Lyubomirsky, S. (2009) Enhancing Well-Being and Alleviating Depressive Symptom with Positive Psychology Interventions: A Practice-Friendly Meta-Analysis. *Journal of Clinical Psychology*, **65**, 467-487.
http://dx.doi.org/10.1002/jclp.20593

[25] Mitchell, J., Stanimirovic, R., Klein, B. and Vella-Brodrick, D. (2014) A Randomized Controlled Trial of a Self-Guided Internet Intervention Promoting Well-Being. *Computers in Human Behavior*, **25**, 749-760.
http://dx.doi.org/10.1016/j.chb.2009.02.003

15

The Effect of a Psycho-Educational Program on Psychiatric Symptoms, Drug Attitude and Treatment Satisfaction of Patients with Schizophrenia

Yueren Zhao[1], Yuko Yasuhara[2], Tetsuya Tanioka[2], Sakiko Sakamaki[2],
Masahito Tomotake[2], Beth King[3], Rozzano C. Locsin[2], Nakao Iwata[1]

[1]Fujita Health University, Toyoake, Japan
[2]Tokushima University, Tokushima, Japan
[3]Florida Atlantic University, Boca Raton, USA
Email: taipeeyen+SciRes@gmail.com

Abstract

The purpose of this study was to determine the effect of a Comprehensive Psycho-Educational Approach and Scheme Set (COMPASS) for patients with schizophrenia who were treated with risperidone long-acting injectable (RLAI), on their psychiatric symptoms, drug attitudes, and treatment satisfaction levels. Participants were sixty-five patients at thirteen hospitals in Japan who met ICD-10 F2 criteria for schizophrenia or schizo-affective disorder and were treated with RLAI. A correlational study design was used to measure the effect of the COMPASS on the psychiatric symptoms, drug attitudes, and treatment satisfaction levels of patients treated with RLAI. Using the following evaluation indicators: The Subjective Satisfaction to Treatment Scale (SSTS), Brief Psychiatric Rating Scale (BPRS), Global Assessment of Functioning (GAF), Drug-Induced Extrapyramidal Symptoms Scale (DIEPSS), and Drug Attitude Inventory-10 (DAI-10), measurements were taken at the beginning of the program (baseline), at the end of the program, and six months after (endpoint). Data analysis included descriptive statistics, Mann-Whitney U test or Wilcoxon signed-rank test, and Spearman's rank correlation coefficient. Significant differences were observed in BPRS total ($p < 0.001$), sub-scales of BPRS positive ($p < 0.001$), BPRS negative ($p < 0.01$), BPRS affective ($p < 0.01$), and GAF ($p < 0.001$). However, there was no significant change in subscale of BPRS manic, DAI-10, DIEPSS, or SSTS but significant positive correlations were found between SSTS and DAI-10 and GAF at baseline; a negative correlation was found between SSTS and BPRS. The findings of the study suggested the benefit of using the COMPASS in conjunction with RLAI to decrease patients' psychiatric symptomatology and improve treatment satisfaction. In addition, patient satisfaction was found to be an important factor to be considered by the psychiatrist.

Keywords

Schizophrenia, Long-Acting Injection, Psycho-Education, COMPASS (Comprehensive Psycho-Educational Approach and Scheme Set), Adherence, Satisfaction Level

1. Introduction

Non-adherence to medication is a major problem in the treatment of schizophrenia. One of the most important treatment methods for patients with poor medication adherence to antipsychotics is the use of long-acting injectable (LAI) medications [1]. LAI has proven to be beneficial in assisting with the prevention of relapse, reduction of readmission rates and alleviation of suicide attempts for patients diagnosed with schizophrenia and poor medication adherence [2] [3]. Similarly, psycho-educational programs for both patients and family members have been found to be effective in preventing relapse [4] [5] and promoting emotional expression [6].

In a randomized study by Guo *et al.* [7], they compared 2 groups of patients diagnosed with early stage schizophrenia. One group received medication only and the other group received medication and a psychosocial intervention program. Those patients receiving both medication and psychosocial intervention had a lower rate of treatment discontinuation or change, a lower risk of relapse, and improved insight, quality of life (QOL), and social functioning. Swelieh *et al.* [8] studied medication adherence and treatment satisfaction of 131 patients diagnosed with schizophrenia. The findings revealed a correlation between treatment satisfaction level, psychiatric scores and medication adherence. Depot antipsychotic drugs are thought to reduce relapse rates by improving adherence [9]. Lee *et al.* [10] revealed that combined therapy with a psychosocial intervention for relapse prevention could be effective in maintaining medication compliance, and that discontinuation of long-acting atypical antipsychotics might be predictive of the next relapse.

Further research is needed to validate the benefits and impact of administering a psycho-education program such as Comprehensive Psycho-educational Approach and Scheme Set (COMPASS) to patients with schizophrenia who are treated using LAI antipsychotics. The COMPASS was developed by Zhao *et al.* [11] for patients diagnosed with schizophrenia and who were treated with RLAI. This is an original psychoeducational program supporting treatments with RLAI and evaluating subjective treatment satisfaction, transition of symptoms, and effectiveness in preventing symptomatic relapse.

The aim of this study was to determine the effect of COMPASS a psycho-educational program for patients with schizophrenia, who were treated with RLAI and the patient's psychiatric symptoms, drug attitude and level of treatment satisfaction.

2. Methods

2.1. Research Design

A correlational study was designed with defined variables focused on the effect of the COMPASS on the symptomatology, attitudes, and satisfaction of sixty-five participants completing the process for data collection.

2.2. Procedure for Data Collection

A complete description of all procedures was provided to the patients who were informed of the goal of treatment (return to everyday life with biweekly administration of RLAI), the need for administration of oral medication during the first four weeks after initiation of RLAI, and the potential risk of adverse events with RLAI. This effect was similar to that works on the balance of chemical substances which act on the nervous system in patient's brain. Both RLAI and oral medication are administered at the beginning of treatment in an effort to quickly decrease symptomatology. Each patient was informed of the costs of RLAI and other important information. Informed consent was obtained from each of the participants. Patients were followed for a 6-month period. During this time the COMPASS program was continuously implemented throughout the transition phase (introduction of RLAI) and to the observation phase which was done six months after the introduction of the RLAI.

2.3. Setting and Subjects

Twelve psychiatric hospitals were private and one was a University hospital in Japan.

Criteria for participant selection included: Patients diagnosed with schizophrenia or schizoaffective disorder based on International Statistical Classification of Diseases and Related Health Problems, Tenth Revision (ICD-10) F2 criteria; were between the ages of 20 - 70 years old; had no systemic or neurologic diseases, including disturbances of hematopoiesis; had no history of electroconvulsive therapy within the past 6 months prior to study enrollment; were not pregnant; were not dependent on any substances other than nicotine during the 5 years before enrollment; had no communication difficulty; and could not be switched to RLAI monotherapy. No patient was excluded from the study because of a medical condition at baseline.

Of the 113 patients who qualified for the study, 48 failed to complete the procedure for data collection, or had exacerbation of psychiatric symptoms.

2.4. Description of the Psycho Educational Program

The name *COMPASS* was created by combining letters from the words, *COM* prehensive *P*sycho-educational *A*pproach and *S*cheme *S*et (The COMPASS is free to download from http://j.mp/COMPASS-eng).

This is comprised of three chapters: *Chapter one* is targeted for patients in the acute phase. In this chapter, disease symptomatology (positive and negative symptoms, cognitive dysfunction), characteristics of conventional treatment (oral medication) and treatment using RLAI are discussed. The strength of the treatment with RLAI in preventing relapse is emphasized. *Chapter two* focuses on the recovery phase. This chapter addresses self-awareness of physical condition (including symptoms of schizophrenia and treatment-related adverse events), mental condition (self-assessment for screening of depression), and coping strategies to prevent relapse. *Chapter three* relates to those preparing to be discharged. In this chapter, patients reconfirm the advantages and disadvantages of treatment with RLAI, learn about social resources which will support daily life in the community, discuss concrete ways in which they could participate in their community, and prioritizes their own hopes and dreams.

All patients in the study had to complete chapter one prior to proceeding to RLAI monotherapy. Furthermore, in order to enhance the patients understanding of the material, clinicians adjusted the teaching times of chapters two and three to meet the learning needs of individual patients.

2.5. Evaluation Indicators

Several instruments were used as indicators to measure the effects of the COMPASS as a psycho-educational program on the psychiatric symptomatology, treatment satisfaction, and patient attitudes towards treatment. Measurements were taken at study baseline (time point when the patient's transition of prescription to RLAI monotherapy was completed) and over the following 6 months (observation period for evaluating treatment continuation of RLAI).

- *Subjective Satisfaction Treatment Scale (SSTS)*. The SSTS was developed by Zhao, one of the researchers in the study. This scale measures, from zero to seven from 1 (completely dissatisfied) to 7 (completely satisfied), using the following four questions: 1) One's perception of the efficacy of RLAI, 2) the difficulty due to side effects of RLAI, 3) Daily life activities, and 4) overall satisfaction to RLAI treatment. This self-administered questionnaire was completed by both the patients and clinicians.
- *Brief Psychiatric Rating Scale (BPRS)*. The BPRS assesses positive, negative and affective symptoms including 18 symptom constructs (*i.e.* hostility, suspiciousness, hallucination, grandiosity). The clinicians rate the patient's behavior and enters a number that ranges from 1 (not present) to 7 (extremely severe) for each symptom construct.
- *Global Assessment of Functioning Scale (GAF)*. Clinicians used the GAF scale to rate a person's overall level of functioning from 1 to 100, using a numeric score to represent the severity of that person's psychological symptoms and/or daily functioning. The three areas examined by the GAF are: Psychological—obsessions, panic attacks, etc. Social and Interpersonal—maintaining friendships, personal hygiene, etc. and Occupational—work attendance, ability to follow directions, etc.
- *Drug-Induced Extrapyramidal Symptoms Scale (DIEPSS)* [12]. Clinicians used the DIEPSS to assess drug induced movement disorders. This consists of questions aimed to detect nine representative symptoms of Parkinsonism including sialorrhea, gait disturbance, hesitation to start walking (freezing), bradykinesia,

muscle rigidity, tremors, loss of vital facial expression (*i.e.*, mask-like face), akathisia and dyskinesia. Questions on the questionnaire used non-technical words. Patients' self-assessment for each item of the questionnaire (*i.e.*, the presence or absence of the symptoms and their severity) was scored using a 5-point scale.

- *Drug Attitude Inventory*-10 (*DAI*-10). The DAI-10 consists of 10 questions rated by a patient to evaluate an individual's perception of their medication and correlating experience. This was modified in this study like the following question: "I feel more normal on medication" (from DAI-10), to the question item of the DAI-10 like "I feel more normal when I am on RLAI treatment".

2.6. Ethical Considerations

The research study design and procedures followed the clinical study guidelines and were approved by the Ethics Committees of Fujita Health University. All patients and clinicians provided informed consents to participate this study.

2.7. Statistical Analysis

Analyses of data included comparing the means and standard deviations of the BPRS, GAF, DIEPSS, DAI-10 and SSTS scores at baseline, prior to the administration of the COMPASS and at end point of the study. Those scores that changed from baseline to the 6-month endpoint with differences between improved and non-improved adherence groups were tested using the Mann-Whitney U test or Wilcoxon signed-rank test. Spearman's rank correlation coefficient was used to test the association between the SSTS and these previously described scores. The level of significance was set at $p < 0.05$.

3. Results

A total of 65 patients comprised the sample of the study. Average age was 44.13 (SD = 3.81) years old: There were 32 women and 33 men. Women patients' average age was 47.48 (SD = 13.86) years old, and 40.97 (SD = 13.19) years old for men.

3.1. Change of Evaluation Indicators

Analysis comparing the baseline scores prior to the COMPASS and initiation of RLAI, and at endpoint (6-months following the program and RLAI treatment) showed that the means and standard deviations of the Evaluation Indicators (BPRS, GAF, DIEPSS, DAI-10, SSTS) indicated a significant decrease in the Total BPRS ($p < 0.001$), sub-scale of BPRS positive ($p < 0.001$), BPRS negative ($p < 0.01$), BPRS affective ($p < 0.01$), and increase in GAF ($p < 0.001$). However, there were no significant changes in the BPRS Manic, DAI-10, DIEPSS, and SSTS total (see **Table 1**).

Table 1. Change of the evaluation indicators before and after implementation.

		Baseline (N = 65)		Endpoint (N = 65)			
		Mean	SD	Mean	SD	Z	p
BPRS	Total	38.57	14.18	32.28	10.16	-4.65	0.00
	Positive	11.78	5.28	9.29	4.03	-3.07	0.00
	Negative	10.22	3.97	8.49	3.41	-2.50	0.01
	Affective	8.28	3.27	6.74	2.69	-2.77	0.01
	Manic	4.29	2.67	3.88	2.32	-1.30	0.19
GAF		49.60	13.62	57.95	15.62	-3.23	0.00
DIEPSS		2.55	3.59	1.91	2.67	-0.76	0.45
DAI-10		5.51	4.44	5.23	5.03	-0.08	0.94
SSTS total		28.57	12.00	31.92	9.30	-1.10	0.27

Mann-Whitney U test. Brief Psychiatric Rating Scale (BPRS), functioning was evaluated using Global Assessment of Functioning (GAF), and extrapyramidal side effects were evaluated using Drug-Induced Extrapyramidal Symptoms Scale (DIEPSS), and Drug Attitude Inventory-10 (DAI-10) were rated by clinical senior psychiatrists at baseline and 6 months study endpoint. Subjective Satisfaction to Treatment Scale (SSTS) in patient was evaluated by patient.

3.2. Relations between Each Evaluation Indicator and Improved Situation in DAI-10

The patients whose scores improved on the DAI-10 following the COMPASS ($p < 0.01$) were classified as the improved group. However, within this group, no significant difference was observed in the BPRS, GAF, DIEPSS and SSTS total at the endpoint (see **Table 2**).

3.3. Correlation between DAI-10 and Evaluation Indicators before and after the Implementation of COMPASS

At baseline, prior to the COMPASS, significant positive correlations were found between DAI-10 and SSTS total ($p < 0.01$), and GAF ($p < 0.01$) and a significant negative correlation was recognized between DAI-10 and BPRS total ($p < 0.01$), and between SSTS total and BRPS total ($p < 0.05$).

Six months later, at the completion of COMPASS intervention, a significant positive correlation was observed between DAI-10 and SSTS total ($p < 0.01$) and between SSTS total and GAF ($p < 0.05$). Significant negative correlations were found between SSTS total and BPRS total ($p < 0.01$) and DIEPSS ($p < 0.05$) (see **Table 3**).

Table 2. Relations between each evaluation indicators and improved situation in DAI-10.

	Improved (N = 24)		Not improved (N = 41)			
	Mean	SD	Mean	SD	Z	p
BPRS total	32.54	7.61	32.13	11.37	−0.81	0.42
GAF	55.46	15.85	59.41	15.30	−1.48	0.14
DIEPSS	1.67	2.78	2.05	2.60	−1.13	0.26
DAI−10	7.42	3.31	3.95	5.38	−2.80	0.01
SSTS total	34.46	6.03	30.44	10.43	−1.59	0.11

Mann-Whitney U test. Brief Psychiatric Rating Scale (BPRS), functioning was evaluated using Global Assessment of Functioning (GAF), and extrapyramidal side effects were evaluated using Drug-Induced Extrapyramidal Symptoms Scale (DIEPSS), and Drug Attitude Inventory-10 (DAI-10) were rated by clinical senior psychiatrists at baseline and 6 months study endpoint. Subjective Satisfaction to Treatment Scale (SSTS) in patient was evaluated by patient.

Table 3. Correlation between DAI-10 and evaluation indicators before and after implementation (N = 65).

Baseline	DAI-10	SSTS total	DIEPSS	BPRS	GAF
DAI-10	1.000				
SSTS total	0.354**	1.000			
DIEPSS	0.047	−0.102	1.000		
BPRS total	−0.294*	−0.263*	0.129	1.000	
GAF	0.360**	0.326**	−0.106	−0.559**	1.000
Endpoint	DAI-10	SSTS total	DIEPSS	BPRS	GAF
DAI-10	1.000				
SSTS total	0.584**	1.000			
DIEPSS	−0.184	−0.253*	1.000		
BPRS total	−0.24	−0.359**	0.080	1.000	
GAF	0.189	0.260*	−0.071	−0.585**	1.000

Spearman rank correlation coefficient; *$p < 0.05$, **$p < 0.01$; Brief Psychiatric Rating Scale (BPRS), functioning was evaluated using Global Assessment of Functioning (GAF), and extrapyramidal side effects were evaluated using Drug-Induced Extrapyramidal Symptoms Scale (DIEPSS), and Drug Attitude Inventory-10 (DAI-10) were rated by clinical senior psychiatrists at baseline and 6 months study endpoint. Subjective Satisfaction to Treatment Scale (SSTS) in patient was evaluated by patient.

month period, forty-eight participants failed to comply with the protocol resulting in their disqualification. This drop-out rate can be avoided.

Limitations

The findings of the study indicate the need to further study the benefit of the COMPASS by comparing medication adherence, re-hospitalization and quality of life of patients who received only RLAI treatment.

The generalizability of the study was limited by the sample size and lack of a control group, which would have strengthened the ability to determine the impact of the COMPASS. Furthermore, the DAI-10 rating scale is typically used with patients receiving oral treatment and not for hypodermic medication administration.

One of the immediate findings of the study is the consideration of providing treatment individualized for each patient to evaluate degree of satisfaction. It became clear that different psycho-educational approaches based on drug attitudes could not be assured.

Acknowledgements

We would like to express deep gratitude to the patients, family members, attending psychiatrists and other healthcare providers who participated in this study, and to psychiatrists and healthcare providers of Fujita Health University Hospital, Holy Cross Hospital, Jindai Hospital, Kitabayashi Hospital, Kokubu Hospital, Kyowa Hospital, Okehazama Hospital Fujita Kokoro Care Center, Mikawa Hospital, Matsusaka Kosei Hospital, Tado Ayame Hospital, Yatsushiro Kosei Hospital, Yuge Hospital, and Meisei Hospital who made profound contributions to development of the original COMPASS psycho-educational tool.

Disclosure

The authors report no conflicts of interest in this work.

References

[1] Burns, T. (2009) Knowledge about Antipsychotic Long-Acting Injections: Bridging That Gap. *British Journal of Psychiatry. Supplement*, **52**, S5-S6. http://dx.doi.org/10.1192/bjp.195.52.s5

[2] Patel, M.X., de Zoysa, N., Bernadt, M. and David, A.S. (2008) A Cross-Sectional Study of Patients' Perspectives on Adherence to Antipsychotic Medication: Depot versus Oral. *Journal of Clinical Psychiatry*, **69**, 1548-1556. http://dx.doi.org/10.4088/JCP.v69n1004

[3] Kane, J.M. (2011) Improving Treatment Adherence in Patients with Schizophrenia. *Journal of Clinical Psychiatry*, **72**, e28. http://dx.doi.org/10.4088/jcp.9101tx2c

[4] Burton, S.C. (2005) Strategies for Improving Adherence to Second-Generation Antipsychotics in Patients with Schizophrenia by Increasing Ease of Use. *Journal of Psychiatric Practice*, **11**, 369-378. http://dx.doi.org/10.1097/00131746-200511000-00003

[5] Lincoln, T.M., Wilhelm, K. and Nestoriuc, Y. (2007) Effectiveness of Psychoeducation for Relapse, Symptoms, Knowledge, Adherence and Functioning in Psychotic Disorders: A Meta-Analysis. *Schizophrenia Research*, **96**, 232-245. http://dx.doi.org/10.1016/j.schres.2007.07.022

[6] Yamaguchi, H., Takahashi, A., Takano, A. and Kojima, T. (2006) Direct Effects of Short-Term Psychoeducational Intervention for Relatives of Patients with Schizophrenia in Japan. *Psychiatry and Clinical Neurosciences*, **60**, 590-597. http://dx.doi.org/10.1111/j.1440-1819.2006.01563.x

[7] Guo, X., Zhai, J., Liu, Z., Fang, M., Wang, B., Wang, C., Hu, B., Sun, X., Lv, L., Lu, Z., Ma, C., He, X., Guo, T., Xie, S., Wu, R., Xue, Z., Chen, J., Twamley, E.W., Jin, H. and Zhao, J. (2010) Effect of Antipsychotic Medication Alone vs Combined with Psychosocial Intervention on Outcomes of Early-Stage Schizophrenia: A Randomized, 1-Year Study. *Archives of General Psychiatry*, **67**, 895-904. http://dx.doi.org/10.1001/archgenpsychiatry.2010.105

[8] Sweileh, W.M., Ihbesheh, M.S., Jarar, I.S., Sawalha, A.F., Abu Taha, A.S., Zyoud, S.H. and Morisky, D.E. (2012) Antipsychotic Medication Adherence and Satisfaction among Palestinian People with Schizophrenia. *Current Clinical Pharmacology*, **7**, 49-55. http://dx.doi.org/10.2174/157488412799218761

[9] Leucht, C., Heres, S., Kane, J.M., Kissling, W., Davis, J.M. and Leucht, S. (2011) Oral versus Depot Antipsychotic Drugs for Schizophrenia—A Critical Systematic Review and Meta-Analysis of Randomised Long-Term Trials. *Schizophrenia Research*, **127**, 83-92. http://dx.doi.org/10.1016/j.schres.2010.11.020

[10] Lee, S.H., Choi, T.K., Suh, S., Kim, Y.W., Kim, B., Lee, E. and Yook, K.H. (2010) Effectiveness of a Psychosocial

Intervention for Relapse Prevention in Patients with Schizophrenia Receiving Risperidone via Long-Acting Injection. *Psychiatry Research*, **175**, 195-199. http://dx.doi.org/10.1016/j.psychres.2008.06.043

[11] Zhao, Y., Kishi, T., Iwata, N. and Ikeda, M. (2013) Combination Treatment with Risperidone Long-Acting Injection and Psychoeducational Approaches for Preventing Relapse in Schizophrenia. *Neuropsychiatric Disease and Treatment*, **9**, 1655-1659. http://dx.doi.org/10.2147/NDT.S52317

[12] Inada, T. (1996) Evaluation and Diagnosis of Drug-Induced Extrapyramidal Symptoms. In: Yagi, G., Ed., *Commentary on the DIEPSS and Guide to Its Usage*, Seiwa Publishers, Toyko, 3-54. (In Japanese)

[13] Galuppi, A., Turola, M.C., Nanni, M.G., Mazzoni, P. and Grassi, L. (2010) Schizophrenia and Quality of Life: How Important Are Symptoms and Functioning? *International Journal of Mental Health Systems*, **4**, 31. http://dx.doi.org/10.1186/1752-4458-4-31

[14] Kurtz, M.M., Bronfeld, M. and Rose, J. (2012) Cognitive and Social Cognitive Predictors of Change in Objective versus Subjective Quality-of-Life in Rehabilitation for Schizophrenia. *Psychiatry Research*, **200**, 102-107. http://dx.doi.org/10.1016/j.psychres.2012.06.025

[15] Kim, J.H. and Kim, M.J. (2009) Association of Adverse Drug Effects with Subjective Well-Being in Patients with Schizophrenia Receiving Stable Doses of Risperidone. *Clinical Neuropharmacology*, **32**, 250-253. http://dx.doi.org/10.1097/WNF.0b013e3181a5d08c

[16] Helldin, L., Kane, J., Karilampi, U., Norlander, T. and Archer, T. (2008) Experience of Quality of Life and Attitude to Care and Treatment in Patients with Schizophrenia: Role of Cross-Sectional Remission. *International Journal of Psychiatry in Clinical Practice*, **12**, 97-104. http://dx.doi.org/10.1080/13651500701660007

[17] Xia, J., Merinder, L.B. and Belgamwar, M.R. (2011) Psychoeducation for Schizophrenia. *Cochrane Database of Systematic Reviews*, **6**, Article ID: CD002831. http://dx.doi.org/10.1002/14651858.CD002831.pub2

[18] Aki, H., Tomotake, M., Kaneda, Y., Iga, J., Kinouchi, S., Shibuya-Tayoshi, S., Tayoshi, S.Y., Motoki, I., Moriguchi, K., Sumitani, S., Yamauchi, K., Taniguchi, T., Ishimoto, Y., Ueno, S. and Ohmori, T. (2008) Subjective and Objective Quality of Life, Levels of Life Skills, and Their Clinical Determinants in Outpatients with Schizophrenia. *Psychiatry Research*, **158**, 19-25. http://dx.doi.org/10.1016/j.psychres.2006.05.017

[19] Medina, E., Salvà, J., Ampudia, R., Maurino, J. and Larumbe, J. (2012) Short-Term Clinical Stability and Lack of Insight Are Associated with a Negative Attitude Towards Antipsychotic Treatment at Discharge in Patients with Schizophrenia and Bipolar Disorder. *Patient Prefer Adherence*, **6**, 623-629. http://dx.doi.org/10.2147/PPA.S34345

16

Training Needs of International Medical Graduates [IMGs] in Psychiatry*

Milton Kramer

Psychiatry Department, College of Medicine, University of Cincinnati, Cincinnati, Ohio, USA
Email: milton1929@yahoo.com

Abstract

The potential shortage of psychiatrists over the next 5 - 10 years has focused attention on the need to recruit more IMGs to fill the needs rather than use nurse practitioners or physician assistants. IMGs make up about 1/3 of first year psychiatry residents. These individuals have been found to provide services to the poor, the elderly and the psychotic. The quality of their medical work has been found to be satisfactory. The training needs of these physicians require an understanding on the part of their teachers that they come from cultures with different values that we have. The extended families of these primarily Asian residents clash with our strong commitment to individualism. It leads to a We-self rather than our I-Self. This difference coupled with the stress of leaving to come to a new culture is a great stress. Their exposure to psychiatry has been limited. They request and need more interview demonstration and practice, ore feedback and examinations. They should have help in accent reduction. They should be exposed to the working of the hospital by sitting on departmental and hospital committees. The faculty should extend their social opportunities and work as mentors on joint projects. Courses on the history of American culture should be taught. Psychotherapy for them should be encouraged as well as teaching medical ethics. They must become the major educational concern for the department that they are in.

Keywords

International Medical Graduates, Psychiatric Residents, Education

1. Introduction

We are at a time in American Medicine when we will be experiencing an extreme shortage of physicians [1]. The consensus is that we will be 90,000 physicians short by 2020 and 200,000 short by 2025. We had an esti-

---

*Presented 2014 at APA IMG Summit: Global Psychiatric Education and Practice: Role of IMGs in American Psychiatry; Panel II: IMGs in the U.S.

mated 45,000 psychiatrist in 2000 and would need an additional 34,700 psychiatrists to reach an optimal level for a population of 310,000,000 [2]. The physician shortage can only be addressed by increasing the number of training positions available and allowing more International Medical Graduates [IMGs] to enter the United States.

The recommendation for seeking a solution to our manpower needs by increasing IMGs entry into our medical system, particularly in psychiatry, is enhanced by the unique roles IMGs which have played in psychiatry: they serve the underserved both as trainees and practitioners meeting the needs of specific, primarily immigrant populations but also the poor, the psychotic, and the elderly [3]. And they are an increasing percentage of psychiatrists in the United States [4]. IMGs are 26% of the members of the American Psychiatric Association and 33% of psychiatric residents [5]. It is not that American psychiatry is just becoming a specialty with more women, it is becoming international as well [6]. It is essential that we be particularly concerned with the learning processes of IMGs in psychiatry because of the contributions that they make to patient care.

2. Discussion

Recognizing the special needs of IMGs encourages training programs to consider techniques to meet the needs of this growing number of residents and future colleagues. The recommendation of IMGs to their teachers [7] is for more structured teaching with verbal recitation of assigned reading along with the liberal use of demonstrations, supervision, examinations and feedback. I believe that the introduction of psychological concepts early in the training program and in every doctor-patient interaction may facilitate a greater awareness of these issues earlier in training before evaluative patterns become fixed and patients are seen only from a biological perspective.

A series of caveats are in order before proceeding with a discussion of IMGs in psychiatry. It is important to recognize that IMGs are not a homogeneous group [6]. It has been estimated that 41% are from Asia. The quality of the medical skills of more recent IMGs has improved as measured by the scores they obtain on the Clinical Skills Assessment (CSA) examination and has begun to approach that of U.S. medical school graduates (USMGs), 89% compared to 80% [8]. In practice, they provide services comparable in effectiveness to USMGs [9] [10].

The learning needs of IMGs must be individualized. We need to keep in mind that these residents have come from very different cultures with very different values. Their conceptualizations of the nature of man may present unique problems and challenges in the learning process [11] [12].

Suggesting that a group has special needs unfortunately implies that the group is being seen as inferior rather than as different and immediately raises the specter of bias, especially if done by a nonmember of the group. This makes a discussion of the issues difficult, if not, at times, impossible. To put the problem in perspective, it is essential for Americans to be reminded that almost all the major innovations in psychiatry were made by non-Americans [13]-[15]. Ramon y Cajal, a Spaniard, described the network rather than syncytial nature of the central nervous system. Convulsive therapy was first described by Meduna, a Hungarian, and Cerletti and Bini, both Italians. Psychopharmacology was inaugurated by the observations of Denniker and Delay in France. Freud, an Austrian, and Pavlov, a Russian, introduced the bases for psychodynamic and behavioral therapies. Humane treatment approaches were introduced by Pinel in France and Tuke in England, while community psychiatry and treatment were developed in Belgium at Gheel. Understanding the role of neurotransmitters in psychiatric illness was dependent on the discovery of intracellular staining techniques by Dahlstrom and Fuxe in Sweden. It was the impact of the immigrant European analysts, mostly IMGs, before and after the Second World War that determined the nature of psychoanalysis and psychodynamic psychotherapy in the United States. And lastly, the work of Kraeplin, a German, was the intellectual base for the turn to biological psychiatry around 1970. The educational problems we are addressing have to do not with issues of intelligence or creativity, but with the demands of learning how to view the world differently in a new cultural context [16]. Very little has been written about the educational issues that may be unique for IMGs [17]. The focus has been on the barriers that exist for IMGs who come for training and remain to practice in the U.S. These barriers are formidable and have been the focus of significant effort by many individuals to remove or reduce them [4] [18].

It is important to point out at the outset of our discussion of the educational problems that confront IMGs that they and USMGs have a great deal in common [4] [19] [20]. Both groups have completed medical school, are of above average intelligence, persevering and ambitious, and upwardly mobile in their aspirations. IMGs, however, have a series of concurrent personal issues [4] [19]-[21] having to do with immigration, such as feeling lonely and socially isolated, experiencing a decrease in status with its accompanying diminishment of self-esteem, concerns related to the family they left behind and the family by marriage that they may have brought with them, lack of money, and worries related to the vagaries of their visa status. Salman Akhtar [16] discusses with great sensitivity the psychosocial impact of immigration on the immigrant's identity. Group and individual social interaction of residents with faculty is enormously valuable in reducing the sense of isolation.

The specific concerns that have been expressed about IMGs include the quality of their medical education and especially their limited psychiatric experience and knowledge [4] [19] [20]. The contact with psychiatric patients may be as little as a one-day visit to a mental hospital. They may have had little on-service responsibility in medical school, with psychiatric exposure being for some IMGs only a series of lectures. The idea of being part of a team is not congenial to residents who come from hierarchically ordered cultures. IMGs are said to be poor at relating to other disciplines and less effective than USMGs in teaching medical students. They believe they cannot complain or they will be terminated, which for many would lead to a forced return home because of their visa status. IMGs feel powerless because they have only themselves to rely on in their working with patients who may be afraid of them, challenge them, or reject them. IMGs have their identity problems compounded by the loss of medical rituals (e.g., white coats and ward rounds).

The ideal psychiatric resident is seen as warm, friendly, open, active, independent, and inquisitive, whereas the prototypical IMGs is seen as passive, inhibited, reserved, and rigid, with greater difficulty in allowing the use of their imagination [20]. These unfortunate stereotypes have a basis in the value system of American culture. IMGs are often treated as second-class trainees and educationally neglected [20]. They may be overtly rejected and used only to meet service needs, with the rationalization that they should be grateful they were given a position. A more subtle but equally pernicious rejection is to provide very little education on the basis that not much can be expected from IMGs. At the other end of the spectrum, there are those who deny the reality of difference and see IMGs as like all other residents and without special needs. They ignore or minimize the struggles that IMGs experience rather than help to ameliorate them. Teachers must help integrate their trainees into the mainstream of American psychiatry, e.g. by encouraging their going to professional meetings and seeing they are appointed to departmental and hospital committees.

The central role of language and culture lies at the heart of the learning problems that IMGs have in general in becoming psychiatrists in the American context and more particularly in learning psychological theory and therapy. Without a mastery of the language, both formal and informal (*i.e.*, slang and idioms), and a reduction in accent so that their spoken communication is readily understood, IMGs may not understand their patients and teachers and not be understood by them.

Knowledge of the culture in which the exchange takes place often is essential for understanding as Hirsch and colleagues (2002) pointed out in their book, *The New Dictionary of Cultural Literacy*: "They (IMGs) may have the words but not the meaning". The lyrics but not the melody.

In some other cultures, the role of parents and the nature of the child-parent relationship are different from what we hold as the norm orideal in the U.S. Attitudes toward authority and the constraints of obedience vary significantly. Gender roles and inter gender behaviors may be different from ours. The aged are seen as a source of wisdom and entitled to respect. America has been described by an IMG as dangerous, the people as materialistic and self-absorbed, caught up in superficial relationships and neglectful of the poor, children, and the elderly [4]. IMGs may have a different view of the nature of man, a different value system, a different Weltanschauung.

It is the special focus on the individual and individualism that may be said to characterize American if not all of Western society, but developed to its fullest in the U.S., The demand on each of us is to develop ourselves to the fullest. The clarion call to the young is to "follow your bliss" [22]. *The Culture of Narcissism*, by Christopher Lasch [23], may be more than just a book title and the narcissistic personality may be more than just a *DSM* 5 classification (2013). A heightened narcissism may capture something central to our cultural values, which is expressed in our psychology. Many IMGs do not come from cultures that share our commitment to individualism. They view behavior and achievement from a different perspective.

Vozzola [23] has summarized, from a psychological point of view, the major foundational moral themes of several societies. The *American moral themes* are personal liberty, privacy and equality. In contrast, The *Indian themes* are sanctity/pollution, chastity and respect. *China's* moral themes are historically Confucian, namely that humans are born good, not the Christian view of man being born with original sin. The Chinese Communist party fosters obedience and that behavior should foster economic development. Chinese culture is shame based, as are other Eastern cultures, with no emphasis to promote critical thinking or meeting individual needs. For

Muslims faith and moral behavior are the same. God disclosed forbidden [Haram] and permitted behavior [Halal]. Moral education is not to develop personal autonomy but to carry out Muslim law [Sharia], and to submit [Islam]. *Latin America's* civil morality was shaped by the independence struggles of the early 20th century. Morality is social customs and traditions and ethics is a reflection of those traditions. In sub-Saharan Africa, *Afro-communitarianism* is the alternative to Western justice and care. A person is a person through other persons. Morality is relational. We punish for retribution and deterrence, they prescribe reconciliation or reparation of broken relationships. Must be concerned about others and the self is defined that encompasses that encompasses morality for everyone as part of a group. "I am because we are". It is clear that no single value appears that is morality for everyone although do no harm and act that you care come very close.

In understanding our trainees, one needs to understand the structure and vicissitudes of their family constellation. The family constellation that is described in the West is the nuclear family. However, for many of our trainees, the model is the extended family, not the nuclear family. The extended family structure, which is the mode in Asia, leads to intense emotional interconnectedness that deeply affects their members. These intimate relationships in the extended family are hierarchical in nature, in which the superior is expected to be nurturing and responsible and the subordinate is deferential and obedient. In these circumstances, the expectation that the student therapist will see the learning relationship to his or her supervisor as egalitarian seems hopelessly naïve. The supervisor is expected to be nurturing, empathically responsive, responsible, and supportive of the student's self-esteem. Maintenance of self-esteem may take precedence over the truth in what may be seen as a contextual conscience. The supervisor may be seen as a family elder, a mentor, or a teacher who is expected to give advice and is hard to criticize directly [24]-[28].

From such an extended family constellation with its attendant expectations and experiences arises a self-structure that is of a familial-group nature and not an individualized self. It is more a We-self than the I-self that is seen in the West. When the self is of a we-type, there are increased concerns about self-esteem, greater dependency and interdependency, a dual self-structure, social and secret, which supports the highly situational conscience of the We-self with its contextual construction of truth. The search for individuality, self-fulfillment, and freedom from parental control that might be seen as a general goal of therapy is going to be seen as selfish, irresponsible, and disobedient by IMG residents with the values that accompany being raised in an extended family. The confrontations with one's own beliefs necessary to becoming a psychiatrist/therapist are more difficult as access to the secret self, make holding contrary views less disturbing and a commitment to the unity and consistency of the personality less necessary.

Roland [25] believes we listen to our patients, and I would add our trainees, based on our own culture. Our norms may view Asian values such as dependency and interdependency, deference and receptivity to superiors, communication by indirect techniques, maintaining and enhancing self-esteem at all costs, and seeing truth as situational as inferior. We may cling to our values of independence and autonomy, self-assertiveness and self-promotion in egalitarian relationships, verbal articulateness and forthrightness, and frank criticism in expressing the truth as superior.

Given the extent to which individualism and the nuclear family are defining themes of American culture, not understanding this centrality may become a stumbling block for many IMGs in internalizing a system of values at odds with their core beliefs. The awareness of these issues by supervisors of residents from cultures with extended families may alert the supervisor to some of the sources of the learning problems his supervisee's may be having in becoming a psychiatrist.

How might we attempt to meet the educational challenge that IMGs present in psychiatric residency? The participation of psychologically informed psychiatrists as paid and volunteer faculty in residency programs is to be promoted. Residency programs need to become more receptive to the participation of volunteer faculty.

The psychiatric resident needs more experience in treating patients in psychodynamic-psychotherapy and needs more supervision informed by a recognition of the cultural dissonance the IMGs may be experiencing. A psychotherapeutic experience for residents is to be encouraged. Psychological theory and understanding need to be introduced from the start of the residents' experience and applied in non-psychotherapy contexts (e.g., medication follow-ups and inpatient care). Residents must be provided with courses in American culture that deal with the values and beliefs that underpin the attitudes and behaviors of Americans and that are linked to the history of the American people. Language adequacy and accent reduction must be guaranteed. Structured instruction with verbal recitation, written exams, and explicit feedback, the value of which was demonstrated in a program helping individuals who failed the boards to pass them [29] needs to be coupled with an increase in demonstration and practice interviews. It is incumbent upon us to understand the cultural sources of the values and needs of our residents to enhance their learning experience.

Mentoring by interested faculty is to be encouraged with the goal of facilitating the residents' entry into the mainstream of American psychiatry. Mentoring which involves working together on a joint project is extremely valuable For example, my Maimonides experience-working together over a 4 years period with 27 residents lead to 31 local talks, 6 regional presentations and 19 national ones and 9 publications. Six of the groups are currently in academic careers.

3. Conclusion

Professionalism, one of the core competencies that residents must achieve, requires special attention in the training of IMGs. Not all countries have the same standards and do not share the same values. Those from Asia [30] and Africa [31] are least likely to aspire to the same medical values while those from the English speaking countries [32] are more likely to have values similar to ours. We are at a time when our own standards are in flux making the understanding even more difficult. The literature is directed at professionalism education for medical students more than to residents. In clinical practice the primacy of the patient is not a universally held view, but in resident education the primacy of the student-resident must be our view.

Conflict of Interest

The author states that there is no conflict of interest.

References

[1] Alberti, M. (2013) Warnings of Doctor Shortage Go Unheeded/Remapping the Debate: Asking Why and Why Not. http://www.remappingdebate.org./article warning-doctor shortage-go-unheeded-1-3

[2] Carlat, D. (2010) 45,000 More Psychiatrists, Anyone. *Psychiatric Times.* http://psychiatrictimes.com/blog/couchincrisis/content/article/10168/1566084

[3] Blanco, C., Carvalho, C., Olfson, M., Finnerty, M. and Pincus, H. (1999) Practice Patterns of International and U.S. Medical Graduate Psychiatrists. *American Journal of Psychiatry*, **156**, 445-450.

[4] Rao, N. (1999) International Medical Graduates. In Kay, J., Silberman, E. and Pessar, L., Eds., *Handbook of Psychiatric Education and Faculty Development*, American Psychiatric Association, Washington, DC, 125-142.

[5] American Psychiatric Association (2013) Diagnostic and Statistical Manual of Mental Disorders. 5th Edition, APPI Press, Washington, DC.

[6] Gangure, D. (2002) International Medical Graduates in American Training Programs. *XII World Psychiatry Congress of Psychiatry.*

[7] Knoff, W., Oken, D. and Prevost, J. (1976) Meeting Training Needs of Foreign Psychiatric Residents in State Hospitals. *Hospital and Community Psychiatry*, **27**, 35-37.

[8] Whelan, G., Gary, N., Kostis, J., Boulet, J. and Hallock, J. (2002) The Changing Pool of International Medical Graduates Seeking Certification in US Graduate Medical Education Programs. *JAMA*, **288**, 1079-1084. http://dx.doi.org/10.1001/jama.288.9.1079

[9] Mick, S. and Comfort, M. (1997) The Quality of Care of International Medical Graduates. How Does It Compare to That of U.S. Medical Graduates. *Medical Care Research and Review*, **54**, 379-413. http://dx.doi.org/10.1177/107755879705400401

[10] Norcini, J., Boulet, J., Dauphinee, W., Opalek, A., Kranz, I. and Anderson, S. (2010) Evaluating the Quality of Care Provided by Graduates of International Medical Schools. *Health Affairs*, **29**, 1461-1468. http://dx.doi.org/10.1377/hlthaff.2009.0222

[11] Kramer, M. (2005) The Educational Needs of International Medical Graduates in Psychiatric Residency. *Academic Psychiatry*, **29**, 322-324. http://dx.doi.org/10.1176/appi.ap.29.3.322-a

[12] Kramer, M. (2006) Educational Challenges of International Medical Graduates in Psychiatric Residencies. *The Journal of the American Academy of Psychoanalysis and Dynamic Psychiatry*, **34**, 163-171. http://dx.doi.org/10.1521/jaap.2006.34.1.163

[13] Alexander, F. and Selesnick, T. (1966) The History of Psychiatry. Harper and Row, New York.

[14] Kandel, E. and Schwartz, J. (1985) Principles of Neural Science. 2nd Edition, Elsevier, New York.

[15] Shorter, E. (1997) A History of Psychiatry. Wiley, New York.

[16] Akhtar, S. (1999) Immigration and Identity. Aronson, Northvale.

[17] Weintraub, W. (1997) International Medical Graduates as Psychiatric Residents: One Training Director's Experience. In: Husain, S., Munoz, R. and Balon, R., Eds., *International Medical Graduates in the United States*, American Psychiatric Press, Washington DC, 53-64.

[18] Balon, R. (2000) Practice Patterns of International Medical Graduates. *American Journal of Psychiatry*, **157**, 485. http://dx.doi.org/10.1176/appi.ajp.157.3.485-a

[19] Brody, E., Modarressi, T., Penna, M., Jegede, R. and Arana, J. (1971) Intellectual and Emotional Problems of Foreign Residents Learning Psychiatric Theory and Practice. *Psychiatry*, **34**, 238-247.

[20] Char, W. (1971) The Foreign Resident: An Ambivalently Valued Object. *Psychiatry*, **34**, 234-238.

[21] Beaubrun, M. (1971) Foreign Medical Training and the "Brain Drain". *Psychiatry*, **34**, 247-251.

[22] Campbell, J. (1988) The Power of Myth. Doubleday & Co., New York, 117.

[23] Lasch, C. (1991) The Culture of Narcissism. Norton, New York.

[24] Vozzola, E. (2014) Moral Development: Theory and Applications. Routledge, New York.

[25] Roland, A. (2003) Psychoanalysis across Civilizations: A Personal Journey. *The Journal of the American Academy of Psychoanalysis and Dynamic Psychiatry*, **31**, 275-295. http://dx.doi.org/10.1521/jaap.31.2.275.22118

[26] Desai, P. and Coelho, G. (1980) Indian Immigration in America: Some Cultural Aspects of Psychological Adaptation. In: Seran, P. and Eames, E., Eds., *The New Ethics: Asian Indians in the United States*, Praeger, New York, 363-386.

[27] Desai, P. (1982) Learning Psychotherapy: A Cultural Perspective. *Journal of Operational Psychiatry*, **13**, 82-87.

[28] Lijtmaer, R. (2001) Countertransference and Ethnicity: The Analyst's Psychic Changes. *Journal of the American Academy of Psychoanalysis*, **29**, 73-83. http://dx.doi.org/10.1521/jaap.29.1.73.17194

[29] Rao, N. (2005) Personal Communication One Day Training to Help Pass Psychiatric Boards. Unpublished Paper.

[30] Plotnikoff, G. and Amano, T. (2007) A Culturally Appropriate, Student Centered Curriculum on Medical Professionalism. Successful Innovations at Keio University in Tokyo. *Minnesota Medicine*, **90**, 42-43.

[31] Van Rooyen, M. (2004) The Views of Medical Students on Professionalism in South Africa. *South African Family Practice*, **46**, 28-31. http://dx.doi.org/10.1080/20786204.2004.10873030

[32] Campbell, J., Roberts, M., Wright, C., Hill, J., Greco, M., Taylor, M. and Richards, S. (2011) Factors Associated with Variability in the Assessment of U.K. Doctor's Professionalism: Analysis of Survey Results. *British Medical Journal*, **343**, d6212. http://dx.doi.org/10.1136/bmj.d6212

17

Interprofessional Communication and Relationships in the Management of "Difficult to Treat" Depression: Perceptions of the Role of General Practitioners

Kay M. Jones*, Leon Piterman

Office of the Pro Vice-Chancellor, Peninsula Campus, Monash University, Frankston, Australia
Email: *kay.jones@monash.edu

Abstract

Background: Team based care is an essential ingredient of chronic disease management including chronic mental illness. Effective health care teams include members who have defined, yet intersecting roles, where mutual respect characterises professional interaction and the patient's wellbeing is central. The aim was to explore the perception of psychologists, psychiatry registrars and psychiatrists with respect to GPs' role in managing difficult-to-treat-depression (DTTD). Methods: A previously developed semi-structured interview schedule comprising six questions was used. Thirty-two health professionals participated. Data were analysed using the Framework method. Findings: Four main themes emerged: 1) The team approach was important, particularly to ensure information accuracy and/or when responding to patient needs and pressures; 2) Referrals, usually generated by GPs can be a vehicle for other health professionals to provide advice to the GP; 3) Availability and accessibility often depended on health professionals work location and knowing how to navigate the system; 4) Limited availability of government funding impacts on patients' accessibility to health professionals. Discussion: Interprofessional relationships were described as paramount. Appropriate and timely referrals are integral to patient management, regardless of challenges. Ongoing challenges include program funding, workforce numbers and costs to patients. Improvement to mental health care access was noted, even for patients among relatively disadvantaged groups and those receiving Medicare Benefits Schedule-subsidised services. Conclusion: Despite adequate GP/specialist communication, the delivery of optimal team based care to patients with difficult-to-treat depression is compromised by lack of access to specialised services and inadequate funding.

---

*Corresponding author.

Keywords

Depression, Perceptions, Psychiatry

1. Background

Team based care is an essential ingredient of chronic disease management [1] including the management of chronic or relapsing mental illness, major depression and difficult to treat depression (DTTD) falling into this category. Effective health care teams are those whose members have defined, yet intersecting roles, where mutual respect characterises professional interaction. In all cases, the patient's well-being should be at the centre of team based decision making and care.

While legal, ethical and professional requirements may vary, interpersonal relationships between general practitioners (GPs) and care team professionals are contextually and systematically determined [2]. Thus, many factors may influence the success, or otherwise, of inter-professional/multidisciplinary service provision including the structure of the care delivery pathway, funding models, practice culture, types of information, activities, and services or funding exchanges as well as the relationship governance in terms of accountability, professionalism, autonomy and power [3]. Although issues such as lack of time and inter-professional communication difficulties may arise [4]-[6], health professionals have reported beneficial changes in attitudes and knowledge as a result of experience gained from working with other professionals, understanding their roles and knowledge, communication and administrative systems [6].

Referrals are an important form of communication between the GP and other health professionals. They require a clear explanation of the problem with adequate patient history from the GP, a response outlining diagnosis and management, justification for the course of action from the care team professional/s; and the patient expects a clear explanation that describes the diagnosis, treatment and follow-up requirements. When this information is not provided, some or all involved in the process may become dissatisfied [7].

In Australia, team-based models of primary care have emerged in response to health system changes and challenges such as complex patient profiles, patient expectations and health system demands [8]. Overwhelmingly, the introduction by the Australian Government of the Better Access to Psychiatrists, Psychologists and General Practitioners (GPs) (the Better Access initiative) [9], has made services more accessible and more affordable for individuals who experience mental health disorders. GPs are providing more mental health services than in the past; patients now have access to psychological services that were previously less affordable and/or accessible, and there have been some changes to the way some psychiatrists provide care, including partnerships between the public and private psychiatric services [9]-[12]. In 2010-2011, $6.9 billion was spent in Australia on mental health for national and state programs and initiatives [13].

Depending on the patient's needs, a care team may include a psychologist, psychiatry registrar and/or psychiatrist, social worker, counsellor to whom patients may have been referred by a GP. Apart from work previously published by this team [14]-[16], no literature could be found describing care team members' thoughts about GPs' role in the management of patients diagnosed with DTTD, or about care team members' interactions.

The aim of this qualitative research was to explore the perception of psychologists, psychiatry registrars and psychiatrists with respect to GPs' role in managing DTTD.

2. Methods

For the purpose of this paper, the description of DTTD as "most often conceptualized in terms of repeated failures to ameliorate depressive symptoms" is used [17].

2.1. Sample Recruitment

A convenience sample was recruited via emails which were forwarded to GPs in 2011, psychologists and psychiatry registrars in mid-2012, and psychiatrists early in 2014. All had links to Monash University, and/or the Monash Medical Centre (a public hospital in Melbourne, Australia). When potential participants responded and agreed to participate, they provided and/or confirmed their contact details (email) to the research team for the purpose of the research team advising time, date and venue for the focus group [18] [19].

2.2. Data Collection and Analysis

A semi-structured interview schedule comprising six headings was developed for interviews and/or focus groups with GPs [14], psychologists [16] psychiatry registrars [15] and psychiatrists.

Data were collected in Melbourne in late 2011(GPs), mid 2012 (psychologists and psychiatry registrars) and early 2014 (psychiatrists). The interviews lasted approximately thirty-to-forty five minutes; the focus groups lasted approximately ninety minutes. All were audio-taped and transcribed verbatim. Apart from gender, profession and workplace experience (public/private, urban/rural) no other demographic data were collected.

Data were analysed using the Framework Method [20] to understand participants' perspectives. Data were analysed manually and independently by the investigators. When there was a difference of opinion, the issues were discussed and agreement reached [20]. Findings, including discussion are reported under the interview schedule's six headings. Comments are reported for GPs as GPFG 1-5 and GPIV 1-5, for psychologists as P1-P7, for psychiatry registrars as PR 1-10, and for psychiatrists as PS1-5.

Ethics approval to conduct the study was obtained from Monash University Human Research Ethics Committee (MUHREC) and Monash Health.

3. Findings

Findings are reported under the four main themes that emerged from the data.

3.1. Participants

Group	Females	Males	Experience in public (Pu)/private (Pr)	Experience in urban (U)/rural (R)
GPs	3	7	10 (Pu & Pr)	8 (U) 2 (R)
Psychologists	5	2	7 (Pu & Pr)	5 (U) 2 (R)
Psychiatry registrars	6	4	10 (Pu)	10 (U)
Psychiatrists	0	5	5 (Pu & Pr)	5 (U)
Total	**14**	**18**		

1) *Significance of relationship between the GP and other health professionals*

"The relationship between the GP and other health professionals is vital, and for the patient: it's a matter of the GP finding the right professional for the patient" (GPIV2).

Psychologists reported working in both the public and private sections of the health system in Australia and receive referrals and patient histories from GPs and other health professionals who may be involved in the patient's primary care. When clarification was needed, the most important starting point for the psychologist was usually the GP, for example, contacting the GP to check if the GP has tried different medications, because the patient may be treatment resistant was considered important. However, conflicting with the importance of the interaction between professionals was their availability:

"GPs can't always be readily accessed, particularly those who work in multiple clinics, thus setting up meetings with the GP, psychologist and psychiatrist can be difficult" (P5).

The psychiatry registrars described GPs as knowing the patients and building a relationship with them, and that GPs are holistic practitioners who see a range of people, have a sense of what else may be going on, can often clearly say what's happening and who are often really good for connectedness with the patient and it's that connectedness and that can help. But again:

"Time constraints and busy schedules were identified as difficulties for some GPs" (PR6).

Psychiatry registrars revealed insights into the difficulties experienced by GPs. They felt that GPs may be challenged by some patients' behaviour, such as those at risk of suicide and those who make demands for prescription drugs or referrals, adding pressure for the GP either because of time constraints or the GP not wanting to be seen to be doing nothing. Subsequently, for GPs or any health professional in a care team, patient pressures and lack of time can impact on relationships with patients and interactions with other health professionals because:

"More often than not, by the time the patient gets to the psychiatry registrar's clinic, private or public, they've already been treated by the GP and sometimes have also seen a psychologist" (PR2).

Psychiatrists also described the importance of the team approach:

"We work in conjunction with the GP and the team might include a psychologist or a social worker or other allied health professionals such as an occupational therapist" (PS4).

2) Referring and management

"Referrals are usually from GPs to care-team health professionals with GPs often receiving regular feedback from their patients about the specialists to whom they were referred" (GPIV5).

From the psychologists perspective co-morbidities might impede the psychologist's ability to engage the patient, particularly patients with progressive illness, progressive degenerative illness such as early dementia or Parkinsons or MS where there's a cognitive element that might be contributing biologically to a lack of motivation that may impact on treatment. While psychologists may refer a patient on to a psychiatrist, generally they would go back to the referrer who is usually the GP with a recommendation for the particular patient. Psychologists also noted that in some instances, referrals need to be made in a specific way, for example via a mental health care plan in order to access a government subsidised service, and to work collaboratively and support GPs:

"Some psychologists may write to the GP advising what services are available and how the GP can refer, because some GPs have no idea about these services and don't have time, so the psychologist's input makes it easier for the GP to refer" (P7).
"It's about finding the balance of being able to give the GP the information, or pointing them in the direction and making a recommendation" (P4, P5).

From the psychiatry registrars' perspective, it was the referring GP who knows and builds a relationship with the patient and understands their life, their paths, their psycho-social stressors and the way the patient relates to others, including the GP:

"I find that if I have been asked to see somebody by another member of the medical team and then I call the GP, the GP can often very clearly say what and why this is happening" (PR5).
"But, by virtue of being a psychiatry registrar in a public hospital, we're the second line already" (PR10).

In addition to receiving referrals from GPs, psychiatrists may refer to other health professionals including psychologists, occupational therapists and social workers in public as well as private practice. Hence they are:
"Inextricably linked to the GP through the referral and health system" (PS5).
3) Availability and accessibility of health professionals

"Deinstitutionalisation of mental health patients in Australia in the late 1980's and 1990's resulted in significant numbers of patients with a mental health diagnosis being placed in the community without the resources there to support them: this resulted in some hard times in the 1990's in just trying to pick up the pieces there for a while" (GPIV1).

More recently, while GPs endeavour to manage patients via access to primary mental health teams to provide support and assist with patients' treatment, availability and accessibility can depend on whether the health professional is working in the public or private sector of the health system in Australia. Currently, not all patients are referred to psychiatrists for a range of reasons:

"Including lack of availability and difficulty in getting an appointment, whether in the public or private sectors and particularly in the rural areas" (GPIV 1, GPIV4).

Psychologists also found difficulty accessing various services, but acknowledged that mental health support and services have been more accessible in recent years because of the Medicare rebate available via the "Better

Access" initiative. With more psychologists and social workers working in the community there are significantly more health professionals to access for the patient management and treatment. Nonetheless challenges remain within the systems, for example:

"There's a certain language that needs to be used with triage to either speed up the referral or to ensure that referral's heard and I think that's still a difficulty" (P3).
"Sometimes you have to be pretty assertive and that's pretty hard" (P1).

While most services have clear admission criteria requirements, sometimes stigmatising can preclude some patients such as those with co-morbidity or substance abuse. Thus, regardless the best endeavours and support of all health professionals involved:

"Making those referrals is actually more difficult because the person's not particularly attractive for the accepting service to pick up. That still happens, yep" (P5).

From the psychiatry registrars' perspective it's not about availability and accessibility because, for them, some of the social issues can be delegated to the social workers and:

"Being psychiatry registrars in a public hospital we're second line already" (PR3).

Psychiatrists raised the issue of containment:

"Rather than availability and accessibility or management options, sometimes for psychotic patients it's about containment, whether it's in the community or in a patient unit using medication" (PS3).

4) *Funding/financial issues*
Sustainable government supported funding models are essential for effective care delivery.
Changes in government funding and programs in Australia have impacted on initiatives delivered in the community and on the health professionals involved:

"Our general practice was part of a primary health team initiative (the Better Access program), a psychologist came to the practice once every three to four weeks for around two years, but the funding and program closed and subsequently, the service discontinued" (GPIV 1).

Psychologists raised similar issues including queries around government funded consultations with psychologists and psychiatrists, and the limits on the number of visits under the Medicare "Better Access" program:

"There's always some patients who can't afford the cost, which can result in patients deciding to stop seeing the psychologist and probably end up back at the GP" (P3, P6, P7).

Psychiatry registrars and psychiatrists expressed concerns about the nexus between hospital and community based treatment. If government subsidised community based services are not available, discharge planning may be delayed:

"In some suburbs it is more difficult again because of patients' limited resources which would factor into decision making about discharging a patient" (PR5).
"Despite funding for various electronic forms of communication, such as psychiatry on line or telephone counselling service, which are government supported, few utilise these options" (GPFG3, GPFG5).

3.2. Summary of Key Findings

Four main themes emerged:
   1) The team approach is paramount, particularly to ensure information is accurate and/or when responding to patient needs and pressures.
   2) Referrals are usually generated by GPs; they can be a vehicle for other health professionals to provide advice to the GP, and may need to be made in a specific way in order to access a particular service.
   3) Availability and accessibility often depended on where the health professional works (public or private), knowing how to navigate the system, and being aware that some patients may be stigmatised and some may need containment.

4) Changes in government <u>funding</u> and programs, particularly the limited availability of "bulk-billing" impacts on patients' accessibility to health professionals, resulting in patients some being treated by the GP only.

4. Discussion

This paper is one of few that describes the thoughts of health professionals about GPs' role in the management of patients diagnosed with difficult-to-treat depression or about the care team member's interactions [14]-[16].

As previously reported [5] [8] [9] [11], participants in this research also identified the GP as usually being the most accessible medical resource in the community and the first point of professional contact for many people seeking help with mental health problems. Similarly, the interprofessional relationship between the GP and other health professionals was described as paramount, particularly when multiple health professionals are involved in a patients' management.

In the past, access to mental health services was limited due to workforce shortage, uneven geographical distribution and access barriers including affordability [5] [10]. For example, prior to June 2008, only GPs could refer patients to the "Access to Allied Psychological Services (ATAPS)" (a component of the Better Outcomes initiative) but in June 2008, policy changes included the introduction of the Suicide prevention program and extending "who" could refer to ATAPS to include mental health services and psychiatrists [11]. Outcomes described in the "Better Access" initiative evaluations [9]-[11] [13] were reflected in participants responses, particularly the provision of support for GPs, referral pathways for appropriate treatment by psychologists, psychiatrists and other appropriately trained mental health professionals, the benefits of the team approach and improving affordable access for patients to services.

General consensus was that appropriate and timely referral was integral to patient management, regardless of challenges such as patients not responding to psychological or psychiatric management [14]. Specific issues identified as impacting on referral process included accessibility and communication. Previous research suggests that communication can be improved by utilising formal and informal meetings [12], improving letter writing skills [4] particularly for referrals [7] and utilising networking and interprofessional education which may help these professionals work more effectively in team based care [8] [9] [12].

All noted that the availability and accessibility of GPs, psychologists, psychiatry registrars and psychiatrists, particularly in rural areas, were described as ongoing challenges [5] [10] [13] [14]. Tied to availability and accessibility, are the costs for the patient and program funding by the government, but despite the gap between fee and rebate, improvement to access of mental health care was noted, even for patients among relatively disadvantaged groups in the community and those receiving Medicare Benefits Schedule-subsidised services, including bulk-billing (government supported fees) [9] [10] [13].

5. Conclusion

While the generalisability of this study may be limited because of the small number of participants, this study is the first to contribute to gaining some insight into care team members' thoughts about the GPs' role in the management of patients diagnosed with DTTD, or about care team members' interactions. Psychiatrists, psychiatry registrars and psychologists all acknowledged the pivotal role of GPs in managing mental illness. Whilst in relative terms the Australian health care system is working, significant constraints related to accessibility and funding to support specialized care and team based care compromise care for patients with mental illness in particular those with major depression or DTTD. Regardless of the level and content of interprofessional communication and relationships, more funding is needed to make interprofessional communication more meaningful and effective for the fee-for-service health care delivery system in Australia.

Conflict of Interest

None.

References

[1]   Wagner, E.H. (1998) Chronic Disease Management: What Will It Take to Improve Care for Chronic Illness? *Effective Clinical Practice*, **1**, 2-4.

[2]   Piterman, L. and Koritsas, S. (2005) Part 1 General Practitioner—Specialist Relationship. *Internal Medicine Journal*,

35, 430-434. http://dx.doi.org/10.1111/j.1445-5994.2005.00855.x

[3]   Bowers, E.J. (2010) How Does Teamwork Support GPs and Allied Health Professionals to Work Together? PHCRIS.

[4]   Sain, K., Shah, N. and Hasan, S. (2012) GPs' Views on the Content and Quality of Psychiatrists' Clinic Letters. *Progress in Neurology and Psychiatry*, **16**, 6-10. http://dx.doi.org/10.1002/pnp.223

[5]   (2006) Senate Select Committee Mental Health: A National Approach to Mental Health—From Crisis to Community. Final Report. Senate Select Committee, Commonwealth of Australia, Canberra.

[6]   Goldman, J., Meuser, J., Rogers, J., Lawrie, L. and Reeves, S. (2010) Interprofessional Collabaoration in Family Health Teams. *Canadian Family Physician*, **56**, e368-e374.

[7]   Piterman, L. and Koritsas, S. (2005) Part II General Practitioner—Specialist Referral Process. *Internal Medicine Journal*, **35**, 491-496. http://dx.doi.org/10.1111/j.1445-5994.2005.00860.x

[8]   Nacarella, L., Greenstock, L.N. and Brooks, P.M. (2012) A Framework to Support Team-Based Models of Primary Care within the Australian Health Care System. *MJA Open*, **1**, 22-25. http://dx.doi.org/10.5694/mjao12.10069

[9]   Pirkis, J., Harris, M., Hall, W. and Ftanou, M. (2011) Evaluation of the Better Access to Psychiatrists, Psychologists and General Practitioners through the Medicare Benefits Schedule Initiative. Summative Evaluation, Final Report. Centre for Health Policy, Programs and Economics, The University of Melbourne.

[10]   (2010) Department of Health and Ageing: Evaluation of the Better Access Initiative Final Report. Department of Health and Ageing.

[11]   Fletcher, J., King, K., Bassilios, B., Reifels, L., Blashki, G., Burgess, P. and Pirkis, J. (2012) Evaluating the Access to Allied Psychological Services (ATAPS) Program. Centre for Health Policy Programs and Economics, University of Melbourne. https://ataps-mds.com/site/assets/.../19th_interim_evaluation_report.pdf

[12]   Yung, A., Gill, L., Somerville, E., Dowling, B., Simon, K., Pirkis, J., Livingston, J., Schweitzer, I., Tanaghow, A., Herrman, H., *et al.* (2005) Public and Private Psychiatry: Can They Work Together and Is It Worth the Effort? *Australian and New Zealand Journal of Psychiatry*, **39**, 67-73. http://dx.doi.org/10.1080/j.1440-1614.2005.01511.x

[13]   Department of Health and Ageing (2013) National Mental Health Report 2013: Tracking Progress of Mental Health Reform in Australia 1993-2011. Commonwealth of Australia, Canberra.

[14]   Jones, K.M., Castle, D.J. and Piterman, L. (2012) Difficult-to-Treat-Depression: What Do General Practitioners Think? *MJA Open*, **1**, 6-8. http://dx.doi.org/10.5694/mjao12.10566

[15]   Jones, K.M. and Piterman, L. (2014) Difficult-to-Treat-Depression and GPs' Role: Perceptions of Psychiatry Registrars. *Open Journal of Psychiatry*, **4**, 301-308. http://dx.doi.org/10.4236/ojpsych.2014.44037

[16]   Jones, K.M. and Piterman, L. (2014) Difficult-to-Treat-Depression and GP's Role: Perceptions of Psychologists. *Open Journal of Psychiatry*, **5**, 31-38. http://dx.doi.org/10.4236/ojpsych.2015.51005

[17]   Grote, N.K. and Frank, E. (2003) Difficult-to-Treat Depression: The Role of Contexts and Comorbidities. *Society of Biological Psychiatry*, **53**, 660-670. http://dx.doi.org/10.1016/S0006-3223(03)00006-4

[18]   Liamputtong, P. and Ezzey, D. (2005) Qualitataive Research Methods. Oxford University Press, Melbourne.

[19]   Polgar, S. and Thomas, S. (2005) Introduction to Research in the Health Sciences. Elsevier Churchill Livingstone, Sydney.

[20]   Ritchie, J. and Spencer, L. (1994) Qualitative Data Analysis for Applied Policy Research. In: Bryman, A. and Burgess, B., Eds., *Analyzing Qualitative Data*, Routledge, London. http://dx.doi.org/10.4324/9780203413081_chapter_9

18

Cerebral Bioavailability of Silexan— A Quantitative EEG Study in Healthy Volunteers

Wilfried Dimpfel[1], Winfried Wedekind[2], Angelika Dienel[3]

[1]Justus-Liebig-University c/o NeuroCode AG, Wetzlar, Germany
[2]NeuroCode AG, Wetzlar, Germany
[3]Dr. Willmar Schwabe GmbH & Co. KG, Karlsruhe, Germany
Email: angelika.dienel@schwabe.de

Abstract

Background: A quantitative EEG (qEEG) study was performed to investigate the cerebral bioavailability of Silexan. Method: Twenty-four male and female healthy volunteers between 20 and 62 years of age were eligible for participation and received 160 or 80 mg/day Silexan or placebo in randomised order according to a 3-way crossover design. Treatment phases of 14 days were separated by 14-day washout periods. qEEG recordings in conditions "eyes open", "eyes closed", as well as during performance of 3 different cognitive tasks, were performed at 0, 1, 2, 3, and 4 h after drug administration on the first (single-dose assessment) and last day of each treatment period (repetitive dose assessment). Result: Compared with placebo, qEEG analysis revealed a significant increase of spectral power within two hours in the alpha1 range (7.0 - 9.5 Hz), particularly in the fronto-temporal region, where it was more pronounced after administration of Silexan 160 mg/day than after the 80 mg/day dose. Changes in other frequency bands were mainly attributable to circadian rhythm. No EEG changes typically seen during the investigation of sedative drugs (general theta increase) were observed. Cognitive task performance under both doses of Silexan was not inferior compared with that in the placebo period. Conclusions: The study provides evidence that ingredients of the anxiolytic lavender oil preparation Silexan penetrate the blood-brain barrier and induce functional changes in the CNS. The types of changes observed in the qEEG are consistent with the anxiolytic clinical effect of the drug represented by increases of alpha1 spectral power. No sedative effects were observed. Silexan was well tolerated during repetitive administration of doses up to twice the marketed dose.

Keywords

Silexan, Clinical Trial, Cerebral Bioavailability, qEEG, CATEEM

1. Introduction

Herbal preparations are multi-ingredient compounds whose bioavailability is difficult to assess. Bioavailability can depend on chemical complexity of the herb due to synergistic and antagonistic actions of their constituents in promoting absorption, hydrophobic or lipophilic properties influencing the ability to cross luminal wall, gut microflora and hepatic activity of the individual, and chemical modifications of the herbal constituents [1]. This is one reason why establishing the pharmacological basis for efficacy of herbal medicinal products remains a constant challenge [2].

Psychotropic drugs act primarily on the central nervous system (CNS), and thus their cerebral bioavailability is of interest. To be effective in the CNS constituents of a herbal drug have to cross the blood brain barrier. In man, the cerebral bioavailability of psychotropic herbal drugs, like that of any other psychotropic drug, can be assessed using non-invasive methods of quantitative pharmaco-electroencephalography (qEEG; [3]). For decades the technique has been used as a standard procedure for the prediction of whether, where, how, when, and in which dosage the investigated compound acts on the brain [4]. Since their introduction in the 1950s [5] [6], qEEG methods have undergone a still ongoing evolution, supported by the increasing availability of powerful computational resources. In order to obtain an objective quantitative analysis time-dependent voltage level recordings from a pair of electrodes are converted into a spectrogram using Fast Fourier Transformation (FFT) in which pre-defined frequency bands are characterised by their respective electric power.

A major step towards a better understanding of the action of pharmacological substances on the brain was the development of methods of EEG assessments such as Computer-Aided Topographical Electro-Encephalometry (CATEEM®; [7] [8]) which started during the 1990s. In CATEEM® the spectral power of the frequency bands obtained for different electrode locations is transformed into a set of spectral colours that are mixed according to an additive model to generate a brain map that visualises the distribution of the spectral frequencies over the areas of the cerebral cortex. The investigation of spectral frequency changes in different brain regions can be used for assessing the effects of investigational drugs on the electric activity of the brain as well as for comparing the observed frequency patterns with those of other substances, which have a well-characterised clinical effect [9]. In phytopharmaceutical research CATEEM® technology has been used in a rat model for the classification of herbal extracts by means of comparison to spectral EEG signatures induced by synthetic drugs [10] as well as for the analysis of neurophysiological changes following herbal drug administration in humans (e.g., [11]).

Silexan[1], the essential oil produced from *Lavandula angustifolia*, is the active substance of a medicinal product for oral use, which is authorised in Germany for the treatment of restlessness accompanying anxious moods, with a recommended dose of 80 mg once daily. Randomised, double-blind clinical trials have shown that Silexan is a potent anxiolytic drug. In sub-syndromal anxiety disorder Silexan was superior to placebo in reducing the total score of the Hamilton Anxiety Scale (HAMA; [12]) during 10 weeks of treatment [13]. Patients suffering from restlessness, agitation, and disturbed sleep also showed a more pronounced HAMA total score reduction when treated with Silexan than those who received placebo [14]. In patients with syndromal generalised anxiety disorder (GAD) Silexan was superior to placebo and comparably efficacious as paroxetine [15] and as lorazepam [16].

This study was performed to substantiate the psychopharmacological effect of Silexan and to supplement information derived from therapeutic clinical trials, by investigating the bioavailability of the herbal compound in the human CNS using methods of qEEG.

2. Methods

2.1. Design Overview, Ethical Conduct

The study was a double-blind, placebo-controlled, single-centre, 3-period crossover trial during which healthy volunteers received single and repetitive doses of 160 mg/day and 80 mg/day Silexan and placebo in 1 out of 3 randomised sequences.

The study protocol was reviewed and approved by competent authority and by an independent ethics committee (Ethik-Kommission bei der Landesärztekammer Hessen, FF84/2010). All subjects provided written informed consent. The principles of Good Clinical Practice and the Declaration of Helsinki were adhered to.

---

[1]Silexan® (WS® 1265) is the active substance of Lasea® (Dr. Willmar Schwabe GmbH & Co. KG, Karlsruhe, Germany).

2.2. Participants

Study participants were recruited through advertisement. Male and female healthy volunteers between 18 and 65 years of age were eligible for participation. Female participants of childbearing potential were required to have a negative pregnancy test and to use adequate double contraception. Subjects who had participated in any other clinical trial within 3 months before enrolment, who suffered from any acute medical condition, who had a history of diseases of relevant vital organs, of the CNS, or of gastrointestinal disorders that could influence the absorption of orally administered drugs, were excluded. Moreover, subjects with known hypersensitivity to Lavender preparations, with relevantly abnormal safety laboratory values or vital signs, or with massive deviations from normal quantitative EEG parameters were also ineligible.

Smoking up to a maximum of 25 cigarettes per day as well as regular alcohol consumption not exceeding 20 g per day, were permitted. Any medical or recreational drugs, including over-the-counter preparations and dietary supplements, which could have an effect on the CNS or otherwise interfere with the EEG assessments, were prohibited during and within 2 weeks before trial participation.

2.3. Interventions, Blinding, Randomisation

Silexan (WS® 1265) is a patented active substance with an essential oil produced from *Lavandula angustifolia* flowers by steam distillation that complies with the monograph Lavender oil of the European Pharmacopoeia (Ph. Eur.). It exceeds the quality definition of the Ph. Eur. with respect to items important for efficacy and tolerability. The study treatments were available in identical, immediate release soft gelatine capsules. During each treatment phase one capsule of the appropriate study medication was administered at about 8:00 h in the morning with non-sparkling water at room temperature for 14 consecutive days. The study participants received 160 mg or 80 mg Silexan or placebo.

2.4. Study Schedule and Assessments

Following a screening examination which included assessments of medical history, safety laboratory measures, ECG, vital signs as well as a physical examination, eligible subjects were randomised and received the investigational treatments in the allocated sequence. The 3 treatment periods of 14 days' duration were separated by 14-day washout phases. EEG examinations were performed on the first and last day of each treatment period on which the subjects were confined to the investigative unit and received standardised meals. The subjects were questioned for any adverse events during all post-screening visits. A safety follow-up examination was performed within 1 week after study drug discontinuation.

On the examination days the subjects were requested to appear at the experimental unit in time and without prior study medication intake so that the assessments could start at 8 h in the morning. Following a brief introduction and check-up qEEG recordings of 25 minutes' duration were performed at pre-dose as well as at 1 h, 2 h, 3 h, and 4 h post dose (**Figure 1**). During the recordings the subjects sat alone in a separate, quiet room in a comfortable easy chair with light dimmed. A baseline recording of 6 min under the condition of "eyes open"

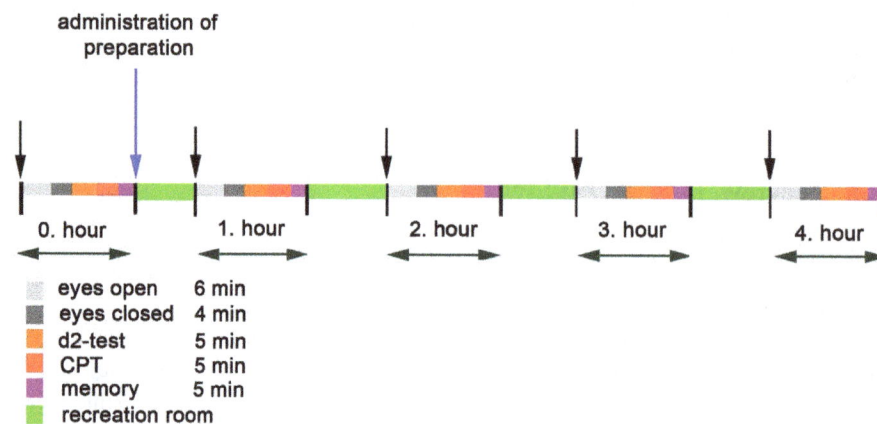

Figure 1. Schedule of EEG recordings during each assessment day.

was followed by a 4-min recording under the condition of "eyes closed", which was in turn followed by 5-min recordings during performance of 3 cognitive tests. The d2 Test of Attention [17] has been validated for the neuropsychological estimation of individual attention and short-term concentration performance. The Concentration Performance Test (Konzentrations-Leistungs-Test, KLT; [18] is a validated measure of vigilance while performing mathematical calculation tasks. Moreover, a Memory Test (MT) was performed to assess short-term retention in a recall task following the presentation of nonsense combinations of letters and numbers.

Bipolar EEG recordings were performed using 17 surface electrodes according to the international 10/20 system, with Cz as physical reference electrode used for calculation of the common average reference. An electrode cap was used for electrode placement. The raw signals were amplified, digitized (2048 Hz/12 bit) and transmitted to the computer via fibre optical devices where they were processed using CATEEM® software (MEWICON CATEEM-Tec GmbH, A-4164 Schwarzenberg, Austria). Artefacts from EEG alterations caused by eye blinks, swallowing, respiration, etc., were rejected using an automated algorithm. An electrooculogram (EOG) was recorded in one channel to facilitate detection of signals superposing the EEG. The artefact rejection set-up was observed for about 5 minutes prior to the start of the recording to ensure that all artefacts were correctly recognized and eliminated from further evaluation. For backup purposes the original raw data (including artefacts) were saved on disk in order to allow a re-evaluation of the artefact rejection if required. The amount of rejected data was determined automatically and given in percent of total recording time. Recording and computer-based automatic artefact rejection were supervised continuously by a trained technician. For each subject settings were kept constant throughout the trial.

In addition to the 17 physical electrodes, signals from 82 additional virtual electrode positions were obtained using Lagrange interpolation, to provide the information required for the generation of high-resolution topographical brain maps. Based on 4-second sweeps of data epochs (Hanning window), the signals from all 99 electrode positions (17 physical and 82 virtual) were FFT transformed into absolute spectral power values in the frequency range between 1.25 and 35 Hz, which was subdivided into the 6 frequency bands of delta (1.25 - 4.50 Hz), theta (4.75 - 6.75 Hz), alpha1 (7.00 - 9.50 Hz), alpha2 (9.75 - 12.50 Hz), beta1 (12.75 - 18.50 Hz), and beta2 (18.75 - 35.00 Hz). Colour coding of the brain maps was achieved by dividing the power spectrum into 140 equidistant frequency ranges with a resolution of 0.25 Hz to which spectral colours from red to dark blue were assigned, followed additive colour mixing to obtain the colours at any given point in the topographical map. The maps show the relative, time averaged changes of electrical brain activity of each recording condition in comparison to the reference period during relaxation with open eyes.

2.5. Random Sequence Generation, Allocation Concealment, Implementation

For the allocation of the patients to the 3 treatment sequences random numbers were generated by a qualified person in the sponsor's bio-statistical department otherwise not involved in the trial, using a validated computer program (RCODE, Dr. Willmar Schwabe GmbH & Co. KG, Karlsruhe, Germany). Randomisation was performed in fixed blocks at a ratio of 1:1:1 with stratification by sex. The study drugs were dispensed to the centre in numbered containers. Upon inclusion into randomised treatment each subject received the medication kit with the lowest available medication number. The block size was withheld from the site personnel until completion of the trial.

2.6. Statistical Methods, Sample Size

Baseline demographic and anthropometric data were compared descriptively between the 3 treatment sequences and were tested for differences using Kruskal-Wallis tests or χ^2 tests as applicable.

For the assessment of spectral power changes in the EEG after drug intake the power values obtained during the "eyes open" and the "eyes closed" conditions at pre-dose were taken as intra-individual reference values and were assumed to represent 100%. All post-dose values were expressed in percent relative to these reference values. Treatment group comparisons for spectral power values as well as for relative change from baseline between Silexan 80 and 160 mg/day on one hand and placebo on the other were performed using non-parametric Sign tests. All p-values are 2-sided and are intended to be descriptive.

No missing data imputation was performed. Subjects were analysed for safety if they had taken at least 1 dose of 1 investigational treatment. They were included into the EEG analysis if they had provided evaluable qEEG data for all 3 treatment periods.

In this exploratory trial a sample size of 24 subjects (8 in each sequence) was chosen based on practical experience from previous trials with a similar design rather than on power considerations.

3. Results

3.1. Recruitment, Participant Flow

The clinical part of the trial was performed between February and July 2011 in a clinical phase I unit in Germany. A total of 32 subjects were screened for participation and 24 were randomised, 8 subjects to each of the 3 treatment sequences. Reasons for non-randomisation were violations of eligibility criteria (5 subjects) and conflicts between the study schedule and the subjects' private calendar (3 subjects). All subjects were evaluated for safety. One subject randomised to sequence Silexan 80 mg-Silexan 160 mg-placebo was withdrawn prematurely on the 8th day of the 1st treatment period due to a non-serious but severe, potentially treatment related adverse event (eructation, nausea, and stomach cramps). All other study participants terminated the trial as scheduled and thus 23 subjects were evaluated in the EEG analysis.

3.2. Baseline Data

Table 1 shows that the treatment groups were essentially comparable with respect to demographic and anthropometric measures. The randomised study participants' medical history and baseline physical examination did not reveal any findings from which interference with the procedures or the outcomes of the trial could be expected. Baseline concomitant medication was limited to hormonal contraceptives (7 subjects), iodine preparations for struma or after thyroidectomy (4 subjects), acetylsalicylic acid for thromboembolic prophylaxis (1 subject), and alendronic acid for osteoporosis.

3.3. Treatment Compliance

Compliance was assessed per treatment period, by comparing the number of unused capsules returned by the subjects to the expected number assuming a fully protocol compliant intake. For all subjects and periods compliance ranged between 93.3% and 100.0%. On the EEG assessment days none of the subjects took the study medication before the 1st or after the 2nd qEEG recording, so that no relevant protocol deviations related to treatment compliance were observed.

3.4. Quantitative EEG Analysis

Table 2 presents the absolute power values for the 17 physical electrodes obtained during pre-dose (baseline) recording on day 1 of each treatment period (*i.e.*, prior to the single dose assessments) in the "eyes closed" condition. For each electrode position and frequency range the data show no baseline differences between placebo on the one hand and one of the doses of Silexan on the other. The same applied to the baseline values for the "eyes open" condition before the first dose of each period as well as to the baseline recordings after repetitive dosing obtained at pre-dose of treatment day 14 of each period in the "eyes open" and "eyes closed" condition (data not shown).

The changes of spectral power in the "eyes closed" condition at 1 h, 2 h, 3 h and 4 h after single dose (acute) administration of the investigational treatments are shown in **Figure 2**. Changes from baseline in the placebo

Table 1. Demographic and other baseline data (EEG analysis set; absolute frequency (%) or mean ± SD).

		Silexan 160 mg-Silexan 80 mg-placebo (n = 8)	Silexan 80 mg-Silexan 160 mg-placebo (n = 7)	Placebo-Silexan 80 mg-Silexan 160 mg (n = 8)	p
Sex	Female	4 (50.0%)	3 (42.9%)	4 (50.0%)	0.95[#]
	Male	4 (50.0%)	4 (57.1%)	4 (50.0%)	
	Age (years)	44.3 ± 10.1	42.3 ± 10.3	48.9 ± 13.6	0.29[§]
	Weight (kg)	74.1 ± 10.3	78.4 ± 15.2	77.3 ± 11.2	0.82[§]
	Height (cm)	170.9 ± 10.2	179.6 ± 11.1	170.5 ± 8.6	0.29[§]

[#]Pearson χ^2-test; [§]Kruskal-Wallis test.

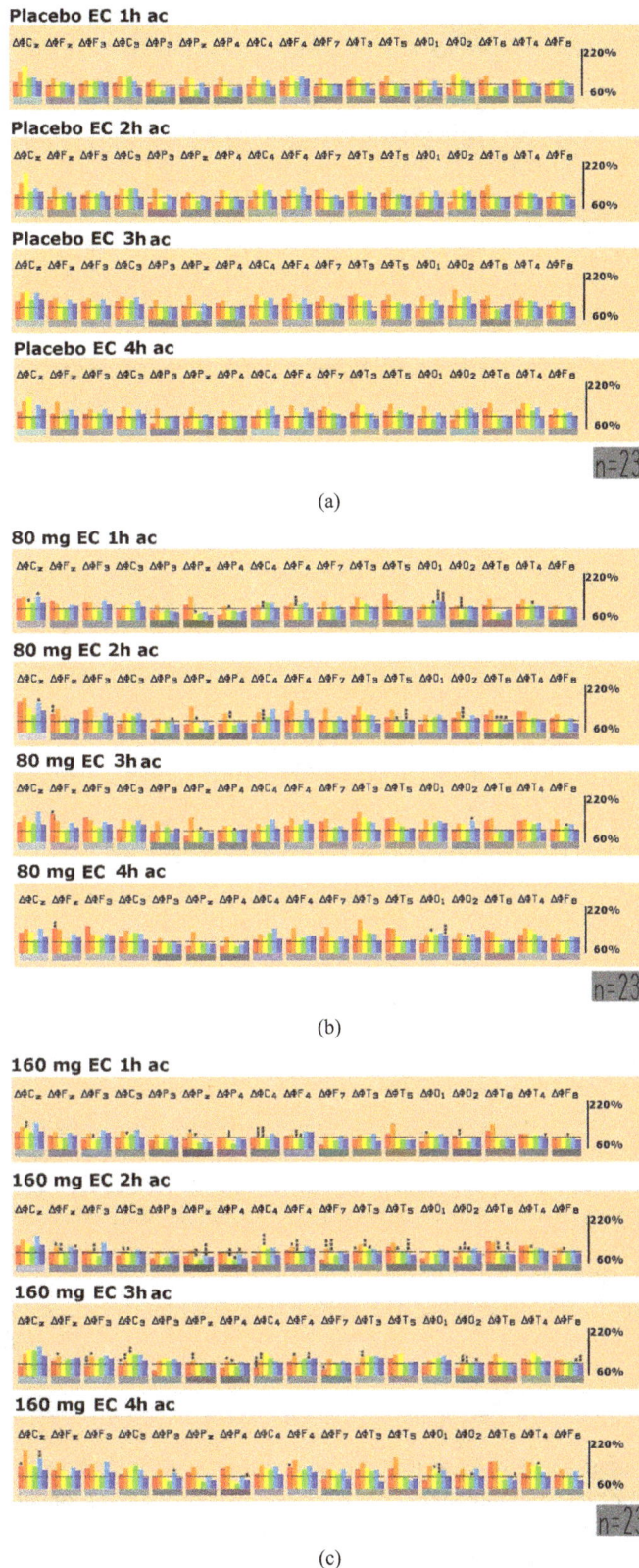

(a)

(b)

(c)

Figure 2. Percent changes in spectral power compared to baseline after single-dose (acute) administration of placebo (a), Silexan® 80 mg (b) and Silexan® 160 mg (c) in condition "eyes closed". Colour coding: red—delta, orange—theta, yellow—alpha1, green—alpha2, light blue—beta1, dark blue—beta2. Comparisons to placebo: *p < 0.10; **p < 0.05; ***p < 0.01.

Table 2. Baseline spectral power (μV^2) for physical electrode locations for placebo (PL), Silexan® 80 mg (80 mg) and Silexan® 160 mg (160 mg) in condition "eyes closed" (M: median values across all locations).

Electrode	n	Delta Pl	80 mg	160 mg	Theta Pl	80 mg	160 mg	Alpha1 Pl	80 mg	160 mg	Alpha2 Pl	80 mg	160 mg	Beta1 Pl	80 mg	160 mg	Beta2 Pl	80 mg	160 mg
Cz	23	2.83	2.49	2.99	0.7	0.73	0.79	1	1.78	1.32	0.99	1.19	0.9	0.82	0.6	0.69	1.07	1.04	0.95
Fz	23	2.91	2.71	2.51	0.85	0.73	0.87	1.33	1.59	1.63	1.02	0.84	0.97	0.67	0.48	0.58	0.72	0.59	0.72
F3	23	2.87	2.22	2.96	0.68	0.65	0.81	1.09	1.48	1.67	0.97	0.87	0.83	0.73	0.55	0.74	0.99	0.74	0.93
C3	23	1.56	1.98	1.57	0.43	0.41	0.46	0.72	0.96	0.98	1.17	0.7	0.88	1.21	0.69	0.81	0.99	0.82	1.02
P3	23	2.22	2.32	2.19	0.5	0.55	0.44	1.44	2.36	1.41	1.85	1.34	1.24	0.93	0.82	0.75	0.59	0.56	0.6
Pz	23	3.03	3.42	2.77	0.82	0.73	0.57	2.53	2.64	1.95	2.99	3.95	2.79	0.81	1.01	0.97	0.55	0.78	0.63
P4	23	2.22	2.94	1.82	0.51	0.61	0.44	2.43	2.03	1.69	1.84	1.81	1.72	1.03	0.81	0.84	0.74	0.57	0.69
C4	23	1.86	2.16	2.18	0.48	0.57	0.53	1.1	1.55	0.9	1.23	0.93	1.14	1.27	0.89	1.11	1.35	1.31	1.34
F4	23	2.43	3.2	2.48	0.65	0.77	0.71	1.17	1.58	1.65	0.98	0.94	1.01	0.73	0.62	0.64	1	0.79	0.85
F7	23	8.07	7.72	10.11	1.27	1.37	1.51	2.8	3.18	3.47	2.3	1.63	2.52	1.3	1.17	0.47	1.7	1.48	1.72
T3	23	3.76	4.68	4.47	0.99	0.85	0.86	2.46	2.25	2.28	1.52	1.59	1.52	1.3	1.27	1.35	1.42	1.29	1.68
T5	23	4.29	4.39	3.88	1.27	1.17	1.29	6.58	5.79	6.79	2.76	2.81	3.11	2.03	1.94	2.08	1.26	1.38	1.17
O1	23	3.86	3.8	3.41	0.81	0.79	0.7	1.27	1.61	1.46	1.99	1.39	1.39	1.39	0.81	0.98	1.22	1.12	1.25
O2	23	3.26	3.96	3.47	0.85	0.9	0.93	1.61	1.54	1.38	1.87	2.01	2.03	1.31	1.29	1.18	1.39	1.42	1.46
T6	23	3.57	5.48	3.11	1.64	1.27	1.09	9.16	8.3	8.47	3.08	2.87	3.21	1.95	1.6	2.12	1.21	1.23	1.3
T4	23	3.89	3.46	3.89	1.04	0.92	0.95	3.02	2.39	2.38	1.8	1.89	1.71	1.6	1.29	1.46	1.48	1.28	1.47
F8	23	8.39	7.96	7.89	1.61	1.52	1.55	2.17	2.58	4.72	2.23	2	2.23	1.68	1.47	1.62	1.93	1.79	1.95
Median	23	3.03	3.42	2.99	0.82	0.77	0.81	1.61	2.03	1.67	1.84	1.59	1.52	1.27	0.89	0.97	1.21	1.12	1.17

period (**Figure 2(a)**) are interpreted to reflect a circadian rhythm as well as random variation. Compared to placebo single dose administration of Silexan 80 mg (**Figure 2(b)**) was associated with increased power in the beta range (notably in the central and occipital regions) and an attenuation in the alpha1 range. Increases of delta and theta power were observed in the frontal and temporal regions. The pattern of differences to placebo in the Silexan 160 mg (**Figure 2(c)**) was similar to that under Silexan 80 mg although the differences to placebo were generally more pronounced after administration of the higher dose. For both Silexan doses statistically meaningful differences to placebo ($p < 0.1$ - $p < 0.001$) were observed already at 1 h after dosing and persisted until the end of the EEG recordings at 4 h.

As an example **Figure 3** shows the colour vision brain maps obtained through electrode interpolation and colour coding and mixing of spectral power for the "eyes closed" condition at 2 h after single dose administration. Note, that the blue to violet shadings (observed mainly after administration of Silexan) indicate a dominance of waves in the beta range whereas the green and yellowish shadings (that were more common during the placebo period) reflect a larger proportion of alpha power. The pattern of differences between Silexan and placebo in the "eyes open" condition after single dose administration of the investigational treatments was comparable to that in the "eyes closed" condition although their magnitude was somewhat less pronounced (data not shown).

EEG assessments for repetitive (chronic) dosing were performed on the last day of each treatment period. **Figure 4** shows the percent differences in spectral power between the post-dose assessments and the pre-dose baseline for the "eyes open" condition. Compared to placebo (**Figure 4(a)**) treatment with Silexan 80 mg/day was associated with an increase in alpha1 power in the temporal lobe and with an increase of beta power in the frontal lobe (**Figure 4(b)**) that were observed during all post-baseline recordings. For Silexan 160 mg/day

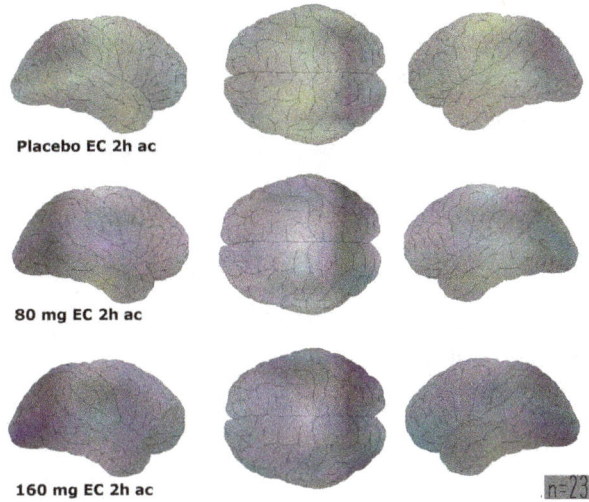

Figure 3. Spectral frequency changes 2 h after single dose (acute) administration of placebo (PL), Silexan® 80 mg (80 mg) and Silexan® 160 mg (160 mg) in condition "eyes closed" (delta through beta2 from red to blue).

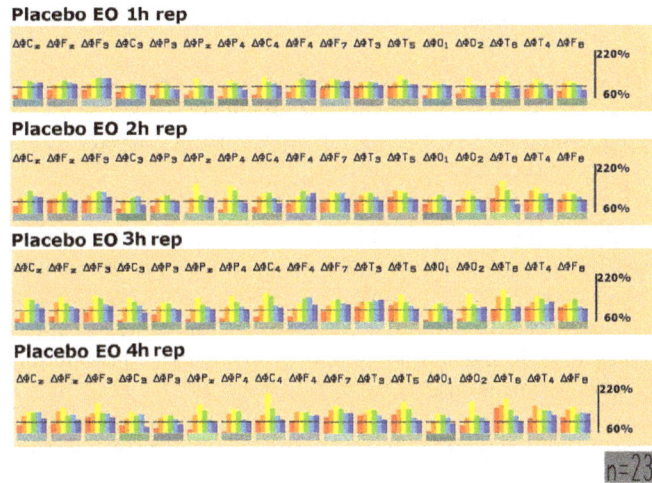

(a)

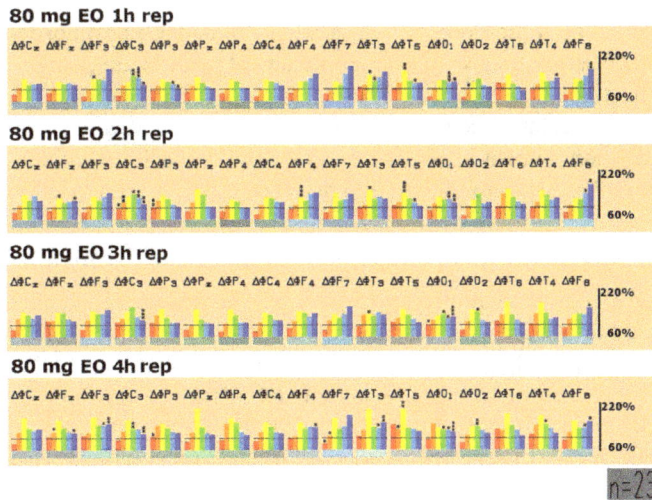

(b)

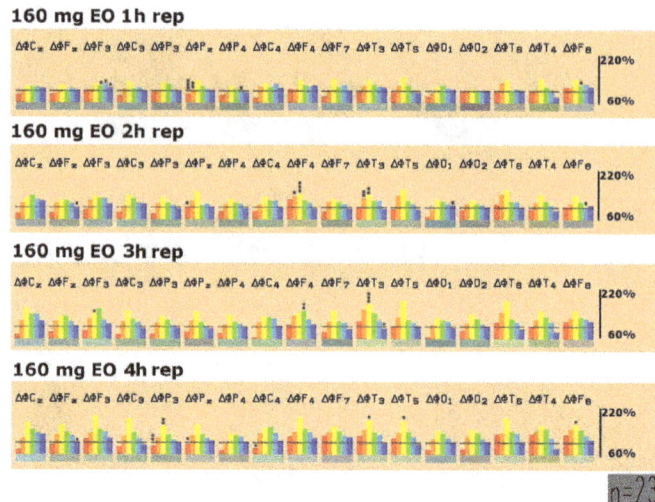

(c)

Figure 4. Percent changes in spectral power compared to baseline after repetitive-dose (chronic) administration of placebo (a), Silexan® 80 mg/day (b) and Silexan® 160 mg/day (c) in condition "eyes open". Colour coding: red—delta, orange—theta, yellow—alpha1, green—alpha2, light blue—beta1, dark blue—beta2. Comparisons to placebo: $^*p < 0.10$; $^{**}p < 0.05$; $^{***}p < 0.01$.

increases of spectral power over the placebo period were observed mainly in the alpha1 frequency band (frontal, temporal, and parietal regions) as well as in the lower frequency ranges in the temporal and parietal regions (**Figure 4(c)**). In recording condition "eyes closed" the differences between Silexan and placebo showed a similar pattern but were less pronounced (data not shown).

Figure 5 and **Figure 6** present the time courses of relative spectral power change from baseline in the fronto-temporal region for recording condition "eyes open" after single and repetitive dosing of placebo in comparison to Silexan 80 mg and 160 mg, respectively (for better legibility the area between the 2 placebo curves for single and repetitive dosing is shaded in grey). Compared to placebo a descriptively significant increase of alpha1 power which persisted throughout the 4-hour recording period was observed after repetitive dosing of Silexan® 160 mg. The results for Silexan® 80 mg confirm an elevation of alpha1 power although the increase over placebo was less pronounced with the lower dose of the herbal drug.

During cognitive performance testing only minor and unsystematic differences in relative spectral frequency power change from baseline were observed between both dosages of Silexan and placebo.

3.5. Cognitive Performance

Across the test administrations at pre-dose as well as at 1, 2, 3, and 4 h post dose moderate improvements in d2 and KLT test performance were observed during all treatment periods after single and repetitive dose administration of the study drugs (including placebo). These changes can most probably be interpreted as a training effect. In the memory test the treatment condition mean values before and at the different time points after dosing showed some minor variation without exhibiting a clear trend. For all 3 cognitive tests only minor differences were observed between both dosages of Silexan and placebo.

3.6. Safety/Tolerability

During and within 2 days after the end of the treatment periods 4 adverse events (AEs) were observed in 4/23 subjects (17.4%) exposed to Silexan 160 mg/day, 13 events were reported by 9/24 subjects (37.5%) during or after the Silexan 80 mg/day period, and 4 events occurred in 4/23 subjects (17.4%) during or after placebo administration. Eleven out of a total of 16 AEs observed under Silexan 80 mg/day or 160 mg/day were gastrointestinal disorders, the most frequent of which was eructation (8 events), whereas no gastrointestinal events were observed in the placebo period. Other events observed in more than one patient within one treatment period were fatigue and increased blood triglycerides both of which occurred in two patients during placebo administration. No serious events were observed.

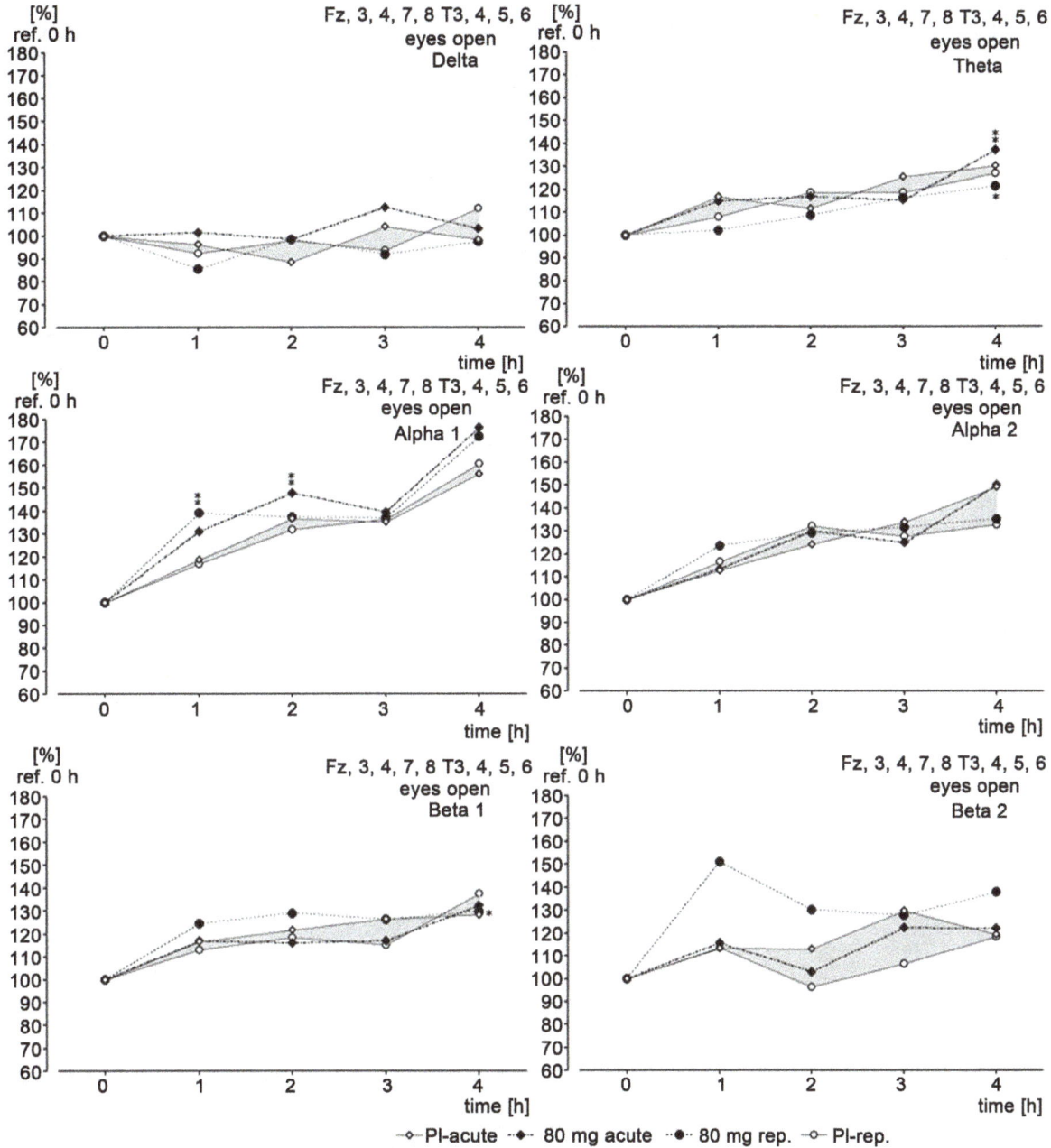

Figure 5. Time course of percent changes in spectral power in the fronto-temporal region compared to baseline after single and repetitive-dose administration of placebo (Pl) and Silexan® 80 mg/day (80 mg) in condition "eyes open". Comparisons to placebo: $^*p < 0.10$; $^{**}p < 0.05$.

4. Discussion

The study indicates that daily doses of 80 and 160 mg Silexan have an objectively verifiable effect in the human brain. The most prominent functional change in the power spectrum associated with the intake of Silexan was an increase of power in the alpha1 range during repetitive administration that persisted until the end of the qEEG recordings at 4 h after dosing. Increased alpha activity of the brain has been associated with a state of relaxed wakefulness (e. g., [19]). In psychotherapy alpha biofeedback has been used successfully in the treatment of anxiety disorders by increasing alpha spectral power [20] [21]. These observations are consistent with the demonstrated clinical efficacy of Silexan as an anxiolytic drug [13] [14] [16] [22].

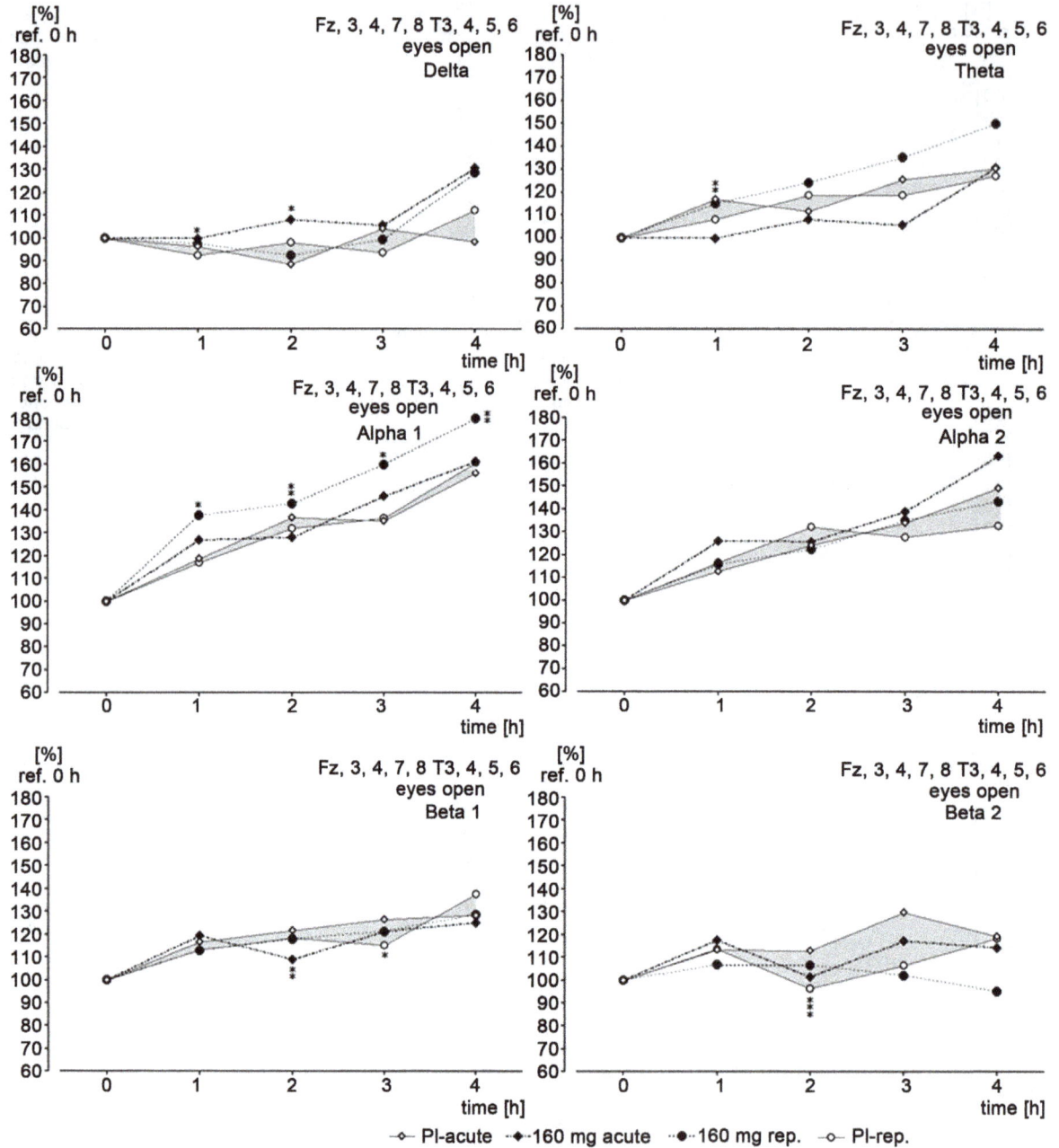

Figure 6. Time course of percent changes in spectral power in the fronto-temporal region compared to baseline after single and repetitive-dose administration of placebo (Pl) and Silexan® 160 mg/day (160 mg) in condition "eyes open". Comparisons to placebo: *p < 0.10; **p < 0.05.

The repetitive administration of Silexan was neither associated with a decrease in absolute and relative alpha power, nor with an attenuation of over-all power, both of which are typically observed following the application of drugs that have a sedative effect, including sedative neuroleptics and benzodiazepines [23]. Whereas benzodiazepines and other sedating drugs have been found to significantly impair cognitive performance, and thus to interfere with essential activities of daily living like driving or operating machinery (e. g., [24]), therapeutic doses of 80 and 160 mg Silexan did not adversely affect the subjects' performance during 3 mental challenges assessing different aspects of cognition and memory. The data of this study therefore do not provide any evidence that Silexan may exert a sedative effect.

Silexan was well tolerated by the healthy volunteers participating in this trial. No dose dependent increase of adverse reactions was observed, and the incidence of AEs during the 160 mg/day period, corresponding to twice the recommended dose according to the marketing authorisation of the drug, was almost entirely on one level with that observed during exposure to placebo. Mild to moderate gastro-intestinal complaints, notably eructation, which constituted the majority of adverse events reported during the administration of Silexan in this trial, may be expected according to the safety profile of the drug and thus do not indicate any previously unknown risks of the herbal essential oil.

5. Conclusion

This study provides evidence that ingredients of the herbal anxiolytic drug Silexan penetrate the blood-brain barrier and induce functional changes in the CNS. The types of changes observed in the qEEG are consistent with the anxiolytic clinical effects of the drug. No sedative effects were observed. Silexan was well tolerated during repetitive administration of doses up to twice the recommended marketed dose.

Acknowledgements

We appreciate the performance of Mrs. Petra Werling with respect to EEG recordings and we thank Mrs. Leonie Schombert for documentation of the results. Mrs. Ingrid Keplinger-Dimpfel is thanked for taking care of the logistics of the study and quality control.

We thank Andreas Völp who provided medical writing services.

References

[1]   Shukla, S.D., Bhatnagar, M. and Khurana, S. (2012) Critical Evaluation of Ayurvedic Plants for Stimulating Intrinsic Antioxidant Response. *Frontiers in Neuroscience*, **6**, 112. http://dx.doi.org/10.3389/fnins.2012.00112

[2]   Bhattaram, V.A., Graefe, U., Kohlert, C., Veit, M. and Derendorf, H. (2002) Pharmacokinetics and Bioavailability of Herbal Medicinal Products. *Phytomedicine*, **9**, 1-33. http://dx.doi.org/10.1078/1433-187X-00210

[3]   Jobert, M., Wilson, F.J., Ruigt, G.S., Brunovsky, M., Prichep, L.S., Drinkenburg, W.H. and Committee, I.P.-E.G. (2012) Guidelines for the Recording and Evaluation of Pharmaco-EEG Data in Man: The International Pharmaco-EEG Society (IPEG). *Neuropsychobiology*, **66**, 201-220. http://dx.doi.org/10.1159/000343478

[4]   Saletu, B., Grünberger, J. and Linzmayer, L. (1983) Quantitative Pharmaco-EEG and Performance after Administration of Brotizolam to Healthy Volunteers. *British Journal of Clinical Pharmacology*, **16**, 333S-345S. http://dx.doi.org/10.1111/j.1365-2125.1983.tb02308.x

[5]   Fink, M. and Shapiro, D.M. (1969) EEG Patterns as an Index of Clinical Activity of Psychoactive Drugs. *Electroencephalography and Clinical Neurophysiology*, **27**, 710. http://dx.doi.org/10.1016/0013-4694(69)91372-8

[6]   Itil, T.M., Ulett, G.A. and Fukuda, T. (1971) Quantitative Pharmaco-Electroencephalography in Early Evaluation of Psychotropic Drugs. *Folia Psychiatrica et Neurologica Japonica*, **25**, 195-202.

[7]   Dimpfel, W., Hofmann, H.C., Prohaska, A., Schober, F. and Schellenberg, R. (1996) Source Density Analysis of Functional Topographical EEG: Monitoring of Cognitive Drug Action. *European Journal of Medical Research*, **1**, 283-290.

[8]   Schober, F., Schellenberg, R. and Dimpfel, W. (1995) Reflection of Mental Exercise in the Dynamic Quantitative Topographical EEG. *Neuropsychobiology*, **31**, 98-112. http://dx.doi.org/10.1159/000119179

[9]   Dimpfel, W. (2003) Preclinical Data Base of Pharmaco-Specific Rat EEG Fingerprints (Tele-Stereo-EEG). *European Journal of Medical Research*, **8**, 199-207.

[10] Dimpfel, W. (2013) Pharmacological Classification of Herbal Extracts by Means of Comparison to Spectral EEG Signatures Induced by Synthetic Drugs in the Freely Moving Rat. *Journal of Ethnopharmacology*, **149**, 583-589. http://dx.doi.org/10.1016/j.jep.2013.07.029

[11] Dimpfel, W., Koch, K. and Weiss, G. (2011) Early Effect of NEURAPAS® Balance on Current Source Density (CSD) of Human EEG. *BMC Psychiatry*, **11**, 123. http://dx.doi.org/10.1186/1471-244X-11-123

[12] Hamilton, M. (1976) Hamilton Anxiety Scale (HAMA). In: Guy, W., Ed., *ECDEU Assessment Manual for Psychopharmacology*, US National Institute of Health, Psychopharmacology Research Branch, Rockville, 193-197.

[13] Kasper, S., Gastpar, M., Müller, W.E., Volz, H.P., Möller, H.J., Dienel, A. and Schläfke, S. (2010) Silexan, an Orally Administered Lavandula Oil Preparation, Is Effective in the Treatment of "Subsyndromal" Anxiety Disorder: A Randomized, Double-Blind, Placebo Controlled Trial. *International Clinical Psychopharmacology*, **25**, 277-287. http://dx.doi.org/10.1097/yic.0b013e32833b3242

[14] Kasper, S., Anghelescu, I. and Dienel, A. (2010) Efficacy of Silexan (WS® 1265) in Patients with Restlessness and

Sleep Disturbance. Annual Congress of the German Society for Psychiatry and Psychotherapy (DGPPN), Berlin.

[15] Kasper, S., Gastpar, M., Müller, W.E., Volz, H.-P., Möller, H.-J., Schläfke, S. and Dienel, A. (2014) Lavender Oil Preparation Silexan Is Effective in Generalized Anxiety Disorder—A Randomized, Double-Blind Comparison to Placebo and Paroxetine. *The International Journal of Neuropsychopharmacology*, **17**, 859-869. http://dx.doi.org/10.1017/S1461145714000017

[16] Woelk, H. and Schläfke, S. (2010) A Multi-Center, Double-Blind, Randomised Study of the Lavender Oil Preparation Silexan in Comparison to Lorazepam for Generalized Anxiety Disorder. *Phytomedicine*, **17**, 94-99. http://dx.doi.org/10.1016/j.phymed.2009.10.006

[17] Brickenkamp, R. (1994) d2-Test. Hogrefe, Göttingen.

[18] Düker, H. and Lienert, G.A. (1965) Der Konzentrations-Leistungstest (KLT). Hogrefe, Göttingen.

[19] Cantero, J.L., Atienza, M., Salas, R.M. and Gomez, C.M. (1999) Brain Spatial Microstates of Human Spontaneous Alpha Activity in Relaxed Wakefulness, Drowsiness Period, and REM Sleep. *Brain Topography*, **11**, 257-263. http://dx.doi.org/10.1023/A:1022213302688

[20] Hardt, J.V. and Kamiya, J. (1978) Anxiety Change through Electroencephalographic Alpha Feedback Seen Only in High Anxiety Subjects. *Science*, **201**, 79-81. http://dx.doi.org/10.1126/science.663641

[21] Rice, K.M., Blanchard, E.B. and Purcell, M. (1993) Biofeedback Treatments of Generalized Anxiety Disorder: Preliminary Results. *Biofeedback and Self-Regulation*, **18**, 93-105. http://dx.doi.org/10.1007/BF01848110

[22] Kasper, S., Dienel, A. and Kieser, M. (2004) Continuation and Long-Term Maintenance Treatment with Hypericum Extract WS® 5570 after Successful Acute Treatment of Mild to Moderate Depression—Rationale and Study Design. *International Journal of Methods in Psychiatric Research*, **13**, 176-183. http://dx.doi.org/10.1002/mpr.173

[23] Saletu, B., Anderer, P. and Saletu-Zyhlarz, G.M. (2006) EEG Topography and Tomography (LORETA) in the Classification and Evaluation of the Pharmacodynamics of Psychotropic Drugs. *Clinical EEG and Neuroscience*, **37**, 66-80. http://dx.doi.org/10.1177/155005940603700205

[24] Takahashi, M., Iwamoto, K., Kawamura, Y., Nakamura, Y., Ishihara, R., Uchiyama, Y., Ebe, K., Noda, A., Noda, Y., Yoshida, K., Iidaka, T. and Ozaki, N. (2010) The Effects of Acute Treatment with Tandospirone, Diazepam, and Placebo on Driving Performance and Cognitive Function in Healthy Volunteers. *Human Psychopharmacology*, **25**, 260-267. http://dx.doi.org/10.1002/hup.1105

19

Differences in Baseline Characteristics of Patients Treated with Olanzapine or Other Antipsychotics in Japanese Patients with Acute Schizophrenia: A 1-Year Observational Study under Routine Clinical Practice in Japan

Michihiro Takahashi[1,2], Shinji Fujikoshi[3], Jumpei Funai[4], Levent Alev[2*], Masaomi Iyo[5]

[1]Takahashi Psychiatric Clinic, Ashiya, Japan
[2]Medical Science, Lilly Research Laboratories Japan, Eli Lilly Japan K.K., Kobe, Japan
[3]Statistical Science, Lilly Research Laboratories Japan, Eli Lilly Japan K.K., Kobe, Japan
[4]Science Communications, Lilly Research Laboratories Japan, Eli Lilly Japan K.K., Kobe, Japan
[5]Department of Psychiatry, Graduate School of Medicine, Chiba University, Chiba, Japan
Email: *alev_levent@lilly.com

Abstract

Objective: Baseline characteristics of acute schizophrenia patients were analyzed to identify differences in the baseline characteristics of patients treated with olanzapine monotherapy compared with those treated with other antipsychotic monotherapies. Methods: This prospective, naturalistic observational study was designed to evaluate discontinuation rates of olanzapine and non-olanzapine antipsychotic monotherapy in Japanese adult patients with acute schizophrenia. Results: A total of 1089 patients were assessed: 578 patients were treated with olanzapine, 487 with non-olanzapine atypical antipsychotics, and 24 with typical antipsychotics. The mean Clinical Global Impression-Severity (CGI-S) Schizophrenia, Brief Psychiatric Rating Scale (BPRS) total, and BPRS positive scores were higher in patients treated with olanzapine compared with most of the non-olanzapine treated patients. The majority of patients with a CGI-S Schizophrenia score of 7 (29/41 patients) as well as patients with a BPRS total score of 90 or higher (14/18 patients) were treated with olanzapine. On the other hand, physicians tended to prescribe antipsychotics other than olanzapine for patients with heavier body weight or diabetes mellitus. Conclusion: The

---

*Corresponding author.

present study demonstrated that olanzapine was more likely to be prescribed to patients with more severe schizophrenia symptoms. However, further studies are warranted to reach a definite conclusion.

Keywords

Schizophrenia, Baseline Characteristics, Olanzapine, Antipsychotics

---

1. Introduction

Atypical antipsychotics have been widely used as a first-line therapy for acute and maintenance phases of schizophrenia. They are essential in the treatment of schizophrenia. However, these medications could be partially ineffective or intolerant for some patients, and a switching strategy is often chosen to address those issues. Today, a number of atypical antipsychotics are available on the market, and selection of antipsychotics is vital to maximize the effectiveness and minimize the risk of undesirable adverse events.

Several studies have investigated the differences in baseline characteristics of patients treated with antipsychotics [1]-[5]. However, Japanese patients with acute schizophrenia treated with antipsychotic monotherapy had not been investigated in a prospective large-scale clinical study with a long-term follow-up period. Previously, we conducted a prospective, naturalistic observational study to evaluate the discontinuation rates of olanzapine and non-olanzapine antipsychotic monotherapies in Japanese patients with acute schizophrenia in a routine clinical practice setting [6]. In the primary evaluation, patients treated with olanzapine monotherapy were found to have a significantly greater chance of continuing the medication than those treated with a non-olanzapine antipsychotic monotherapy, possibly due to the greater efficacy of olanzapine monotherapy and its acceptable tolerability and safety profile. Using this study population, we extended our analysis to a comparison of baseline characteristics of the patients who were treated not only with olanzapine monotherapy but also those treated with other atypical antipsychotic monotherapies (*i.e.*, risperidone, aripiprazole, blonanserin, quetiapine, and paliperidone) as well as typical antipsychotic monotherapies (*i.e.*, haloperidol).

The objectives of the present analysis were 1) to identify specific characteristics of patients with acute schizophrenia who were treated with olanzapine monotherapy, and 2) to identify differences in patient characteristics that might be related to the selection of antipsychotic monotherapy. The findings of the present analysis would be beneficial for selection of antipsychotic treatment.

2. Materials and Methods

2.1. Study Design

This was a prospective, naturalistic multi-center observational study designed to evaluate discontinuation rates of antipsychotic monotherapies in Japanese adult patients with acute schizophrenia. The selection of the medication depended on the investigators, and patients were monitored until discontinuation of the monotherapy or completion of study. Using its cohort data, we investigated the differences between baseline characteristics of patients treated with olanzapine monotherapy and those treated with other antipsychotics.

Oral antipsychotics were prescribed following the dosage and administration approved in Japan. Informed consent was obtained from all patients enrolled in this study. This study was conducted in compliance with guideline of Good Post-marketing Study Practice (GPSP) and the Declaration of Helsinki.

2.2. Patients

The key eligibility criteria for this study were patients who were diagnosed with schizophrenia according to Diagnostic and Statistical Manual of Mental Disorders Fourth Edition (DSM-IV) Text Revision and ≥20 years of age, and who started treatment with oral antipsychotic monotherapy (patients who were treatment-naïve, or who had switched from other antipsychotics or from poly-pharmacotherapy to monotherapy were included), had a Clinical Global Impression-Severity (CGI-S) Schizophrenia score of ≥4 at the start of oral antipsychotic monotherapy, and had acute stage of schizophrenia developed within one month prior to starting oral antipsychotic monotherapy.

2.3. Measures and Statistical Methods

Analysis was performed in patients whose case report forms were collected and who were confirmed to meet all the eligibility criteria. The baseline characteristics of patients treated with olanzapine monotherapy (olanzapine group) were compared with those treated with non-olanzapine atypical antipsychotic monotherapy (non-olanzapine atypical antipsychotic group). The baseline characteristics of patients treated with typical antipsychotic monotherapy (typical antipsychotic group), and those treated with individual antipsychotics that included 20 or more patients (*i.e.*, risperidone, aripiprazole, blonanserin, quetiapine, and paliperidone) were summarized using descriptive statistics, however due to small sample size, no statistical comparison with the olanzapine group was conducted.

In the present study, baseline information for analysis was grouped into four categories: 1) demographic and clinical characteristics of patients (*i.e.*, gender, age, history of schizophrenia, inpatient or outpatient status, living status, prior antipsychotic medication use within one month prior to the initiation of antipsychotic monotherapy, CGI-S Parkinsonism score, use of anti-Parkinsonism agents, antidepressants, antiepileptic agents, or mood stabilizers; 2) severity of schizophrenia (*i.e.*, CGI-S Schizophrenia Score, Brief Psychiatric Rating Scale [BPRS] total score, Positive, Negative, and Anxiety-Depression scores); 3) body weight and body mass index (BMI); and 4) history of diabetes mellitus or presence of diabetes mellitus, and blood glucose level.

Differences in baseline patient characteristics between the olanzapine and non-olanzapine atypical antipsychotic groups were compared using Student's t-test for continuous variables, Fisher's exact test for binary variables, or the Monte Carlo method for other categorical variables. Multiplicity adjustments were not performed.

3. Results

A total of 1124 patients from 72 centers in Japan were enrolled and the study was conducted from January 2010 to November 2012, and assessed for baseline characteristics. Thirty-five patients were not eligible for analysis: 26 for inclusion criteria not met (14, age under 20 years old; 12, concomitant use of multiple antipsychotics) and 9 for lack of case report. Thus, data from 1089 patients were analyzed. Among those, 578 patients were treated with olanzapine, 487 with non-olanzapine atypical antipsychotics (including 160 risperidone, 154 aripiprazole, 67 blonanserin, 44 quetiapine, 40 paliperidone) and 24 with typical antipsychotics (including 13 haloperidol) (**Figure 1**).

The baseline demographic and clinical characteristics of patients in each group are summarized in **Table 1**. Overall, 46.0% of the patients in the olanzapine group and 42.7% in the non-olanzapine atypical antipsychotic group were male (p = 0.293). For the individual antipsychotic groups, more than half of the patients were male in the paliperidone and typical antipsychotic groups (60.0% and 54.2%, respectively) while the majority of patients were women in the other groups. History of schizophrenia (mean duration) was 14.42 years in the olanzapine group, which was comparable to 14.43 years in the non-olanzapine atypical antipsychotic group (p = 0.992). It was the longest in the typical antipsychotic group, with 22.47 years. Although there was no statistically significant difference (p = 0.117), the percentage of inpatients in the olanzapine group (61.8%) was higher than that of the non-olanzapine atypical antipsychotic group (56.9%). With the exception of the risperidone group, inpatient percentages for all other individual antipsychotic groups were lower than that of the olanzapine group.

The percentages of patients with antipsychotic use within one month prior to the start of monotherapy in the olanzapine group (37.9%) was comparable to the 37.2% observed in the non-olanzapine atypical antipsychotic group (p = 0.849).

The mean CGI-S Parkinsonism score in the olanzapine group was 0.8, which was the same as that in the non-olanzapine antipsychotic group (0.8, p = 0.758), but lower than that in the typical antipsychotic group (1.6). Moreover, the percentages of patients with use of any anti-Parkinsonism agent in the olanzapine group (8.7%) were significantly lower than those in the non-olanzapine atypical antipsychotic group (13.3%, p = 0.017). The highest percentage of patients using an anti-Parkinsonism agent was seen in the typical antipsychotic group (41.7%).

There was no statistically significant difference between the percentages of patients who used an antidepressant, antiepileptic agent, or mood-stabilizer in the olanzapine group and the non-olanzapine atypical

Table 1. Baseline demographic and clinical characteristics of patients.

| | | Olanzapine (n = 578) | | Non-olanzapine atypical antipsychotics | | | | | | | | | | | | | Typical antipsychotics overall (n = 24) | |
| | | | | Overall* (n = 487) | | Risperidone (n = 160) | | Aripiprazole (n = 154) | | Blonanserin (n = 67) | | Quetiapine (n = 44) | | Paliperidone (n = 40) | | | |
		n	(%)	n	(%)	n	(%)	n	(%)	n	(%)	n	(%)	n	(%)	n	(%)
Gender	Male	266	(46.0)	208	(42.7)	72	(45.0)	59	(38.3)	27	(40.3)	18	(40.9)	24	(60.0)	13	(54.2)
	Female	312	(54.0)	279	(57.3)	88	(55.0)	95	(61.7)	40	(59.7)	26	(59.1)	16	(40.0)	11	(45.8)
	p-value[F]	0.293															
Age (years)	n	574		484		160		152		67		43		40		24	
	Mean (SD)	46.1	(15.6)	47.1	(15.9)	47.3	(16.0)	46.0	(15.5)	47.0	(16.4)	50.3	(16.9)	46.0	(15.6)	49.2	(14.0)
	p-value[M]	0.295															
History of schizophrenia (years)	n	404		305		95		106		39		29		22		10	
	Mean (SD)	14.42	(14.11)	14.43	(13.80)	15.46	(14.40)	13.06	(12.93)	12.57	(12.38)	17.60	(15.09)	15.22	(16.07)	22.47	(10.69)
	Median	10.00		10.00		10.00		8.54		10.25		12.00		6.13		19.29	
	Min - max	0.0 - 55.0		0.0 - 60.0		0.0 - 60.0		0.0 - 45.5		0.1 - 42.8		0.3 - 53.5		0.1 - 45.0		10.0 - 44.1	
	p-value[S]	0.992															
Inpatient or outpatient status	Inpatient	357	(61.8)	277	(56.9)	113	(70.6)	83	(53.9)	26	(38.8)	24	(54.5)	18	(45.0)	10	(41.7)
	Outpatient	221	(38.2)	210	(43.1)	47	(29.4)	71	(46.1)	41	(61.2)	20	(45.5)	22	(55.0)	14	(58.3)
	p-value[F]	0.117															
Living status	Single-person household	43	(7.4)	37	(7.6)	7	(4.4)	10	(6.5)	10	(14.9)	4	(9.1)	5	(12.5)	3	(12.5)
	Living with family	163	(28.2)	166	(34.1)	38	(23.8)	60	(39.0)	29	(43.3)	16	(36.4)	17	(42.5)	11	(45.8)
	Living with non-family members	14	(2.4)	6	(1.2)	2	(1.3)	0	(0.0)	2	(3.0)	0	(0.0)	0	(0.0)	0	(0.0)
	Others	1	(0.2)	1	(0.2)	0	(0.0)	1	(0.6)	0	(0.0)	0	(0.0)	0	(0.0)	0	(0.0)
	Unknown	357	(61.8)	277	(56.9)	113	(70.6)	83	(53.9)	26	(38.8)	24	(54.5)	18	(45.0)	10	(41.7)
	p-value[M]	0.284															
Antipsychotics use within 1 month prior to the initiation of monotherapy	Yes	219	(37.9)	181	(37.2)	48	(30.0)	63	(40.9)	25	(37.3)	16	(36.4)	21	(52.5)	14	(58.3)
	No	359	(62.1)	306	(62.8)	112	(70.0)	91	(59.1)	42	(62.7)	28	(63.6)	19	(47.5)	10	(41.7)
	p-value[F]	0.849															
CGI-S Parkinsonism Score**	n	401		325		108		106		48		30		20		15	
	Mean (SD)	0.8	(1.5)	0.8	(1.4)	0.9	(1.5)	0.8	(1.3)	0.8	(1.5)	0.8	(1.4)	0.8	(1.3)	1.6	(2.0)
	p-value[S]	0.758															
Use of any anti-Parkinsonism agents**	Yes	50	(8.7)	65	(13.3)	27	(16.9)	13	(8.4)	14	(20.9)	3	(6.8)	4	(10.0)	10	(41.7)
	No	528	(91.3)	422	(86.7)	133	(83.1)	141	(91.6)	53	(79.1)	41	(93.2)	36	(90.0)	14	(58.3)
	p-value[F]	0.017															

Continued

Use of any antidepressants**	Yes	31	(5.4)	28	(5.7)	8	(5.0)	8	(5.2)	1	(1.5)	5	(11.4)	3	(7.5)	3	(12.5)
	No	547	(94.6)	459	(94.3)	152	(95.0)	146	(94.8)	66	(98.5)	39	(88.6)	37	(92.5)	21	(87.5)
	p-value[F)]	0.790															
Use of any antiepileptic agents**	Yes	79	(13.7)	66	(13.6)	18	(11.3)	25	(16.2)	5	(7.5)	9	(20.5)	3	(7.5)	6	(25.0)
	No	499	(86.3)	421	(86.4)	142	(88.8)	129	(83.8)	62	(92.5)	35	(79.5)	37	(92.5)	18	(75.0)
	p-value[F)]	1.000															
Use of any mood stabilizers**	Yes	11	(1.9)	17	(3.5)	3	(1.9)	7	(4.5)	2	(3.0)	4	(9.1)	1	(2.5)	0	(0.0)
	No	567	(98.1)	470	(96.5)	157	(98.1)	147	(95.5)	65	(97.0)	40	(90.9)	39	(97.5)	24	(100.0)
	p-value[F)]	0.125															

*Including patients treated with perospirone (n = 16) and zotepine (n = 6); **At initiation of monotherapy; CGI-S, Clinical Global Impression-Severity of Illness; SD, standard deviation. [S)]Student's t-test; [F)]Fisher's exact test; [M)] Monte Carlo method (vs. olanzapine group).

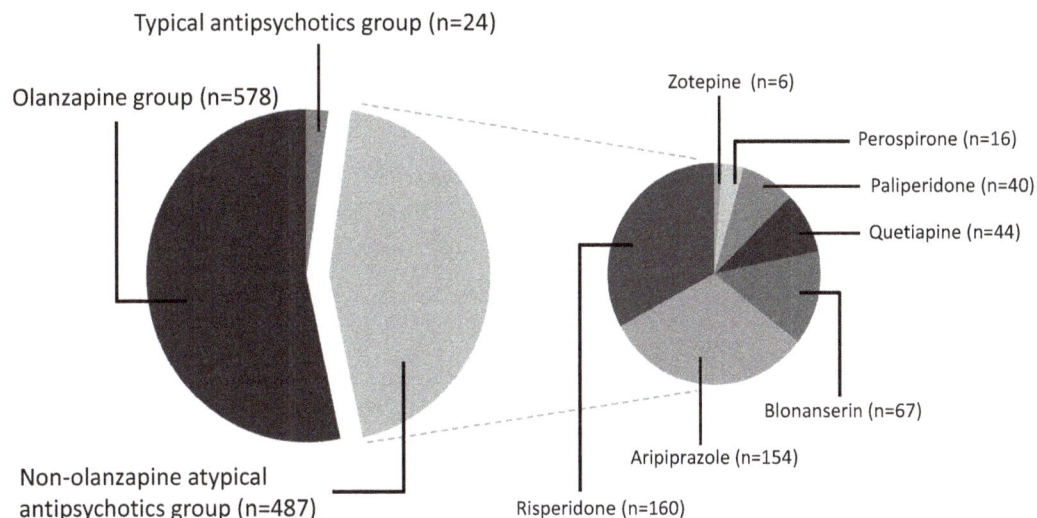

Figure 1. Number of patients in each treatment group.

antipsychotic group. The percentages of patients who used an antidepressant or antiepileptic agent in the typical antipsychotic groups were numerically higher than those in the olanzapine group. On the other hand, there were no significant differences observed for age and living status (single or living together with family or other individuals).

The baseline CGI-S Schizophrenia and BPRS scores are summarized in **Table 2**. The mean CGI-S Schizophrenia score was significantly higher in the olanzapine group than that in the non-olanzapine group (4.9 vs. 4.8; p = 0.015). Although there were no statistically significant differences (p = 0.108 and p = 0.225, respectively), mean BPRS total and BPRS positive scores in the olanzapine group (60.3 and 16.5, respectively) were numerically higher than those in the non-olanzapine atypical antipsychotic group (58.5 and 16.1, respectively). For the individual antipsychotics groups, the scores in the olanzapine group were numerically higher compared with most of the other groups, with the exception of the risperidone group. The scores between the olanzapine and risperidone groups were comparable. On the other hand, mean BPRS Negative and Anxiety/Depression scores were comparable between groups. The majority of patients with a CGI-S Schizophrenia score of 7 (29 of 41 patients) as well as patients with a BPRS total score of 90 or higher (14 of 18 patients) were treated with olanzapine monotherapy. Moreover, the majority of patients with a BPRS positive score of 25 or higher (19 of 31 patients) were also treated with olanzapine monotherapy.

Baseline body weight and BMI are summarized in **Table 3**. With the exception of the quetiapine group, the mean body weight of patients in the olanzapine group (57.70 kg) was numerically lower than those in the

Table 2. Baseline CGI-S and BPRS scores.

| | | Olanzapine (n = 578) | | Non-olanzapine atypical antipsychotics | | | | | | | | | | | | Typical antipsychotics | |
| | | | | Overall* (n = 487) | | Risperidone (n = 160) | | Aripiprazole (n = 154) | | Blonanserin (n = 67) | | Quetiapine (n = 44) | | Paliperidone (n = 40) | | Overall (n = 24) | |
		n	(%)	n	(%)	n	(%)	n	(%)	n	(%)	n	(%)	n	(%)	n	(%)
CGI-S schizophrenia score	n	578		487		160		154		67		44		40		24	
	Mean (SD)	4.9	(0.9)	4.8	(0.9)	5.0	(0.9)	4.7	(0.8)	4.7	(0.8)	4.9	(0.9)	4.9	(0.9)	4.7	(0.8)
	p-value[S)]	0.015															
	4	240	(41.5)	230	(47.2)	63	(39.4)	83	(53.9)	34	(50.7)	19	(43.2)	17	(42.5)	11	(45.8)
	5	165	(28.5)	137	(28.1)	42	(26.3)	43	(27.9)	23	(34.3)	12	(27.3)	12	(30.0)	9	(37.5)
	6	144	(24.9)	108	(22.2)	52	(32.5)	24	(15.6)	9	(13.4)	11	(25.0)	9	(22.5)	4	(16.7)
	7	29	(5.0)	12	(2.5)	3	(1.9)	4	(2.6)	1	(1.5)	2	(4.5)	2	(5.0)	0	(0.0)
BPRS total score	n	354		308		103		101		49		22		21		14	
	Mean (SD)	60.3	(15.5)	58.5	(14.2)	61.8	(15.4)	58.4	(13.2)	54.9	(13.2)	59.0	(13.1)	56.0	(11.8)	54.3	(15.2)
	p-value[S)]	0.108															
	≥20, <30	2	(0.3)	2	(0.4)	0	(0.0)	1	(0.6)	0	(0.0)	0	(0.0)	0	(0.0)	0	(0.0)
	≥30, <40	25	(4.3)	23	(4.7)	5	(3.1)	4	(2.6)	7	(10.4)	2	(4.5)	2	(5.0)	2	(8.3)
	≥40, <50	70	(12.1)	57	(11.7)	20	(12.5)	22	(14.3)	8	(11.9)	3	(6.8)	3	(7.5)	3	(12.5)
	≥50, <60	82	(14.2)	97	(19.9)	28	(17.5)	31	(20.1)	19	(28.4)	6	(13.6)	8	(20.0)	5	(20.8)
	≥60, <70	81	(14.0)	60	(12.3)	16	(10.0)	22	(14.3)	7	(10.4)	8	(18.2)	6	(15.0)	2	(8.3)
	≥70, <80	54	(9.3)	40	(8.2)	18	(11.3)	12	(7.8)	6	(9.0)	1	(2.3)	2	(5.0)	1	(4.2)
	≥80, <90	26	(4.5)	25	(5.1)	13	(8.1)	8	(5.2)	2	(3.0)	2	(4.5)	0	(0.0)	1	(4.2)
	≥90, <100	10	(1.7)	3	(0.6)	2	(1.3)	1	(0.6)	0	(0.0)	0	(0.0)	0	(0.0)	0	(0.0)
	≥100, <110	4	(0.7)	1	(0.2)	1	(0.6)	0	(0.0)	0	(0.0)	0	(0.0)	0	(0.0)	0	(0.0)
BPRS positive score	n	354		308		103		101		49		22		21		14	
	Mean (SD)	16.5	(4.9)	16.1	(4.8)	17.5	(4.7)	16.0	(4.5)	14.5	(4.9)	15.6	(4.7)	15.1	(4.3)	13.5	(5.2)
	p-value[S)]	0.225															
	<5	0	(0.0)	1	(0.2)	0	(0.0)	0	(0.0)	1	(1.5)	0	(0.0)	0	(0.0)	0	(0.0)
	≥5, <10	28	(4.8)	28	(5.7)	6	(3.8)	9	(5.8)	5	(7.5)	3	(6.8)	2	(5.0)	3	(12.5)
	≥10, <15	100	(17.3)	87	(17.9)	23	(14.4)	28	(18.2)	21	(31.3)	5	(11.4)	5	(12.5)	5	(20.8)
	≥15, <20	120	(20.8)	114	(23.4)	35	(21.9)	43	(27.9)	14	(20.9)	10	(22.7)	10	(25.0)	4	(16.7)
	≥20, <25	87	(15.1)	67	(13.8)	34	(21.3)	18	(11.7)	7	(10.4)	3	(6.8)	4	(10.0)	1	(4.2)
	≥25, <30	19	(3.3)	11	(2.3)	5	(3.1)	3	(1.9)	1	(1.5)	1	(2.3)	0	(0.0)	1	(4.2)
BPRS negative score	n	354		308		103		101		49		22		21		14	
	Mean (SD)	10.4	(3.8)	10.6	(3.5)	10.7	(3.8)	10.6	(3.4)	10.5	(3.6)	10.0	(3.3)	11.0	(2.1)	12.0	(3.3)
	p-value[S)]	0.493															
	<5	29	(5.0)	14	(2.9)	4	(2.5)	5	(3.2)	3	(4.5)	1	(2.3)	0	(0.0)	0	(0.0)

Continued

		Olanzapine		Overall		Risperidone		Aripiprazole		Blonanserin		Quetiapine		Paliperidone		Typical	
≥5, <10		107	(18.5)	110	(22.6)	37	(23.1)	37	(24.0)	18	(26.9)	7	(15.9)	6	(15.0)	3	(12.5)
≥10, <15		166	(28.7)	136	(27.9)	42	(26.3)	43	(27.9)	20	(29.9)	12	(27.3)	14	(35.0)	7	(29.2)
≥15, <20		49	(8.5)	48	(9.9)	20	(12.5)	16	(10.4)	8	(11.9)	2	(4.5)	1	(2.5)	4	(16.7)
≥20, <25		3	(0.5)	0	(0.0)	0	(0.0)	0	(0.0)	0	(0.0)	0	(0.0)	0	(0.0)	0	(0.0)
≥25, <30		0	(0.0)	0	(0.0)	0	(0.0)	0	(0.0)	0	(0.0)	0	(0.0)	0	(0.0)	0	(0.0)
BPRS anxiety/ depression score	n	354		308		103		101		49		22		21		14	
	Mean (SD)	12.6	(4.9)	12.0	(4.0)	11.8	(4.6)	12.4	(3.8)	11.8	(3.3)	11.6	(3.9)	12.3	(3.8)	12.8	(3.9)
	p-value[S]	0.093															
	<5	17	(2.9)	5	(1.0)	3	(1.9)	0	(0.0)	1	(1.5)	0	(0.0)	0	(0.0)	0	(0.0)
	≥5, <10	80	(13.8)	82	(16.8)	37	(23.1)	22	(14.3)	9	(13.4)	8	(18.2)	3	(7.5)	3	(12.5)
	≥10, <15	145	(25.1)	151	(31.0)	37	(23.1)	53	(34.4)	30	(44.8)	10	(22.7)	15	(37.5)	6	(25.0)
	≥15, <20	77	(13.3)	54	(11.1)	19	(11.9)	20	(13.0)	9	(13.4)	3	(6.8)	1	(2.5)	4	(16.7)
	≥20, <25	29	(5.0)	16	(3.3)	7	(4.4)	6	(3.9)	0	(0.0)	1	(2.3)	2	(5.0)	1	(4.2)
	≥25, <30	6	(1.0)	0	(0.0)	0	(0.0)	0	(0.0)	0	(0.0)	0	(0.0)	0	(0.0)	0	(0.0)

[*]Including patients treated with perospirone (n = 16) and zotepine (n = 6). CGI-S, Clinical Global Impression-Severity of Illness; BPRS, Brief Psychiatric Rating Scale; SD, standard deviation. [S]Student's t-test (vs. olanzapine group).

Table 3. Baseline body weight and body mass index.

		Olanzapine (n = 578)		Non-olanzapine atypical antipsychotics												Typical antipsychotics	
				Overall[*] (n = 487)		Risperidone (n = 160)		Aripiprazole (n = 154)		Blonanserin (n = 67)		Quetiapine (n = 44)		Paliperidone (n = 40)		Overall (n = 24)	
		n	(%)	n	(%)	n	(%)	n	(%)	n	(%)	n	(%)	n	(%)	n	(%)
Body weight (kg)	n	313		217		80		69		36		16		11		5	
	Mean (SD)	57.70	(11.99)	59.62	(14.88)	58.87	(14.09)	62.02	(15.41)	60.09	(16.45)	52.70	(12.52)	59.75	(12.21)	66.48	(21.71)
	Median	57.00		57.00		57.00		60.00		57.00		53.63		63.00		67.60	
	Min - max	0.101															
BMI (kg/m²)	n	288		204		78		62		36		14		11		5	
	Mean (SD)	21.99	(3.85)	23.03	(4.76)	22.87	(4.26)	24.16	(5.49)	23.18	(4.85)	19.88	(3.12)	21.75	(3.70)	24.72	(7.05)
	Median	21.50		22.41		22.24		23.20		23.06		20.54		20.63		24.24	
	Min - max	14.1 - 37.5		13.8 - 43.0		16.6 - 42.7		16.3 - 40.6		16.9 - 43.0		13.8 - 25.0		15.9 - 27.6		16.4 - 33.4	
	p-value[S]	0.008															
	≥18.5	49	(8.5)	32	(6.6)	11	(6.9)	8	(5.2)	6	(9.0)	4	(9.1)	2	(5.0)	1	(4.2)
	≥18.5, <25	177	(30.6)	117	(24.0)	46	(28.8)	32	(20.8)	21	(31.3)	10	(22.7)	6	(15.0)	2	(8.3)
	≥25, <30	54	(9.3)	39	(8.0)	16	(10.0)	13	(8.4)	7	(10.4)	0	(0.0)	3	(7.5)	1	(4.2)
	≥30	8	(1.4)	16	(3.3)	5	(3.1)	9	(5.8)	2	(3.0)	0	(0.0)	0	(0.0)	1	(4.2)

[*]Including patients treated with perospirone (n = 16) and zotepine (n = 6); SD, standard deviation; BMI, body mass index. [S]Student's t-test (vs. olanzapine group).

non-olanzapine atypical antipsychotic group (59.62 kg, p = 0.101). The mean BMI of patients in the olanzapine group (21.99 kg/m^2) was significantly lower than those in the non-olanzapine atypical antipsychotic group (23.03 kg/m^2, p = 0.008). With the exception of the quetiapine and paliperidone groups, the mean BMI for the olanzapine group was lower than each of the other non-olanzapine atypical antipsychotic groups. Moreover, fewer patients with BMI of 30 kg/m^2 or higher were treated with olanzapine (8/25 patients).

Only one patient with diabetes mellitus was treated with olanzapine and no patient with diabetes mellitus was treated with quetiapine. On the other hand, the percentage of patients with diabetes mellitus in the non-olanzapine atypical antipsychotic group was 8.4%, which was statistically significantly higher than those in the olanzapine group (p < 0.001). Percentages of patients whose blood glucose levels categorized as diabetic type were 0.3% (2/578 patients) in the olanzapine group and 0% (0/9 patients) in the quetiapine group, however 3.7% (18/487 patients) in the non-olanzapine atypical antipsychotic group which was significantly higher than those in the olanzapine group (p < 0.001).

4. Discussion

The present study was a large prospective, naturalistic multi-center observational study providing data on the baseline characteristics of more than 1000 Japanese patients with acute schizophrenia. Of those patients, 578 were treated with olanzapine monotherapy, 487 with non-olanzapine atypical antipsychotic monotherapy, and only 24 with typical antipsychotic monotherapy. We analyzed the cohort data to identify differences in the baseline characteristics between the patients with olanzapine monotherapy and those with other antipsychotic monotherapies.

It is thought that the severity of schizophrenia is related to the severity of positive symptoms. The mean CGI-S Schizophrenia score as well as mean BPRS total and positive scores for patients treated with olanzapine and risperidone were higher than those treated with other antipsychotics. Most of the patients with severe symptoms, characterized by a CGI-S Schizophrenia score of 7 or a BPRS total score of 90 or higher, were treated with olanzapine monotherapy. A large-scale observational study (SOHO study, 8519 patients) conducted in 10 European countries also showed that olanzapine was frequently administered to patients with severe symptoms [1]. Moreover, with the exception of risperidone, olanzapine was administered more often to inpatients than other antipsychotics in the present study. Our primary evaluation showed that discontinuation due to the lack of efficacy was significantly less frequent for olanzapine monotherapy than for non-olanzapine antipsychotic monotherapies [6]. Moreover, a previous study conducted in Japan showed that adherence of olanzapine and risperidone were superior to quetiapine and aripiprazole for acute treatment of psychosis in hospitalized patients [7]. Taken together, these results suggest that it would be reasonable to select olanzapine monotherapy, a highly efficacious antipsychotic, for such patients with severe symptoms of schizophrenia or hospitalized patients who might have difficulties in recovering from severe symptoms.

On the other hand, olanzapine was less likely to be prescribed to patients with heavier body weight and those with higher BMI. Similar results were reported in the SOHO study [1]; where patients treated with olanzapine monotherapy had a lower baseline mean BMI compared with those treated with other antipsychotics. One of the potential adverse events of olanzapine is weight gain, so physicians might have hesitated to prescribe olanzapine to patients with heavier body weight to avoid that risk. On the other hand, as a post-marketing surveillance of olanzapine reported that patients with lower body weight gained more weight than other patients following olanzapine administration [8], individual differences in changes of body weight during antipsychotic treatment should also be taken into account. The selection of antipsychotics should be made based on the risk-benefit balance. When olanzapine is selected, body weight of the patient should be regularly monitored as well as other metabolic variables. For patients with diabetes mellitus or higher blood glucose levels, antipsychotics other than olanzapine and quetiapine were more likely to be selected, most likely because olanzapine and quetiapine are contraindicated in patients with diabetes mellitus in Japan [9] [10].

The mean CGI-S Parkinsonism score in patients treated with olanzapine was lower than those treated with risperidone and typical antipsychotics, moreover the proportion of patients who used anti-Parkinsonism agents was lower than those treated with other antipsychotics. On the other hand, the mean CGI-S Parkinsonism score was the highest in patients treated with typical antipsychotics, and anti-Parkinsonism agents were frequently prescribed to those patients. Olanzapine has a relatively low risk of extrapyramidal adverse events, thus concomitant use of anti-Parkinsonism agents may not be necessary for olanzapine treated patients.

5. Limitations

This was a non-randomized, naturalistic observational study in which treatment decisions were made by investigators. Although the present study showed essential clinical data analyzing the baseline characteristics of more than 1000 patients with acute schizophrenia in a routine clinical practice setting, it was difficult to generalize our data for patients treated with typical antipsychotics because typical antipsychotics were administered to only 24 patients.

Acknowledgements

This study was sponsored by Eli Lilly Japan K. K. (Kobe, Japan).

Disclosure of Interest

MT was a past employee of Eli Lilly Japan K.K.; SF, JF and LA are employees of Eli Lilly Japan K.K.; MI received honoraria from Eli Lilly Japan K.K.

References

[1]   Haro, J.M., Novick, D., Belger, M. and Jones, P.B. (2006) Antipsychotic Type and Correlates of Antipsychotic Treatment Discontinuation in the Outpatient Treatment of Schizophrenia. *European Psychiatry*, **21**, 41-47. http://dx.doi.org/10.1016/j.eurpsy.2005.12.001

[2]   Bitter, I., Treuer, T., Dyachkova, Y., Martenyi, F., McBride, M. and Ungvari, G.S. (2008) Antipsychotic Prescription Patterns in Outpatient Settings: 24-Month Results from the Intercontinental Schizophrenia Outpatient Health Outcomes (IC-SOHO) Study. *European Neuropsychopharmacology*, **18**, 170-180. http://dx.doi.org/10.1016/j.euroneuro.2007.08.001

[3]   Karagianis, J., Novick, D., Pecenak, J., Haro, J.M., Dossenbach, M., Treuer, T., Montgomery, W., Walton, R. and Lowry, A.J. (2009) Worldwide-Schizophrenia Outpatient Health Outcomes (W-SOHO): Baseline Characteristics of Pan-Regional Observational Data from More than 17,000 Patients. *International Journal of Clinical Practice*, **63**, 1578-1588. http://dx.doi.org/10.1111/j.1742-1241.2009.02191.x

[4]   Kuramochi, M., Ono, H., Fujikoshi, S., Tokimoto, T., Nishiuma, S. and Takahashi, M. (2009) Safety and Efficacy of Olanzapine in Patients with Schizophrenia in Acute Phase: Analysis Based on the Starting Dose of Olanzapine. *Japanese Journal of Clinical Psychopharmacology*, **12**, 1179-1197.

[5]   Ye, W., Nakahara, N., Takahashi, M. and Ascher-Svanum, H. (2011) Characteristics of Outpatients Initiated on Olanzapine versus Risperidone in the Treatment of Schizophrenia in Japan: A Healthcare Database Analysis. *The Japanese Society of Clinical Neuropsychopharmacology*, **2**, 1-8. http://dx.doi.org/10.5234/cnpt.2.1

[6]   Takahashi, M., Fujikoshi, S., Nakahara, N. and Iyo, M. (2013) The Continuation Rate of Monotherapy with Olanzapine or Other Antipsychotic Drugs in Patients with Acute-Phase Schizophrenia—A 1-Year Observational Study in Routine Clinical Practice. *Japanese Journal of Clinical Psychopharmacology*, **16**, 1649-1660.

[7]   Hatta, K., Sato, K., Hamakawa, H., Takebayashi, H., Kimura, N., Ochi, S., Sudo, Y., Asukai, N., Nakamura, H., Usui, C., Kawabata, T., Hirata, T. and Sawa, Y. (2009) Effectiveness of Second-Generation Antipsychotics with Acute-Phase Schizophrenia. *Schizophrenia Research*, **113**, 49-55. http://dx.doi.org/10.1016/j.schres.2009.05.030

[8]   Nishiuma, S., Takagaki, N., Sakaridani, M., Fujikoshi, S., Takahashi, M. and Yagi, G. (2008) Final Report of the Post-marketing Prospective Study in Patients with Schizophrenia Using Olanzapine. *Japanese Journal of Clinical Psychopharmacology*, **11**, 1107-1124.

[9]   Seroquel® Package Insert. (2015) Astellas Pharma, Inc. Tokyo, Japan.

[10]   Zyprexa® Package Insert. (2015) Eli Lilly Japan K.K. Kobe, Japan.

20

Iranian Medical Staff's Perception of the *All Saints* TV Series

Arsia Taghva[1], Masoud Azizi[2*], Mohammad Reza Hatami[1], Vahid Donyavi[1]

[1]Department of Psychiatry, AJA University of Medical Sciences, Tehran, Iran
[2]Department of English Language, Amirkabir University, Tehran, Iran
Email: *m.azizi@ut.ac.ir

Abstract

The present study was an attempt to explore the Iranian medical staff's perception of the *All Saints* TV series. 199 participants including doctors, nurses, interns, and paramedics took part in this survey study which was done in 2011. A 17-item Likert scale questionnaire was developed by the team of researchers to gather further evidence on the issues raised by the participants in the focus group which was formed in order to delve into their thoughts, attitudes, and feelings about the mentioned program. The supportive and non-blaming nature of the working relationship among the treatment team, their respect for the patients, their strong team work, the accuracy and precision of the presented medical information, and the discipline and sense of responsibility on the part of the medical staff were among the most frequent issues being mentioned and noticed by the participants. In addition, the majority of the participants considered the demonstrated model for providing healthcare services to be an efficient one; however, they believed that it was not possible to apply that model in the Iranian hospitals mainly due to the cultural differences between the two contexts and the current regulations in Iran. The participants were also observed to be only moderately satisfied with the system they were working in. It seems that healthcare systems in the developed countries can be used as models to identify the problems with the existing healthcare system in Iran. Authorities need to take appropriate measures to resolve such problems. The possible solutions and actions have been suggested in the present article.

Keywords

All Saints TV Series, Iranian Medical Staff, Perceptions

---

*Corresponding author.

1. Introduction

For professions other than one's own job, each individual has an image of what it looks like. This image is formed as a result of his or her life time experience of living in the society, being in interaction with others including the ones in those professions, and what he or she hears from others. The media have a very strong effect on the image we build for everything including others' professions [1]. Sometimes these images are formed based on reliable information and are accurate as a result; however, sometimes they are shaped as a result of false or incomplete information we receive and are illusions rather than accurate images [2].

For instance, one's image of what doctors, nurses, and other hospital staff do can be shaped by a number of sources of information. One's visit to hospitals as a patient or visitor, what others say or have said about these professions, the internet, the news, and the TV programs and movies featuring these people and their professions. Due to their short duration, all these sources help shape this image bit by bit during time, and it is their repetition that helps build this image. However, when a TV program and more specifically a TV series is made revolving around a profession, one's image can be heavily affected either positively or negatively depending on the accuracy of the information presented [3].

Popular images can even affect people's decisions for choosing a particular profession [3]. Many high school students are observed to choose to be doctors or engineers in Iran as a result of the popular image of these professions in the public. Such images can also impact students' perception of what they must do as individuals in that profession. Fictional characters in the medical TV programs may affect the way real people in the same professions may behave. For instance, watching a doctor in ER may affect the way one perceives real doctors' roles, behaviors, and responsibilities [4]. These images can help shape students' expectations of medical ethics, identity, and practice [3]. In a study on medical students in Iran, participants reported that movies were the most influential tool in shaping their attitudes toward mentally-ill patients [5].

Therefore, studies exploring the medical staff or students' perception of their public image presented on the media have been the focus of attention over the past few years. A number of studies have examined the kind of image being presented by the medical dramas. For example, it was observed that in American medical dramas, men nurses were often shown in ways which involved with explicit and implicit stereotypes which were sometimes even reinforced by those TV programs [6]. [7], examining 484 undergraduate nursing students' perceptions of the nursing image being shown on TV, observed that the students were concerned about the kind of image which was being presented, though they also recognized some educational value in TV programs. [2] observed that due to sometimes inaccurate information being presented about medical practice, students with more clinical experience tended to have a more negative attitude towards these programs.

Medical dramas also can play an efficient role in education. Many TV series can be used to teach medical students issues in different areas. For example, clips from ER and Scrubs are said to be good for teaching and learning while episodes of House and Grey's Anatomy are good for teaching ethics and team working [8]. However, [9] believes that Scrubs is more successful in teaching ethics than bioethics classes.

While some scholars believe that such programs can positively affect students [2] [10], some think otherwise [11] [12]. Such programs, for instance, were observed to help teach ethics [9] [13] [14] and improve students' communication skills [15].

These programs can also be used to teach the general audience to affect their health beliefs. The "Family House" medical TV series, for instance, was produced in Egypt to disseminate key health messages in an entertaining context to affect Egyptians' health behaviors, beliefs, and attitudes [1].

The Present Study

In addition to the importance of the image such programs present, examining how this image is presented from the medical staff's point of view and their perceptions and attitudes toward such programs are of great importance. This image affects the general audience's attitude towards these professions and the people involved. Therefore, when a TV series is produced in one country and is supported to be broadcasted in another country, there may be mismatches between the image intended for the country in which the program was produced and the image appropriate for the country in which it is being broadcasted. The image the general audience form based on an ideal or at least standard healthcare system will enhance their expectations, which is two-folded. It can be problematic since such expectations may not be met due to infrastructural shortcomings or any other reasons, which will end up with the patients' dissatisfaction with the services they receive. However, at the same time, these mismatches can be used to identify the shortcomings in the present healthcare system in order to improve the system itself and the quality of the services being provided.

Regarding the hospital staff, a number of TV series have been produced. *All Saints*, *House M. D.*, *ER*, and *Grey's Anatomy* are only some of them. These TV programs, due to their length and details, can be said to have the strongest effects on the image the general audience may form in their mind about the importance, difficulties, sensitivity, and responsibilities in those professions.

Among these TV series, *All Saints* invested more in the working environment and the relationship among the medical staff than their personal life. In addition, it is the only one which was broadcasted on the Iranian national TV. As such, the extent to which it presented an accurate image of this profession from Iranian medical staff's point of view is important and needs to be investigated.

All Saints, an Australian medical drama first aired in February 1998 on the 7th Network, revolved around the incidents in Ward 17 which received the overflow of other wards in the fictional Western General Hospital. In 2004, the story shifted to the incidents in the Emergency Department (ED) in order to attract more audience. Also in February 2009, a Medical Response Unit was added to the story line. The last episode, which was the 493rd episode, was aired on October 27, 2009.

All Saints presents the audience an in-depth view of nurses' life at hospitals. It pictures their good and bad days with moments of happiness, sadness, and frustration. It demonstrates their working relationship with others and their interaction with the patients. It also portraits the kind of healthcare and managerial system they were working in. *All Saints* was broadcasted in many countries including United Kingdom, Ireland, and Belgium. After the exclusion of the scenes which did not conform to the Iranian Islamic context and rules, the *All Saints* was also aired on the Iranian National TV Channel 1 under the title of "Nurses", which received a lot of popularity.

In the present study, the *All Saints* TV series was examined in terms of the impression it had on the Iranian medical staff. Their attitudes and thoughts about this program were studied using a questionnaire which was developed based on a focus group formed to delve into the extent to which the participants could communicate with this TV series.

2. Method

2.1. Participants

199 participants (84 male and 115 were female) working in the health care system in military hospitals in Tehran took part in this survey study. Their age ranged from 20 to 45 with a mean of 30.32 (SD = 6.5) and an average working experience of 11.51 years (SD = 6.6, range = 1 - 26). All participants were selected using convenience sampling.

2.2. Data Collection Tool

In order to collect data, a researcher-made questionnaire was used. It included two sections, with the first part gathering participants' demographical information and the second section gathering information on their opinion and attitude about the *All Saints* TV program. The second section included 17 items (16 five-point Likert scale items and one multiple-choice question) examining three factors: *Satisfaction* (with 4 items asking respondents about the extent to which they were satisfied with the system in which they were working), *Comparison* (with 4 Likert scale and one multiple-choice items asking respondents for their opinion about the extent to which the shown Health System corresponded with the one they were working in), and *Realism* (with 4 items asking respondents for their opinion about the extent to which the TV series matched the realities of their job). In the later analyses it was observed that two items did not load under any of the three identified factors and two items showed very low communalities. As such, these items were excluded from data analysis.

2.3. Procedure

Before developing the questionnaire, a focus group was formed, inviting the medical staff working at two hospitals to participate and share their opinion about the mentioned TV program. The meeting was held in the library at the Army Psychiatry Hospital with the presence of 13 medical staff (6 male and 7 female). The group consisted of a psychiatrist, two psychologists (one PhD holder and one MA holder in Clinical Psychology), four medical interns, five nurses (1 MA holder and 4 BA holders in Nursing), and two clinical assistants. The participants' opinions were later used to develop a checklist by each researcher.

After a checklist on the related issues was prepared by each researcher, all the items were pooled together, and the team of researchers evaluated each item. The repetitive and inappropriate items were excluded then. In the next step, a team consisting of the faculty members at the psychology and psychiatry departments, consisting of 3 psychiatrists and a psychologist (PhD in Clinical Psychology) helped analyze the questionnaire. As a result, a number of items were added and some were excluded from the final version of the questionnaire.

The final version of the questionnaire consisted of 17 items. One of the items was of multiple choice type, probing the reason why they had answered a particular question in a particular way (see below). The rest of items were of five-point Likert scale intended to measure three different factors of interest to the researchers: participants' opinion about the accuracy and reality of the medical and non-medical issues presented on the TV program, the extent to which the healthcare system shown on this TV show matched with or could be incorporated into the Iranian hospitals, and finally, the extent to which the participants were satisfied with the healthcare system they were working in.

The 16 Likert scale items were subject to principal component analysis (PCA) using SPSS Version 17. The suitability of the data for factor analysis was checked prior to the analysis. The KMO value was 0.62 with the Bartlett's Test of Sphericity reaching statistical significance, supporting the factorability of the correlation matrix.

The PCA revealed the presence of six components with eigenvalues above 1; however, the screeplot showed a clear break after the third component. This was further supported by the results of Parallel Analysis, showing only three components with eigenvalues exceeding the corresponding criterion values for a randomly generated data matrix of the same size (16 variables × 199 respondents).

The three-component solution explained a total of 42.66% of the variance with each component contributing 16.25%, 13.81%, 12.60% of the total variance, respectively. Since the correlation among the components was very low, the results of Varimax and Oblimin rotation were very similar. The three component model as intended by the researchers was confirmed by the results of the PCA, with 2 items (items 8 & 11) not loading under any of these three components and 2 other items (items 4 & 10) showing very low communalities, which resulted in their deletion from later analyses. **Table 1** presents the related statistics for a three factor solution oblimin rotation PCA.

Table 1. The pattern & structure matrix for PCA with oblimin rotation of three factor solution.

Item	Pattern coefficients			Structure coefficients			Communalities
	Comp. 1	Comp. 2	Comp. 3	Comp. 1	Comp. 2	Comp. 3	
Q1	0.198	−0.043	0.703	0.269	-0.046	0.724	0.565
Q2	0.025	0.061	0.790	0.109	0.052	0.792	0.632
Q3	−0.191	0.247	0.703	−0.110	0.232	0.680	0.557
Q4	0.136	0.415	−0.077	0.184	0.440	−0.112	0.216
Q5	0.153	0.669	−0.052	0.171	0.675	−0.045	0.480
Q6	0.072	0.523	0.101	0.100	0.524	0.102	0.291
Q7	−0.193	0.650	0.014	−0.169	0.643	−0.014	0.451
Q8	0.117	0.206	−0.058	0.140	0.227	−0.072	0.067
Q9	−0.010	−0.386	0.399	0.018	−0.391	0.403	0.311
Q10	0.021	0.099	−0.405	0.014	0.142	−0.414	0.182
Q11	0.344	0.156	−0.073	0.360	0.206	−0.071	0.161
Q12	0.571	0.067	0.155	0.589	0.085	0.213	0.375
Q13	0.787	0.168	−0.080	0.785	0.196	−0.001	0.651
Q14	0.787	0.098	−0.170	0.772	0.127	−0.090	0.635
Q15	0.640	−0.363	0.156	0.643	−0.342	0.226	0.571
Q16	0.083	0.566	0.109	0.113	0.567	0.110	0.342

Note: items no. 17 was a multiple choice question probing the reason why participants believed that the model presented in that TV show was not applicable to the Iranian context.

The internal consistency of the three components identified in the researcher-made questionnaire was checked using Cronbach alpha. The obtained reliability coefficient for Satisfaction was 0.67. It was 0.50 for Comparison and 0.56 for the Realism component. The low observed reliability coefficients could be due to the low number of items in each component. In addition, since the three components showed a very low correlation with each other, with the highest correlation coefficient being only 0.11, no reliability coefficient was calculated for the whole questionnaire because the three components could not be regarded as constituting a unified whole.

2.4. Data Analysis

Since the number of items was low and due to the nature of each item which was probing an almost different issue indicated by the participants in the focus group, the main type of statistics used was descriptive statistics in order to analyze the patterns of responses for each item. However, as minor questions probing more into the factors affecting the participants' opinion, inferential statistics were used, too. In order to check the effect of sex and experience on the three components examined in this study, a number of two-way between subjects ANOVA were run. Moreover, to check the effect of age, one-way between subjects ANOVA was used.

3. Results

3.1. The Focus Group

Very interesting issues were raised in the focus group meeting. Participants were asked about different aspects of the program, and the responses they provided helped shape the questionnaire in order to further delve into the same issues raised in that session. In fact, the questionnaire was used in order to confirm the points pointed out by the medical staff participating in the focus group.

The participants were asked about the points and issues in *All Saints* which were attractive to them. The intimacy present among the characters; the intimacy the audience could feel while watching that TV program; the specificity of working domains for each member of the medical team; the close and supportive working relationship among the treatment team and more specifically between doctors and nurses; the observed working discipline; the presentation of true and accurate information about medical issues; the possibility for each member of the treatment team to express their feelings in the highly stressful situations and being supported by other members; and the separation of staff's job and personal life were among the most important points mentioned by the participants. As the psychologist of the group stated, "*All Saints* did in fact reveal all our psychological and mental needs and desires."

The interns stated that in that program the patients looked quite real. In addition, the educational nature of the TV program, the non-blaming nature of the relationships among the treatment team, the staff's feeling of consciousness, and the respect they had for the patients and the kind of work they were doing were other points emphasized by them.

In the case of the differences between the two working environments, a number of discrepancies were mentioned. The medical staff in that program did their best to complete their responsibilities despite all the problems they might have faced. In addition, when a problem arose, instead of looking for somebody to blame, the treatment team tried to find a solution. The nurses believed that in comparison with what was going on in their working environment, one could see a more significant role for the head nurses in that TV series. Being in charge did not mean staying away from being involved in actions; instead the head nurses worked more than others. In addition, patients were respected more. More team working could be observed. Each member in the treatment team was emotionally supported by other members. The number of patients each nurse had to take care of was lower. They did not have to work in multiple shifts. Regulations rather than relations were important, and finally, despite all the difficulties, the medical staff were still cheerful and satisfied with their job.

Regarding the extent to which they could communicate with the program, the participants stated that it seemed as if their problems in the Iranian context were being filmed in *All Saints*. In response to whether this program could teach something to the participants, they stated that *All Saints* was instructive in terms of having more and better interaction with patients especially on the part of doctors. A major point emphasized by the nurses was the respect for each member's opinion in the treatment team and the permanent and instructive presence of the doctors in the ward. They believed that this presence could reduce the risk of malpractice and help other staff feel more secure. One of the nurses said that in that program she could see all the ideals she had in mind about this profession.

The characters' personality growth and cognitive development during the time in that TV series was another strong point noticed by the participants. The interesting point was that this growth happened in the hospital and in interaction with their colleagues and patients during time rather than overnight. It was better seen in the case of Luke, the surgeon, and Scott, the young ambulance staff. The participants also liked the fact that in that TV program the medical staff were not shown as mere medical service providers to the patients. Patients were also shown to bring about something new to the ward with their presence there. Even four of the participants stated that unlike some other programs by which they felt offended, *All Saints* made them feel proud of their profession.

Regarding the extent to which this program could affect their practice, the majority of the participants used the term "a lot." The psychologist of the group stated that "we had already heard a lot about the type of interaction we should have with patients, but we had not seen such a good demonstration of that. It was very difficult to find a problem with the type of interactions presented in that TV program as a model."

3.2. The Questionnaire

According to **Table 2**, the participants believe that the two systems do not differ that much in terms of the responsibilities and job-related issues (M = 9.24). However, regarding the extent to which the demonstrated medical issues were scientifically accurate and matched the realities of their profession, the participants were quite positive (M = 14.80). Finally, the participants' level of satisfaction with the system they were working in was not found to be high (M = 11.17). They were only moderately satisfied with the healthcare system they were working in.

Due to the fact that each item was developed in response to an issue raised in the focus group meeting and in order to collect more evidence on that subject, the individual items were of more interest to the researchers than the main factors. **Table 3** presents the descriptive statistics for each item on the questionnaire.

Table 2. Descriptive statistics for participants' responses for the 3 factors.

	N	Minimum	Maximum	Mean	Std. deviation
Comparison	184	4	16	9.24	3.24
Realism	194	5	18	14.80	2.54
Satisfaction	199	4	20	11.17	3.63

Table 3. Descriptive statistics for participants' responses to each item.

Items	N	Minimum	Maximum	Mean	Std. deviation
Q1	198	1	3	2.73	0.54
Q2	198	1	5	4.25	1.07
Q3	195	1	5	3.37	1.05
Q4	198	1	5	1.59	0.98
Q5	189	1	3	1.56	0.67
Q6	196	1	5	2.58	1.71
Q7	197	1	5	3.54	1.71
Q8	198	1	5	2.45	1.76
Q9	199	1	5	4.45	1.23
Q10	198	1	5	1.44	0.97
Q11	190	1	5	3.78	1.59
Q12	199	1	5	3.29	1.49
Q13	199	1	5	2.34	1.17
Q14	198	1	5	2.24	1.18
Q15	199	1	5	3.33	1.33
Q16	199	1	4	1.57	0.80

Regarding the comparison between the two working environments and healthcare systems, the majority of the participants believed that the relationships among the members of the treatment team on the TV program were quite different from those in the Iranian context. They also believed that while the shown nursing practice expectations were a little higher than those in the Iranian context (M = 3.54, with the maximum possible score being 5 and the minimum possible score being 1 for all items), the responsibilities the medical team in Iran have are much heavier, and the level of stress they experience is higher, too.

The majority of the participants believed that it is very difficult to apply the presented model on the TV program in the Iranian hospitals. For the reason why they believed so, 43.8 percent of the participants considered cultural differences as the main obstacle. The problems with present regulation stood as the second reason with 28.4 percent. A number of participants (18.3 percent) considered doctors' resistance to the shown model as the main problem in this regard. Fewer people (7.1 percent) blamed nurses' lack of professional commitment. However, 4 participants (2.4 percent) believed that the shown model was harmful for the Iranian hospitals.

The participants considered the demonstrated medical issues to be scientific and correspond the realities of their job (M = 4.25). They also found the approach to hospital management on *All Saints* to be quite different from the ones running in Iran (M = 4.45). In addition, more than 80 percent of the participants believed that the TV program was not offensive, with less than 20 percent perceiving it to be somewhat insulting to them as the medical staff.

Regarding the extent to which they were satisfied with the system in which they were working in, it was observed that the participants were only moderately satisfied with their job (M = 3.29) and colleagues (M = 3.34). Their level of satisfaction was even lower regarding their working environment (M = 2.34) and their managers (M = 2.24).

As complimentary questions, the effect of participants' age, sex, and working experience was checked on their responses to the items in the questionnaire. The effect of age was also checked on the participants' attitudes toward the program. However, the results of the one-way between subjects ANOVA did not show any significant differences among different age groups in any of the three factors: $F_{Satisfaction}$ (2, 195) = 0.24, $p = 0.78$, $F_{Comparison}$ (2, 179) = 1.48, $p = 0.23$, and $F_{Realism}$ (2, 189) = 1.21, $p = 0.30$.

In order to check the effect of sex and working experience on participants' opinion regarding the *All Saints* TV series and the related issues, a two-way between subjects analysis of variance was run for each factor. The variable *Experience* was binned into three groups using SPSS visual binning procedure, with those with 7 or less than 7 years of experience being in group one, those with 8 to 15 years of experience in group two, and those participants with 16 or more years of experience in the third group. The only significant difference was found in the case of the *Comparison* factor. For the other two, no significant difference was observed between male and female participants and among different experience groups.

As it is presented in **Table 4**, women tended to perceive the shown health system on the mentioned TV program to be more compatible with the system they were working in (M_{female} = 9.06, M_{male} = 8.77). Among the

Table 4. Descriptive statistics for sex and experience variables on the comparison factor.

Sex	Experience	Mean	Std. deviation	N
Male	≤7	9.36	3.18	22
	8 - 15	7.57	3.30	14
	16+	9.09	3.86	11
	Total	8.77	3.40	47
Female	≤7	10.56	2.89	25
	8 - 15	8.43	3.29	35
	16+	8.46	3.50	26
	Total	9.06	3.35	86
Total	≤7	10.00	3.06	47
	8 - 15	8.18	3.28	49
	16+	8.65	3.57	37
	Total	8.96	3.36	133

three experience groups, as in the case of the other two factor, group one (those with 7 or less years of experience) had a more positive attitude towards the compatibility of the two systems (M = 10.00). However, based on each group's mean score, it seems that both male and female participants in all experience groups did not believe that much in the compatibility of the shown health system with the one in the Iranian hospitals.

While the interaction between Sex and Experience was not statistically significant F (2, 127) = 0.76, p = 0.47, the main effect for experience was found statistically significant F (2, 127) = 3.91, p = 0.02 with a moderate effect size (Partial Eta Squared = 0.06). However, the main effect for Sex was not found to be significant F (1, 127) = 0.59, p = 0.44. The post hoc comparisons using Tukey HSD test revealed that the observed difference in the case of Experience was between Group one (M = 10.00, SD = 3.06) and Group Two (M = 8.18, SD = 3.28).

Regarding the compatibility of the two systems, those participants who believed in the inapplicability of the shown health system model in the Iranian hospitals were asked for the reason why they believed so through answering a multiple choice question. **Table 5** summarizes participants' answers to this question.

4. Discussion

The present study was an attempt to evaluate the impression the *All Saints* TV series had on the Iranian audience who were involved in the Iranian healthcare system. The results of the focus group and the follow-up survey study revealed a number of major points in this regard.

The most important subject expressed very extensively and emphasized by the majority of the participants was the kind of working relationship observed among the treatment team on that TV program. The intimacy among the medical staff and the supportive and non-blaming nature of their relationships were of great importance to the participants. They liked the way each member of the treatment team expressed her feelings and was emotionally supported by others. The participants also pointed out the good team work they had on the show, which was due to the kind of relationship among the staff and their approach to hospital management especially by those who were in charge of each department or ward. The way head nurses were involved in action and worked even more than other staff, as mentioned by participants in the focus group, can be an instance of this approach.

In addition, the kind and amount of interaction between the medical staff and patients was largely noticed by the participants. Patients were seen to be respected more in that system and their questions and concerns were paid more attention. This could be due to the better development and practice of medical ethics in the developed countries. In Iran, medical ethics is also being practiced and is of great importance. However, since it is only a few years that this concept has been largely introduced and emphasized, its practice is still far from the ideals.

The self-discipline, sense of responsibility, and keeping the work and personal life apart on the part of the medical staff on *All Saints* were among other issues attractive to the participants. The level of details and accuracy of the information presented regarding the medical problems and practices in all the scenes was largely noticed and liked by the participants. This indicates that a strong medical team supported the production of this TV series, which could be the reason why this program was successful in communicating with the general audience and more specifically the audience working in the healthcare system.

The presentation of the difficulties the medical staff had to face in everyday work and the significance and sensitivity of their job caused the participants to feel proud of their profession when watching this TV program rather than feel offended due to the demonstration of their occasional mistakes in the treatment process.

Table 5. Participants' answers for the reason for the inapplicability of the presented model.

Options	N	Percentage
Cultural differences	74	43.8
Problems with present regulations	48	28.4
Doctors' resistance to the shown model	31	18.3
Nurses' lack of professional commitment	12	7.1
The harmfulness of their model for Iranian hospitals	4	2.4
Total	169	100.0

While the majority of the participants considered the demonstrated hospital management to be an acceptable and efficient model to be used, they believed that applying this model in the Iranian hospitals is a very difficult task mainly due to cultural differences. These differences are not only in the way the hospitals are run, but they are also in the way people think, behave, and live. As one of the interns in the focus group mentioned, even the patients are different. People are more patient-wise in the more developed countries. A second obstacle in this regard was the current regulations in Iran, changing which is a difficult and time-consuming task.

All these could be the reason why the participants were only moderately satisfied with the healthcare system they were working in. Working multiple shifts, experiencing more stress, receiving less support from colleagues, and observing that in that context, unlike their working environment, those in charge work even more than others and are directly involved in action can give a clue to why the participants were not that much satisfied with their job, managers, colleagues, and working environment.

The authorities should be aware that the medical staff are the backbone in any healthcare system and the success and efficiency of any system is determined by the efficiency of the medical staff working in that system. When these individuals are not satisfied with their job or the environment they are working in, for sure the type of service they provide cannot be the one intended and approved by the system. Therefore, identifying and resolving the major problems with this system is of utmost importance. The results of the present study and the type of model presented on *All Saints* TV program can help achieve this goal.

The participants' emphasis and paying attention to the way patients were respected and treated indicates the importance of practicing and teaching medical ethics. Unfortunately, the practice of ethics in the Iranian hospitals is still far from the standards. It is not a long time that teaching medical ethics has been incorporated in the educational curriculum. More emphasis on that and its inclusion in the curriculum of all fields related to medicine seems to be quite necessary. In addition to medical ethics, courses in psychology need to be included in the educational curriculum of all fields whose graduates are supposed to be in interaction with other people and more specifically patients. This is a gap extensively felt in such fields in Iran.

An important implication the result of the present study has is the necessity of working on people's culture. This extremely hard but important task must target all individuals and more specifically those at very young ages. Team working should be taught and internalized. The type of education people receive in Iran is mainly individualistic and is not strong in helping them learn and internalize team working. It is quite necessary that the authorities need to revisit this system of education.

5. Conclusion

Another aspect of culture which needs to be worked on is concerned with the kind of relationship among the members of a team. All members need to learn to value each other's opinion and regard each teammate to be an important asset of the group who has a lot to contribute to the success of the team. Unfortunately, a common objection especially by the nursing staff is that the majority of the doctors tend to regard the nursing staff to lack the necessary knowledge to have an active participation in the treatment process. They believe that nurses are only supposed to follow their orders. However, they need to learn that the nursing staff, as members of the treatment team, have the knowledge and experience which can be quite helpful in the treatment process. Individuals from very young ages need to learn that when working in a group, each member's opinion is valuable and needs to be respected. Two heads are better than one.

References

[1]   Elkamel, F. (1995) The Use of Television Series in Health Education. *Health Education Research*, **10**, 225-232. http://dx.doi.org/10.1093/her/10.2.225

[2]   Czarny, M.J., Faden, R.R., Nolan, M.T., Bodensiek, E. and Sugarman, J. (2008) Medical and Nursing Students' Television Viewing Habits: Potential Implications for Bioethics. *The American Journal of Bioethics*, **8**, 1-8. http://dx.doi.org/10.1080/15265160802559153

[3]   Weaver, R. and Wilson, I. (2011) Australian Medical Students' Perceptions of Professionalism and Ethics in Medical Television Programs. *BMC Medical Education*, **11**, 1-6. http://dx.doi.org/10.1186/1472-6920-11-50

[4]   O'Connor, M.M. (1998) The Role of the Television Drama ER in Medical Student Life: Entertainment or Socialization? *JAMA*, **280**, 854-855. http://dx.doi.org/10.1001/jama.280.9.854

[5]   Amini, H., Majdzadeh, R., Eftekhar Ardabili, H., Shabani, A. and Davari-Ashtiani, R. (2013) How Mental Illness Is

Perceived by Iranian Medical Students: A Preliminary Study. *Clinical Practice & Epidemiology in Mental Health*, **9**, 62-68. http://dx.doi.org/10.2174/1745017901309010062

[6]   Weaver, R., Ferguson, C., Eilbourn, M. and Salamonson, Y. (2014) Men in Nursing on Television: Exploring and Reinforcing Stereotypes. *Journal of Advanced Nursing*, **70**, 833-842. http://dx.doi.org/10.1111/jan.12244

[7]   Weaver, R., Salamonson, Y., Koch, J. and Jackson, D. (2013) Nursing on Television: Student Perceptions of Television's Role in Public Image, Recruitment and Education. *Journal of Advanced Nursing*, **69**, 2635-2643. http://dx.doi.org/10.1111/jan.12148

[8]   Hirt, C., Wong, K., Erichsen, S. and White, S. (2013) Medical Dramas on Television: A Brief Guide for Educators. *Medical Teacher*, **35**, 237-242. http://dx.doi.org/10.3109/0142159X.2012.737960

[9]   Spike, J. (2008) Television Viewing and Ethical Reasoning: Why Watching Scrubs Does a Better Job than Most Bioethics Classes. *The American Journal of Bioethics*, **8**, 11-13.

[10] Strauman, E. and Goodier, B.C. (2008) Not Your Grandmother's Doctor Show: A Review of Grey's Anatomy, House, and Nip/Tuck. *Journal of Medical Humanities*, **29**, 127-131. http://dx.doi.org/10.1007/s10912-008-9055-3

[11] Wicclair, M.R. (2008) The Pedagogical Value of House, M.D.: Can a Fictional Unethical Physician Be Used to Teach Ethics? *The American Journal of Bioethics*, **8**, 16-17. http://dx.doi.org/10.1080/15265160802478503

[12] Hallam, J. (2009) Grey's Anatomy: Scalpels, Sex and Stereotypes. *Medical Humanities*, **35**, 60-61.

[13] White, G.B. (2008) Capturing the Ethics Education Value of Television Medical Dramas. *The American Journal of Bioethics*, **8**, 13-14. http://dx.doi.org/10.1080/15265160802568782

[14] Wicclair, M.R. (2008) Medical Paternalism in House M.D. *Medical Humanities*, **34**, 93-99. http://dx.doi.org/10.1136/jmh.2008.000372

[15] Wong, R., Saber, S., Ma, I. and Roberts, J.M. (2009) Using Television Shows to Teach Communication Skills in Internal Medicine Residency. *BMC Medical Education*, **9**, 1-9. http://dx.doi.org/10.1186/1472-6920-9-9

Appendix

A Survey on "*All Saints*" TV Series

Sex: Male Female   **Age:** .... years   Experience: .... years

Job: ....   Workplace: .... Hospital; .... Ward

TO WHAT EXTENT DO YOU AGREE WITH THE FOLLOWING STATEMENTS?

1 = LOW   3 = MEDIUM   5 = HIGH

	Items	1	2	3	4	5
1	As a health care provider, I think the dialogues were very strong.					
2	The medical information presented on this TV show were accurate.					
3	The kind of relationship among the medical staff looked appropriate to me.					
4	I think the type of relationships among the treatment team were similar to those in the Iranian context.					
5	I think the medical staff's responsibilities were similar to those in the Iranian hospitals.					
6	I think the shown job stress was comparable with that in the Iranian hospitals.					
7	I think the nurses' responsibilities were very similar to those in the Iranian hospitals.					
8	I believe that one of the drawbacks in the presented working relationship was the eradication of power hierarchy.					
9	I found the presented hospital management system very different from those in the Iranian hospitals.					
10	I didn't feel offended because of the shown weaknesses with the medical staff.					
11	In case this TV show was to be produced in Iran, I would agree with showing the possible weaknesses with the medical staff.					
12	I am happy with my job.					
13	I am happy with my workplace.					
14	I am happy with my boss.					
15	I am happy with my colleagues.					
16	I think the model for such relationships as presented in that TV show is applicable to the Iranian hospitals.					
17	In case you do not find that model applicable to the Iranian hospitals, what do you think is the reason? a) Cultural differences b) Problems with present regulations c) Doctors' resistance to the that model d) Nurses' lack of professional commitment e) The harmfulness of their model for Iranian hospitals					

21

Prevalence of Depression and Anxiety Disorders in Peri-Natal Sudanese Women and Associated Risks Factors

Abdelgadir H. Osman[1*], Taissier Y. Hagar[2], Abdelaziz A. Osman[2], Hussein Suliaman[3]

[1]Department of Psychiatry, Faculty of Medicine University of Khartoum, Khartoum, Sudan
[2]Formerly Registrar in Sudan Medical Council, Currently Specialists in Saudi Arabia
[3]Khartoum Neuropsychiatric Centre, Khartoum, Sudan
Email: *abdelgadir1159@yahoo.com

Abstract

The purpose of this study was to estimate a point prevalence of depression and anxiety disorders among Sudanese peri-natal women attending ant-natal and postnatal clinics in the capital city of Sudan. Simultaneously, to examine the associated risks factors. Participants were 945 peri-natal women in two main women antenatal and post natal clinics in the Capital City of Sudan screened consecutively. They were divided into two groups. The first group was of, Four Hundreds eighty (480) women in their third trimester, and the second group consisted of Four Hundreds Sixty Five (465) women in the first 10 week of postnatal period. All participants were screened, using Beck Depression Inventory (BDI), Hospital Anxiety and Depression scale (HADS), and Personal information Questionnaire (PIQ) for collecting socio-demographic, personal, medical, social and family history data. Routine urine and blood results were recorded. Results: 59% of prenatal and 46% of postnatal women suffered from high levels of distress in the form of mixed anxiety and depressive symptoms. However, only 20.9% of peri-natal women suffered of moderate to severe depression. Over 90% of the depressed women were not formally diagnosed or received psychiatric help. Poor marital relationship, physical co-morbidity, positive family history and past psychiatric history of depression were the main significant risk factors associated with perinatal depression and anxiety. Conclusion: Contrary to the commonly held views that perinatal women are mainly plighted with depression as the main mental illness, this study confirms initial findings that, anxiety disorder is far more prevalent and more distressing to this vulnerable group. Moreover, psychiatric morbidities in both prenatal and postnatal periods attract high prevalence rates in low income countries. Maternal health policies in low income countries must incorporate routine screening for mental health status, basic support and interventions for mental illnesses in perinatal women. Depression and emotional disorders in perinatal women should be seen as important public health priority.

Keywords

Prenatal, Postnatal, Peri-Natal, Depression, Anxiety, Psychiatric Morbidities, Risks Factors

1. Background

Symptoms of anxiety and depressive disorders in perinatal women have received considerable attention in high income countries over the last three decades. However, little attention and limited resources, if any, were directed to this group, in low income countries. Only a few prevalence studies were conducted in low income countries to examine the prevalence of the common mental disorders in perinatal women and especially so in Africa, Sudan included [1] [2].

Peri-natal depression has long been recognized to be associated with a number of risks factors such as genetic vulnerability, hormonal changes, major life events, psychosocial stressors and past and present medical complication [3]-[5]. High stress during pregnancy can increase susceptibility to maternal infections by mechanisms that inhibit components of the immune system, also lead to premature delivery and post natal complications [5]-[7]. Post natal depression however, has been associated with low infant body weight, higher infant physical morbidity including diarrhea, vitamin deficiencies weaker mother baby bond and risk of maternal suicide [8]-[12].

Despite all the high maternal and infant morbidity as a consequence to maternal mental health problems, yet the total number of all the prevalence studies that were conducted in Africa did not exceed a total of 11,000 cases, at a recent systemic review of prevalence of depression in perinatal women in Africa [1] [13] [14]. Most studies on perinatal women and mental health disorders have focused on depression and depressive disorders in this sensitive period, rightly so. However, little attention has been given to high rate and distressing symptoms of anxiety which has by itself significant consequences to both mother and baby's health. This can only be unraveled, by using appropriate tools to pick up this condition [15]-[17].

Prevalence findings for anxiety disorders in prenatal and postnatal women attracted rates between 10% - 20% which can either be purely anxiety disorder or mixed anxiety depressive symptoms with anxiety features predominating the psychiatric presentation. Therefore, both anxiety and depression warrant appropriate attention and investigation by researchers and women's mental health strategists [18] [19].

There is conflicting evidence as to whether or not symptoms of anxiety deserve separate attention in the perinatal period, as it might be seen as part of a depressive spectrum by some researchers [20].

Many recent researchers have investigated the initial reported risk factors by Kendal *et al.* in 1976, with anxiety during pregnancy, viz, poor quality of intimate relationship, previous episodes of depression and anxiety, perinatal obstetric complications, positive family history of depression, past history of depression and general low annual income [21] [22]. However, many studies consistently found that past psychiatric history of depression, strong family history of depressive disorder and poor quality of intimate relationship or violence were the strongest risk factors for perinatal depression and mostly so for post natal depression. However, some other risk factors such as presence of high anxiety symptoms during pregnancy as, predictor and risk factor for future development of post natal depression received less attention [23]. Likewise, health factors such as low hemoglobin levels, chronic physical co-morbidity, the number of already born children, job and employment status and presence or absence of family support received less attention in perinatal psychiatric studies [24].

2. Method

2.1. Subjects

Subjects were consecutively collected from two main antenatal clinics at Khartoum Teaching Hospital, and Omdurman antenatal clinic. These two clinics serve a large catchment areas of around 2 million population and overseen by obstetricians, midwives *and senior University consultant obstetricians. Inclusion criteria were designed to include all women who presented to the antenatal clinics in their 3rd trimester in the period between, 1st of June to 30th of September* 2009. Written informed consents to participate in the study in Arabic were obtained. The only exclusion criteria was language barrier for only a few women that didn't speak clear Arabic or

Sudanese dialect leading to clear communication barriers.

Total of 945 consecutive candidate satisfying inclusion criteria were interviewed by trained psychiatric registrars and clinical psychologists.

480 Prenatal women in their third trimester, and 465 postnatal women in the 2nd to 10th week of the postnatal period, had been interviewed in the specified research period.

Separate postnatal clinics exists, serving the same territory, therefore all postnatal women were interviewed at these clinics, as they arrived to see their midwives and health visitors for routine checkup. Most of postnatal women presented between the second and the 10th week of their post natal period (90% were between the 4th to 8th week post delivery).

2.2. Assessments

Six research psychologists and two psychiatrists received three days training on applying interview questionnaires. Most of inter-rater differences were ironed out during training. Then, a pilot phase was carried out in the first two weeks prior to commencement of the study phase which revealed 96.5% of inter-rater reliability for all instruments used for the study. Three instruments were used to collect relevant information.

The first questionnaire was Personal information Questionnaire (PIQ) used to obtain detailed social demographic information about candidates with special reference to, important personal, family, past and present psychiatric history and physical morbidities beside social stressors and circumstances. There was special section for recording hemoglobin and urine results obtained on the same day.

The second questionnaire was a standardized Hospital anxiety and Depression scale (HADS) to report on symptoms of anxiety and depression with this instrument, indicating distress level.

HADS is a self report scale, contains 14 items rated on 4-point Likert-type scale. HADS, has, subscales assess depression and anxiety. The seven-items for either depression or anxiety, yields a score of 0 - 21 that is interrupted with the following cut points: 0 - 7, normal; 8 - 10, mild mood disturbance; 11 - 14, moderate mood disturbance; and 12 - 21, severe mood disturbance [25].

However, a third questionnaire, Beck Depression Inventory (BDI), was used to validate the reported depressive symptoms and obtained by (HADS). The other reason for using BDI was to report on the degree and intensity of the depressive illness. BDI, it's also Likert-type scale, of 21 items, reports symptoms from 0 - 3 (0 meaning symptom not existing, 3, the symptom is sever). BDI, yields score from 0 - 63. The score for moderate depression is 18 - 23, whilst 23 and over indicate severe depression [26].

HADS scale has been validated to be a sensitive instrument to detect symptoms of anxiety and depression, compared with the widely used, Edinburgh Depression Inventory (EDI), which is only sensitive for depressive disorders in perinatal period. Both HADS and BDI instruments have been validated in the Sudanese culture.

The study protocol was approved by the Ethics and research Committee of the University. Written authorizations were obtained from relevant health authorities, beside individual patient's written informed consents.

2.3. Statistical Analysis

All information obtained was entered on the statistical package for social science (SPSS) version 15. Chi square and T-test were calculated for all subjects as per results.

3. Results

3.1. Social Demographic Characteristics

Table 1 gives important socio-demographic characteristics of our participants. 566 (59.9%) of the participants were under the age of 35, 492 (52.1%) finished school before university level while 59 (6.4%) were illiterate. 730 (77.3%) were housewives, that, had previously worked or never worked. 583 (61.7%) of the subjects reported low socio economic background as defined by comparative criteria for an average income in Sudanese community *i.e.* the total family income per year is less than 2500 dollars per year (as defined by Sudanese Social Security and Welfare office). 489 (51.1%) had, had no supporting hand from relatives or other sources to help with the running of the household apart from husbands. While 476 (49%) of the participants had a close relative such as a mother, or a sister, regularly giving them a hand for the household chores and with kids support. It is part of Sudanese culture to have a close relative or senior female relative moving in to live with the pregnant woman prior to giving birth and shortly afterwards to support the family. It is customary that such relative will offer sympathy, and support to the young mother. Most women were of multi-parity (had more than one previously born child), with an average of 2.3 children at the household.

3.2. Clinical Characteristics

Table 2 and **Table 3** show 496 (52.5%) of our perinatal women *i.e.* antenatal and post natal showed high levels of distress (either depression/anxiety, or mixed condition) as reflected by, HADS questionnaire with a threshold above 12 as a cutoff point which denoting clinical threshold from mild to moderate for both anxiety and depression whilst, 449 (47.5%) did not manifest with clinically significant symptoms of anxiety or depression. Prenatal women in particular showed high levels of distress and anxiety (59%) **Table 4**, but only 24% of them presented with clinically significant symptoms of depression as per Becks results, **Table 5** and **Table 6**.

Table 1. Demographics characteristics.

	Number	percentage %
25 - 35 years of age	566	59.9%
Undergraduates	492	52.1%
Illiterates	59	6.4%
Housewives	730	77.3%
Low socioeconomic background	583	61.7%
No helping hand at home apart from the husband	489	51.1%
Average no. of children	2.33	

Table 2. Risks factors leading to high symptoms of mixed anxiety and depression.

	Number of Children		Marital relationship			Past psychiatric		Family history of depression		Physical co-morbidity with pregnancy	
	0 - 4	5 - 10	Good	Average	Poor	Yes	No	Yes	No	Yes	No
Normal	162	34	208	14	1	13	205	13	203	23	174
Mild	185	17	219	4	0	23	202	12	217	21	161
Moderate	205	21	251	18	0	38	233	24	239	38	192
Severe	176	28	184	40	4	42	189	31	188	48	148
Total	728	100	862	76	5	116	829	80	847	130	675

$X^2 = 50.99$ DF = 30 P = 0.010 $X^2 = 51.1$ DF = 6. P = 0000 $X^2 = 15.9$, DF = 3, P = 0.001 $X^2 = 13.8$ DF = 3, P = 0.003

Table 3. Shows distribution of Psychiatric disorder in perinatal period.

	Number	Percentage
HADS	497	52.6%
Beck	198	20.9%

Table 4. Shows prevalence of mixed anxiety and depressive symptoms in prenatal and postnatal period using HADS.

	Prenatal		Postnatal	
	Number	Percentage	Number	Percentage
Normal	87	18.10%	139	30%
Mild	110	22.90%	112	24%
Moderate	149	31%	121	26%
severe	134	28%	93	20%
Total	480	100%	465	100%

Table 5. Positive risk factors for depression with BDI.

	Marital relationship			Past history of depression		Family history of psychiatric illness		Organic illness	
	Good	Average	Poor	Yes	No	Yes	No	Yes	No
Normal	394	18	0	29	384	28	383	42	329
Mild	306	26	0	48	334	27	303	46	226
Moderate	118	18	4	22	140	15	115	30	82
Severe	44	14	0	16	57	10	45	11	38
Total	862	76	4	115	829	89	846	129	675

$X^2 = 55.6$ DF = 6 P = 0.000 $X^2 = 26.9$, DF = 3, P = 0.000 $X^2 = 9.6$ DF = 3 P = 0.023 $X^2 = 17.4$ DF = 3 P = 0.001

Table 6. Shows prevalence of depressive symptoms in prenatal and postnatal period using BECK.

	Prenatal		Postnatal	
	Number	Percentage	Number	Percentage
Normal	182	37.9%	237	51%
Mild-borderline	183	38.10%	149	32%
moderate	81	17%	56	12%
severe	34	7%	23	5%
Total	480	100%	465	100%

3.3. Comparing Prenatal versus Postnatal Morbidities

When, both anxiety and depression were dichotomized to case and non case, taking 12 score as cut off points on the HADS for anxiety and depression, (which were previously validated in Sudanese culture), (**Table 4**), this, revealed that, 383 (59%) of prenatal women showed clinically significant results for both anxiety and depression. On the other hands, 214 (46%), as reflected in HADS, results for postnatal women (**Table 4**).

However, only 115 (24%) of prenatal women presented with clinically significant score for depression of a moderate and severe degree, and 79 (17%) of postnatal women attracted high score results for moderate to severe depression as manifested on the Beck Depression Inventory (BDI), **Table 6**.

3.4. Risk Factors and Associations (Table 7)

Poor marital relationship emerged as a major risk factor for developing both antenatal depression and anxiety as well as post natal, with p-value below 0.0001. Physical co-morbidity with pregnancy came as a second factor especially for a combination of anxiety and depression when it is taken as a spectrum with a p-value of 0.001 as reflected in the HADS test, **Table 7**. Other significant associations were past psychiatric history of depression and anxiety and positive family history for psychiatric illness with a p-value of 0.001, and 0.003 consecutively. Women who had more than 3 children showed higher symptoms for anxiety and depression with a p-value of 0.01, whilst, whether the mother was working or holding a job at the time of her pregnancy or shortly afterwards did not manifest as a major risk factor for depression or anxiety. Educational level whether illiterate or post graduate did not bear any correlation to probability of developing anxiety or depression, nor seen as a protective factor. On the other hand the three most significant factors for developing severe depression for, both pre-natal and postnatal women, were poor marital relationship, past psychiatric illness (both P values below 0.001), and family history of psychiatric illness **Table 7**.

4. Discussion

This study found high prevalence of both anxiety and depression for antenatal (59%) and post natal (46%) women more than previously thought. These disorders were assessed by the HADS test as it was previously noted by O'Hara *et al.* (1990). A diagnosis of depression is only one index of psychological distress which could be rather insensitive and may be more useful to identify psychological distress in the perinatal period with the

Table 7. Collated P values for all risks factors.

Risk Factors	P value against HADS	P value as Per BDI
Poor marital relationship	0.000	0.000
Urine general	0.000	0.009
Co-morbidity with pregnancy	0.001	0.001
Past history of psychiatric illness	0.001	0.000
Family history of psychiatric illness	0.003	0.023
Number of Children	0.010	0.010
Type of co-morbidity	0.020	0.001
Occupation	0.026	
Educational level	0.036	

use of an instrument capable of tapping a common core or psychological impairment. We believe that the HADS test is both sensitive and valid for tapping high levels of distress in perinatal period which reflects the higher result found in this study [27].

Most studies on perinatal psychiatric prevalence didn't take into account the strong co-morbidity between depressive mood and anxiety disorders. Therefore, one of the aims of the present study is to report on the prevalence of these two conditions together and, separate in perinatal periods. Moreover, this study examined a wide range of risk factors that had been noted by different researchers elsewhere.

Principal Findings

This study identified two categories of associated risk factors for perinatal emotional disorders (depression and anxiety), confirmed the widely known risks factors for depression that may occur at any period in a woman's life, such as associated perceived lack of social support or hostility from intimate husband, past psychiatric history of depression or anxiety and family history of depression or anxiety.

However, this study, revealed, a second category of risks factors that are relatively specific to peri-natal emotional disorders such as, physical co-morbidity in the prenatal period, anemia and presence of high psychological distress at the first and second trimester of pregnancy.

Most importantly, we reported, higher rates of psychiatric morbidity, than previously thought, in the form of general distress (stress, anxiety, and depression) at the prenatal period up (59%), and 46% for postnatal period, leading to detrimental health consequence for both the mother and her baby.

Moreover, we were able to discover that, most of this high rates of distress did not receive any formal recognition or treatment via the psychiatric system, (90% of cases) that were found to have moderate to severe mood disorders had not received any formal mental health treatment. Therefore, the distress was endured by the sufferer unrecognized or diagnosed and not treated or supported by mental health team in the developing countries, as was the case in Sudan. Many factors can be cited to this failure, of provisions and recognition for mental ill-health of peri-natal women, not least, due to, stigma associated with mental illness, but, also one can cite other factors, such, as, ignorance, and limitations of resources.

It's worth noting that, contrary to the widely believed vulnerability factor for depression, this study could not detect association of mental morbidity with type of employment or the lack of it, level of education a woman might have attained, or presence or absence of a family support extra to that of the partner. Although, the findings of this paper suggest that dimensional or categorical anxiety is a major risk factor for post natal depression. However, interpretation of the two conditions were hampered by methodological limitations such as, being, relatively small sample size, a cross sectional study, and, lacked adjustment for confounding factors.

Strengths and Weaknesses

This study examined a large number of cases, more that most studies conducted in developing countries, that is to say 945 candidate, and was able to tap on categorical findings of perinatal depression and anxiety.

Among the weaknesses of this study, the inherent problem of being a cross sectional study, one would want to see a longitudinal cohort findings after the initial assessment. Moreover a more structured and standardized assessment tool such as, SCID (Structured Clinical Interview Schedule) would have revealed more elaborate and specific psychiatric diagnosis than HADS and BDI would have allowed.

Declaration of Interest

None.

References

[1]   Sawyer, A., Ayers, S. and Smith, H. (2010) Pre- and Postnatal Psychological Wellbeing in Africa: A Systematic Review. *Journal of Affective Disorders*, **123**, 17-29. http://dx.doi.org/10.1016/j.jad.2009.06.027

[2]   O'Hara, M.W. and Swain, A.M. (1996) Rates and Risks of Postpartum Depression—A Meta-Analysis. *International Review of Psychiatry*, **8**, 37-54. http://dx.doi.org/10.3109/09540269609037816

[3]   Eberhard-Gran, M., Eskild, A., Tambs, K., Samuelsen, S.O. and Opjordsmoen, S (2002) Depression in Postpartum and Non-Postpartum Women: Prevalence and Risk Factors. *Acta Psychiatrica Scandinavica*, **106**, 426-433http://dx.doi.org/10.1034/j.1600-0447.2002.02408.x

[4]   O'Hara, M.W., Schlechte, J.A., Lewis, D.A. and Varner, M.W. (1991) Controlled Prospective Study of Postpartum Mood Disorders: Psychological, Environmental, and Hormonal Variables. *Journal of Abnormal Psychology*, **100**, 63-73. http://dx.doi.org/10.1037/0021-843X.100.1.63

[5]   Faisal-Cury, A., Tedesco, J.J.A., Kahhale, S., Menezes, P.R. and Zugaib, M. (2004) Postpartum Depression: In Relation to Life Events and Patterns of Coping. *Archives of Women's Mental Health*, **7**, 123-131. http://dx.doi.org/10.1007/s00737-003-0038-0

[6]   Fisher, J.R.W., Morrow, M.M., Nhu Ngoc, N.T. and Hoang Anhc, L.T. (2004) Prevalence, Nature, Severity and Correlates of Postpartum Depressive Symptoms in Vietnam. *BJOG*, **111**, 1353-1360. http://dx.doi.org/10.1111/j.1471-0528.2004.00394.x

[7]   Gausia, K., Fisher, C., Ali, M. and Oosthuizen, J. (2009) Magnitude and Contributory Factors of Postnatal Depression: A Community-Based Cohort Study from a Rural Subdistrict of Bangladesh. *Psychological Medicine*, **39**, 999-1007. http://dx.doi.org/10.1017/S0033291708004455

[8]   Patel, V., DeSouza, N. and Rodrigues, M. (2003) Postnatal Depression and Infant Growth and Development in Low-Income Countries: A Cohort Study from Goa, India. *Archives of Disease in Childhood*, **88**, 34-37. http://dx.doi.org/10.1136/adc.88.1.34

[9]   Lack, M.M., Baqu, A.H., Zaman, K., McNary, S.W., Le, K., El Arifeen, S., *et al.* (2007) Depressive Symptoms among Rural Bangladeshi Mothers: Implications for Infant Development. *Journal of Child Psychology and Psychiatry*, **48**, 764-772. http://dx.doi.org/10.1111/j.1469-7610.2007.01752.x

[10] Evans, J., Heron, J., Patel, R.R. and Wiles, N. (2007) Depressive Symptoms during Pregnancy and Low Birth Weight at Term: Longitudinal Study. *The British Journal of Psychiatry*, **191**, 84-85. http://dx.doi.org/10.1192/bjp.bp.105.016568

[11] Orr, S.T., James, S.A. and Blackmore Prince, C. (2002) Maternal Prenatal Depressive Symptoms and Spontaneous Preterm Births among African-American Women in Baltimore, Maryland. *American Journal of Epidemiology*, **156**, 797-802. http://dx.doi.org/10.1093/aje/kwf131

[12] Murray, L., Cooper, P.J., Wilson, A., *et al.* (2003) Controlled Trial of the Short- and Long-Term Effect of Psychological Treatment of Post-Partum Depression: 2. Impact on the Mother-Child Relationship and Child Outcome. *British Journal of Psychiatry*, **182**, 420-427. http://dx.doi.org/10.1192/bjp.182.5.420

[13] Agoub, M., Moussaoui, D. and Battas, O. (2005) Prevalence of Postpartum Depression in a Moroccan Sample. *Archives of Women's Mental Health*, **8**, 37-43. http://dx.doi.org/10.1007/s00737-005-0069-9

[14] Mirza, I. and Jenkins, R. (2004) Risk Factors, Prevalence, and Treatment of Anxiety and Depressive Disorders in Pakistan: Systematic Review. *BMJ*, **328**, 794-797. http://dx.doi.org/10.1136/bmj.328.7443.794

[15] Eberhard-Gran, M., Tambs, K., Opjordsmoen, S., Skrondal, A. and Eskild, A. (2003) A Comparison of Anxiety and Depressive Symptomatology in Postpartum and Non-Postpartum Mothers. *Social Psychiatry and Psychiatric Epidemiology*, **38**, 551-556. http://dx.doi.org/10.1007/s00127-003-0679-3

[16] Klein, D.N., Lewinsohn, P.M., Rohde, P., Seeley, J.R. and Shankman, S.A. (2003) Family Study of Co-Morbidity between Major Depressive Disorder and Anxiety Disorders. *Psychological Medicine*, **33**, 703-714. http://dx.doi.org/10.1017/S0033291703007487

[17] Littleton, H.L., Breitkopf, C.R. and Berenson, A.B. (2007) Correlates of Anxiety Symptoms during Pregnancy and Association with Perinatal Outcomes: A Meta-Analysis. *American Journal of Obstetrics and Gynecology*, **196**, 424-432. http://dx.doi.org/10.1016/j.ajog.2007.03.042

[18] Meades, R. and Ayers, S. (2011) Anxiety Measures Validated in Perinatal Populations: A Systematic Review. *Journal of Affective Disorders*, **133**, 1-15.

[19] Lau, Y. and Keung, D.W. (2007) Correlates of Depressive Symptomatology during the Second Trimester of Pregnancy among Hong Kong Chinese. *Social Science & Medicine*, **64**, 1802-1811. http://dx.doi.org/10.1016/j.socscimed.2007.01.001

[20] Bolton, H.L., Hughes, P.M., Turton, P. and Sedgwick, P. (1998) Incidence and Demographic Correlates of Depressive Symptoms during Pregnancy in an Inner London Population. *Journal of Psychosomatic Obstetrics & Gynecology*, **19**, 202-209. http://dx.doi.org/10.3109/01674829809025698

[21] Husain, N., Bevc, I., Husain, M., Chaudhry, I.B., Atif, N. and Rahman, A. (2006) Prevalence and Social Correlates of Postnatal Depression in a Low Income Country. *Archives of Women's Mental Health*, **9**, 197-202.

[22] Abiodun, O.A., Adetoro, O.O. and Ogunbode, O.O. (1993) Psychiatric Morbidity in a Pregnant Population in Nigeria. *General Hospital Psychiatry*, **15**, 125-128. http://dx.doi.org/10.1016/0163-8343(93)90109-2

[23] Rahman, A., Iqbal, Z. and Harrington, R. (2003) Life Events, Social Support and Depression in Childbirth: Perspectives from a Rural Community in the Developing World. *Psychological Medicine*, **33**, 1161-1167. http://dx.doi.org/10.1017/S0033291703008286

[24] Kumar, R. and Robson, K. (1984) A Prospective Study of Emotional Disorders in Childbearing Women. *The British Journal of Psychiatry*, **144**, 35-47. http://dx.doi.org/10.1192/bjp.144.1.35

[25] Snaith, R.P. and Zigmond, A.S. (1994) The Hospital Anxiety and Depression Scale Manual. Nfer-Nelson, Windsor.

[26] Beck, A.T. (1993) Beck Depression Inventory Manual. Psychological Corporation, San Antonio.

[27] Bjelland, I., Dahl, A.A., Haug, T.T. and Neckelmann, D. (2002) The Validity of the Hospital Anxiety and Depression Scale. An Updated Literature Review. *Journal of Psychosomatic Research*, **52**, 69-77. http://dx.doi.org/10.1016/S0022-3999(01)00296-3

Self-Genital Mutilation and Attempted Suicide by Cut Throat in the Same Patient at Presentation: A Rare Event

Senyo Gudugbe[1], Isaac Asiedu[2], Jonathan Lamptey[1], Mathew Y. Kyei[2], Kenneth Baidoo[3]

[1]Department of Surgery, Korle Bu Teaching Hospital, Accra, Ghana
[2]Urology Unit, Department of Surgery, School of Medicine and Dentistry, College of Health Sciences, University of Ghana, Accra, Ghana
[3]Otolaryngology Unit, Department of Surgery, School of Medicine and Dentistry, College of Health Sciences, University of Ghana, Accra, Ghana
Email: senyomd@gmail.com

Abstract

Genital self-mutilation is an uncommon event that is commonly associated with psychotic disorders. Such injuries have also been reported secondary to complex religious beliefs and delusions regarding sexual guilt. Even though few case reports of male genital self-mutilation are available in literature, it is rare to have a combined self-genital mutilation and attempted suicide by cut throat occurring in the same patient at presentation. We presented the case of a 38-yr-old male who presented to the accident and emergency centre of a tertiary hospital in Accra, Ghana.

Keywords

Self Genital Mutilation, Attempted Suicide, Cut Throat

1. Introduction

Self mutilation has been defined as the deliberate destruction or alteration of body tissue without conscious suicidal intent [1], so though there could be scars on other parts of the body, they are usually from minor superficial lacerations. It has been performed by individuals of all races religions and cultures. The first report in English medical literature of genital self mutilation (GSM) was in 1901 by Strock [2] [3]. The occurrence of genital self mutilation in the absence of psychopathology is extremely rare [4]. Self inflicted genital injuries range from simple lacerations of the external genitalia to more complex injuries such as penile amputation, self castration or a combination of both [5]. Suicide is defined as death due to an intentional act or acts of the deceased who anticipates his or her resultant death [6]. It has been observed that cut throat is the most commonly preferred method for committing suicide [7]. Epidemiological studies have established that, patients with background schizophrenia have an 8.5 fold-increased risk for suicide compared to the general population [8] [9]. In this patient, there was genital self mutilation followed by an attempted suicide by cut throat. This rare presentation and the challenges of management are presented in this case report.

2. Case Summary

38-yr-old male was referred from a primary health facility where he had presented with a history of an attempted suicide having amputated his glans penis and then cut his throat in sequence. He was found in his apartment bleeding and rushed for medical attention. An estimated two hours had elapsed between time of injury and arrival at the accident and emergency centre. Patient was diagnosed of schizophrenia five years earlier but has been non compliant and off his regular medications (Olanzapine) for a month. The Patient alluded to auditory hallucinations beckoning him to commit suicide although this index presentation was his first attempt. He is separated from the wife and lives alone in a suburb of Accra. He is a Christian who works as a carpenter and has no history of illegal substance use.

On physical examination patient was fully conscious, communicating and pale. His oxygen saturation was 95% on room air with a respiratory rate of 30 cycles per minute and a mild inspiratory stridor. His Blood pressure was 110/65 mmHg and the pulse was 92 beats per minute regular with good volume. Neck examination revealed a single transverse incision measuring 8 cm × 2 cm with bleeding edges. The incision extends to the medial edges of both sternocleidomastoids (**Figure 1**).

Examination of the abdomen and perineum revealed an amputated glans penis, bleeding penile stump and an exposed penile urethra. There were two ventral penile shaft lacerations measuring 1 cm × 0.5 cm each, limited to the dermis and located 2 cm and 3 cm from the peno-scrotal junction. The urethra was not lacerated ventrally (**Figure 2**). The amputated stump was not brought to the hospital.

The patient was resuscitated with intravenous crystalloids and started on intravenous antibiotics. He was given tetanus prophylaxis. No foreign bodies or subcutaneous emphysema was demonstrated on Lateral soft tissue neck x-ray. Chest x-ray done was normal. Haemoglobin at presentation was 12.4 g/dl with a Haematocrit of 40%. Patient was sent to theatre within 4 hours of presentation and had emergency neck and penile exploration under general anaesthesia. Neck findings were a single transverse upper neck incision measuring 8 cm × 2 cm, severed strap muscles exposing the laryngeal prominence, the thyroid cartilage and oedematous vocal chords. The oesophagus was not injured. The carotid sheath and its contents were spared on both sides. Penile findings were an amputated glans penis, two ventral penile lacerations limited to the dermis and located 2 cm and 3 cm from the peno-scrotal junction. The urethra was not lacerated ventrally. Surgical procedures performed included laryngeal repair, strap muscle repair and a low tracheostomy by the ENT surgeon. The penile stump was refashioned after a urethral catheter was passed and the ventral lacerations were sutured by the Urologists (**Figure 3**). A nasogastric tube was passed intra operatively.

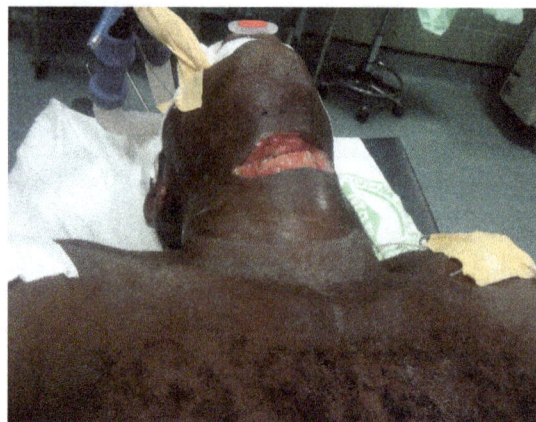

Figure 1. Cut throat.

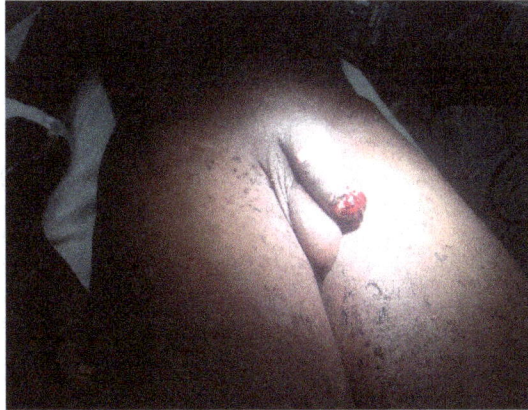

Figure 2. Penile stump,

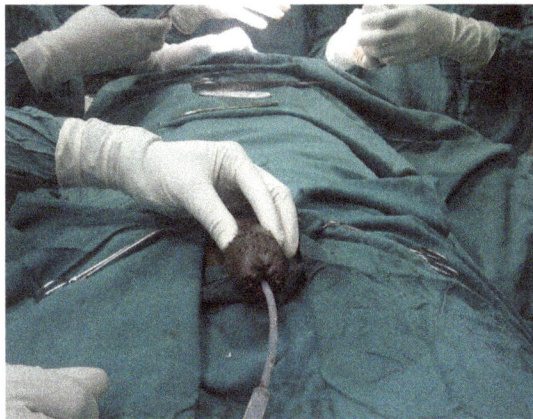

Figure 3. Refashioned Penile stump.

Post operatively patient was fed via the nasogastric tube for the first four days, his neck drain was removed on post operative day (POD) 3 and neck stitches removed POD 5. Flexible laryngoscopy done on POD 6 showed normal vocal cords that abduct and adduct normally, patient had normal breathing and phonation. Patients refashioned penile stump and sutured ventral lacerations healed well, the urethral catheter was removed on POD 6. De-canulation of the tracheostomy was done POD11. Whilst on admission, patient had reassessment by the psychiatrist and the diagnosis of schizophrenia (DSM code 295.3) was confirmed and restarted on Olanzapine. He was discharged home POD 12 after confirming his appointment with the Psychiatrist for the ensuing 3 months.

3. Discussion

Self injurious behaviour is observed in both psychotic and nonpsychotic individuals though the self genital mutilation is usually associated with the psychotic disorders. Patients with command hallucinations, religious preoccupations, substance abuse and social isolation are the most vulnerable [10]. Our patient admits to auditory accusatory hallucinations secondary to schizophrenia. Male sex, young age, higher levels of education, depressive symptoms and active hallucinations have been found to be strongly associated with suicide in schizophrenia [11]. Suicide prediction in schizophrenia is complex and efforts on prevention should also focus on ensuring compliance with medications [6]. An effective multidisciplinary team comprising the Psychiatrist, Urologist, and the ENT surgeon should be involved in the management of patients with a background psychotic disorder, self genital mutilation and an attempted suicide by cut throat.

References

[1]   Coons, P.M. (1992) Self-Amputation of the Breasts by a Male with Schizotypal Personality Disorder. *Hospital &*

Community Psychiatry, **43**, 175-176. http://dx.doi.org/10.1176/ps.43.2.175

[2] Eke, N. (2000) Genital Self-Mutilation. There is no method in this madness. *BJU International*, **85**, 295-298. http://dx.doi.org/10.1046/j.1464-410x.2000.00438.x

[3] Bhattacharyya, R., Sanyal, D. and Roy, K. (2011) A Case of Klingsor Syndrome: When There Is No Longer Psychosis. *Israel Journal of Psychiatry & Related Sciences*, **48**, 30-33.

[4] Mareko, G.M., Othienco, C.J., Kuria, M.W., Kiarie, J.N. and Ndetei, D.M. (2007) Body Dysmorphic Disorder. *Case report. East African Medical Journal*, **84**, 450-452.

[5] Stunnel, H., Power, R.E., Floyd, M. Jnr and Quinlan, D.M. (2006) Genital Self Mutilation. *International Journal of Urology*, **13**, 1358-1360. http://dx.doi.org/10.1111/j.1442-2042.2006.01548.x

[6] Horswell, J. (2000) Suspicious Deaths, Encyclopedia of Forensic Sciences. In: Siegel, J.A., Saukko, P.J. and Knupfer, G.C., Eds., *Crime Scene investigation and Examination*, Academic Press, San Diego, 1, 463.

[7] Marak, F.K. and Singh, Th. B. (2005) Suicidal Cut Throat—A Case Report. *JIAFM*, **27**, 260-262.

[8] Inskip, H.M., Harris, E.C. and Barraclough, B. (1998) Lifetime Risk of Suicide for Affective Disorder, Alcoholism and Schizophrenia. *The British Journal of Psychiatry*, **172**, 35-37. http://dx.doi.org/10.1192/bjp.172.1.35

[9] Harris, E.C. and Barraclough, B. (1997) Suicide as an Outcome for Mental Disorders: A Meta-Analysis. *The British Journal of Psychiatry*, **170**, 205-228. http://dx.doi.org/10.1192/bjp.170.3.205

[10] Tobias, C.R, Turns, D.M, Lippman, S., Parry, R. and Oropilla, T.B. (1988) Evaluation and Management of Self Mutilation. *South Medical Journal*, **81**, 1261-1263. http://dx.doi.org/10.1097/00007611-198810000-00015

[11] Hor, K. and Taylor, M. (2010) Suicide and Schizophrenia: A Systematic Review of Rates and Risk Factors. *Journal of Psychopharmacology*, **24**, 81-90. http://dx.doi.org/10.1177/1359786810385490

23

Fluvoxamine in Treatment of Depression in Russian Patients: An Open-Label, Uncontrolled and Randomized Multicenter Observational Study

Anatoly Boleslavovich Smulevich*, Natalia Alekseevna Ilyina, Victoria Valentinovna Chitlova

National Centre of Mental Health of the Russian Academy of Medical Sciences, Moscow, Russia
Email: *absmulevich@list.ru

Abstract

Background: Fluvoxamine, a selective serotonin reuptake inhibitor is widely used in the treatment of depression, one of the most common disorders prevalent in Russia. However, studies demonstrating its efficacy and safety in routine settings in Russia are scarce. Methods: This prospective, uncontrolled, open-label study was conducted at 11 centers in Russia. Total 293 patients (aged ≥ 18 years), meeting DSM-IV criteria for depression and scoring ≥ 17 on 17-item Hamilton Rating Scale of Depression (HAMD-17) received fluvoxamine 50 - 300 mg for 6 weeks. Primary efficacy measures included change from baseline in the HAMD-17 and Clinical Global Impression (CGI) scores. Secondary efficacy measure was evaluation of sleep quality changes on HAMD-17 subscale. Safety was assessed by monitoring of adverse drug reactions (ADRs). Results: Mean age of patients was 42.7 years and the majority of them were women (72%). At the end of treatment (day 42), clinically significant reduction was observed in mean HAMD-17, CGI-severity of illness and HAMD-17 sleep sub-score from 23.1, 4.5 and 3.9 at baseline to day 42; change from baseline (Δ) was: Δ-17.3 [95% CI: −18.0; −16.7]), Δ-2.1 and Δ-3.4 [95% CI: −3.53; −3.20]), respectively. At day 42, 20.8% patients reported as normal (not at all ill) on the CGI-severity scale and 85% patients reported as "much improved" or "very much improved" on the CGI-change in severity and quality of life scores. Nausea (12.6%) and somnolence (5.1%) were the most frequently reported ADRs. No deaths or serious ADRs were reported but eight patients discontinued treatment due to ADRs. Conclusion: Treatment with fluvoxamine under routine settings showed marked improvement in Russian patients with depression as measured by HAMD-17 and CGI ratings and was thus efficacious as well as safe and well-tolerated.

---

*Corresponding author.

Keywords

Fluvoxamine, Depression, Hamilton Rating Scale of Depression, Routine Settings

1. Introduction

Depression is a complex mental disorder having a long-term negative impact on the health and economic well-being of both individuals and society. Globally, it affects more than 350 million people annually [1] with life time prevalence rates in general population ranging from 10% to 15% [2]. It is projected that by the year 2020 it will rank second for the Disability Adjusted Life Years calculated for all ages [3].

The scenario is similar in Russia where recent studies have indicated the prevalence of lifetime and current depressive disorders to be 30% and 20.7%, respectively [4] with high percentages in both women (44%) and men (23%) [5]. Biochemical, endocrinal, neurophysiological, psychological and social-economical factors are known to play a role in the aetiology of depression. Social circumstances in particular, have a strong influence in increasing human depressive symptoms [6]. This is particularly evident in Russia, where social upheaval over a last few decades have led to high psychological distress and increased incidence of depression and related disorders [5]. Depressive disorders in general population needs immediate attention as it reduces a person's social functioning, ability to work and have a negative impact on the physical health and quality of life [7]. Moreover, its presence as a comorbid medical illness [8] with other prevalent psychotic disorders in Russia such as schizophrenia [9] raises concern as it usually tends to emerge in the form of psychogenic disorders and worsens the course of the primary disease [10]. A high quality of care for patients with depression in primary care settings is, therefore needed in order to minimize the morbidity caused by such a prevalent condition.

Various antidepressants currently dominate the medical management of depressive disorders and amongst different classes (e.g. tricyclic antidepressants [TCA], monoamine oxidase inhibitors, etc.), selective serotonin reuptake inhibitors (SSRIs) are recommended for wider usage around the world [11] [12]. The SSRIs act by selectively inhibiting the reuptake of neurotransmitter serotonin, which improves the transmission of neural signals, thereby reducing depressive symptoms and elevating the state of mind [12]. They are equivalent to TCAs in terms of efficacy, but score better on safety and tolerability [13]. National Institute for Health and Clinical Excellence recommends the use SSRI in generic form after considering potential side effects and patient preferences [14].

Among SSRIs, fluvoxamine is approved for the treatment of depression in many countries [15]. It has suitable pharmacokinetics that supports once-daily dosing [16] and has shown greater therapeutic benefit when compared with imipramine in patients with severe depression [17] [18]. Treatment with fluvoxamine is also associated with improvement in sleep quality [19] and has a lower impact on body weight [20].

Although fluvoxamine-based treatment is widely used for the management of depressive disorders in Russia, there are limited efficacy trials that are conducted in carefully selected populations under controlled conditions [4] [21]-[23]. Information on its efficacy and safety in treating depression under routine, uncontrolled settings, which is intended to have a greater generalizability in Russian population, is scarce. As a part of post-marketing surveillance, the present uncontrolled, multicenter, observational study was conducted to evaluate the efficacy and safety of fluvoxamine-based treatment for management of patients with depression under routine settings in Russia.

2. Methods

2.1. Study Design

This was an open label, observational study conducted at 11 centers in Russia from November 2006 to May 2007. Eligible patients received fluvoxamine 50 - 300 mg once-daily for 6 weeks with study visits scheduled on day 1, 7, 14, 28 and 42 (**Figure 1**). The recommended starting dose was 50 to 100 mg once-daily and if necessary, the dose was increased by 50 mg weekly up to a maximum of 300 mg/day according to the patient's response and was divided in those receiving >150 mg/day.

The study was conducted in accordance with the ethical principles originating in the Declaration of Helsinki

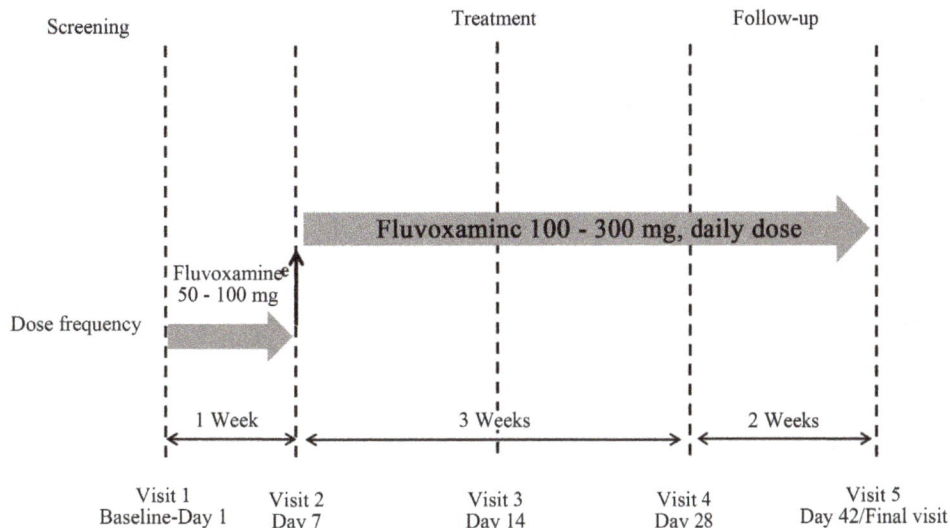

Figure 1. Study design.

and European Good Clinical Practice guidelines, applicable regulatory requirements, and in compliance with the protocol.

2.2. Patients

Adult male or female outpatients of 18 years of age and above with established depression, and who fulfilled the diagnostic criteria defined by the Diagnostic and Statistical Manual of Mental Disorders, 4th edition (DSM-IV) and had a score ≥ 17 on the 17-item Hamilton Rating Scale of Depression (HAMD-17) were included in the study.

Patients with proven hepatic or renal insufficiency and those hypersensitive to the drug were excluded from the study. Other exclusion criteria included treatment with tizanidine or irreversible monoamine oxidase inhibitors within two weeks prior to baseline visit as well as pregnant or lactating women. Various classes of drugs that were not allowed during the surveillance period of the study included; antidepressants other than fluvoxamine, sedatives, tranquillizers, neuroleptics, antipsychotics, narcotics, anticonvulsants, anticoagulants and drugs like cisapride, propranolol, theophylline, cyclosporine, methadone, mexiletine, tacrine, metoprolol, terfenadine and astemizole. All patients were free to withdraw their participation in the study at any time.

2.3. Efficacy Assessments

The primary efficacy end points were the change from baseline in HAMD-17 total score and Clinical Global Impression (CGI). The HAMD-17 total scores were assessed at baseline and study days 7, 14, 28 and day 42 (or upon early withdrawal from the study), while CGI was recorded at baseline and day 42.

The secondary efficacy end point was the change from baseline in the sleep quality as assessed by items 4, 5 and 6 of the HAMD-17 over the six-week period.

2.4. Safety Assessments

Tolerability and safety were assessed through collection and monitoring of any spontaneously reported adverse drug reactions (ADRs), serious ADRs, and physical examination (height and weight). All concomitant medications were also reviewed and vital characteristics such as systolic blood pressure (SBP), diastolic blood pressure (DBP), and pulse rate were measured at baseline and day 42.

2.5. Statistical Analysis

No formal sample size calculation was done. Based on the feasibility, a total number of 300 patients were considered adequate to collect considerable exposure of fluvoxamine. Safety analysis was performed on all patients who received at least one dose of study medication (safety population), whereas efficacy analysis was performed on all patients who were included in the safety sample and had at least one post-baseline assessment of any efficacy measurement (ITT population).

Descriptive statistics were used to summarize the demographic variables. Changes from baseline for all efficacy measures were presented by descriptive statistics, including 95% confidence intervals (CIs) and one-sample t-test. Endpoint refers to the last non-missing observation during a post-baseline visit.

Safety was assessed primarily by reporting of ADR. All reported treatment-emergent ADRs were taken into account, coded according to Medical Dictionary for Regulatory Activities (MedDRA) and presented in summary tables with the number and percentage of patients who reported that ADR.

3. Results

3.1. Patient Disposition, Baseline Demographics and Clinical Characteristics

A total of 293 patients were recruited and treated with fluvoxamine. Total 15 patients withdrew before completion of the six weeks of treatment, reasons were: ADRs (n = 8; nausea being the most frequent [n = 3]), lack of efficacy (n = 3), loss to follow-up (n = 2) and withdrawal of consent (n = 2). No clinically relevant protocol deviations were observed during the study.

The patient's baseline characteristics are listed in **Table 1**. The mean age was 42.7 years with body mass index

Table 1. Patient baseline demographics and clinical characteristics.

Parameter	Value
Age (years)	
N	293
Mean (SD)	42.7 (13.9)
Age category (years), n (%)	
17 - 29	59 (20.1)
30 - 49	138 (47.1)
50 - 64	76 (25.9)
≥65	20 (6.8)
Sex, n (%)	
Men	81 (27.6)
Women	212 (72.4)
Height (cm)	
n	287
Mean (SD)	168.0 (8.6)
Weight (kg)	
n	292
Mean (SD)	70.2 (13.6)
Body Mass Index (Kg/m^2)	
n	287
Mean (SD)	24.9 (4.2)
Diastolic Blood Pressure (mmHg)	
n	292
Mean (SD)	78.0 (9.1)
Systolic Blood Pressure (mmHg)	
n	292
Mean (SD)	123.0 (13.5)
HAMD-17 Total Score	
n	293
Mean (SD)	23.1 (4.6)
CGI-S	
n	293
Mean (SD)	4.5 (0.8)
HAMD-17 Sleep Sub-score	
n	293
Mean (SD)	3.9 (1.3)

CGI-S: Clinical Global Impression Severity, HAMD-17: 17-item Hamilton Rating Scale of Depression, SD: standard deviation.

(BMI) of 24.9 kg/m^2 and majority of them were women (72%). The most frequently reported pre-existing medical conditions were cardiovascular diseases (15%), cranial trauma (13.0%) and psychiatric disorders other than depression (9.9%). Drug/alcohol abuse was recorded in nine patients (3.1%).

The most frequently prescribed concomitant medications were sedatives (23.9%), cardiovascular drugs (12.6%), anti-epileptic drugs (9.6%) and antipsychotics (9.6%). Antidepressant combination therapy was prescribed for seven patients (2.4%).

3.2. Efficacy Variables

3.2.1. HAMD-17 Total Score

A visit-wise plot of mean change in HAMD-17 total score is presented in **Figure 2**. At baseline, the mean (±SD) total HAMD-17 score was 23.1 ± 4.6 and decreased steadily over time and improved to 5.8 ± 4.3 at the final visit on day 42 (change from baseline Δ [95% CI]: −17.3 [−18.0; −16.7]). Overall, a reduction of 74.89% was observed in the mean scores of HAMD-17 from baseline to the final visit on day 42.

3.2.2. HAMD-17 Sleep Sub-Score

The mean (±SD) HAMD-17 sleep sub-score decreased from 3.9 ± 1.3 at baseline to 0.6 ± 0.8 at the final visit on day 42 (change from baseline Δ [95% CI]: −3.4 [−3.53; −3.20]). At endpoint, the mean score was 0.7 ± 1.0 (**Figure 3**).

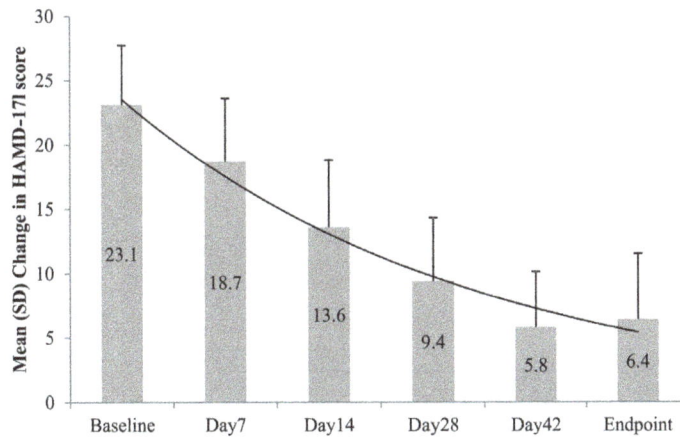

Figure 2. Change from baseline to day 42 in HAMD-17 total score (intent-to-treat analysis set) HAMD-17: 17-item Hamilton Rating Scale of Depression.

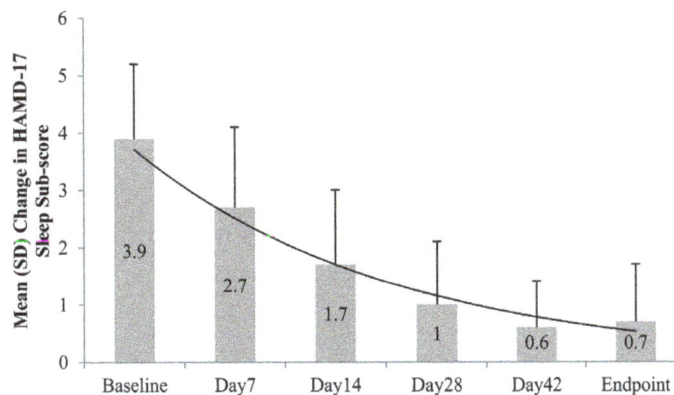

Figure 3. Changes from baseline to day 42 in the HAMD-17 sleep sub-score (intent-to-treat analysis set) HAMD-17: 17-item Hamilton Rating Scale of Depression.

3.2.3. CGI Scores

The mean CGI-severity score decreased from 4.5 (moderately to markedly ill) at baseline to 2.4 (borderline to mildly ill) on day 42. Overall, a reduction of 46.67% was recorded in the mean CGI-scores at the end of treatment (day 42). More than 85% of patients were reported as "much improved" or "very much improved" as per the CGI-change in severity and quality of life scores at day 42 (**Figure 4**).

At the end of treatment (day 42), 20.8% patients (n = 58) were reported as normal (not at all ill) on the CGI-severity scale by the investigator. There was a substantial improvement in patient's clinical condition classified as "borderline mentally ill" when compared to baseline in this category (40.9% vs 0.7%) (**Table 2**). The majority of patients and investigators rated the treatment as good (66.67%) to excellent (20% - 21%).

3.3. Safety and Tolerability

A total of 72 patients (24.6%) experienced at least one ADR during the six-week period (**Table 3**). The majority of ADRs were mild or moderate in severity. Nausea (37, 12.6%) and somnolence (15, 5.1%) were the most frequently reported ADRs. No deaths and serious ADRs were reported, but eight patients discontinued treatment

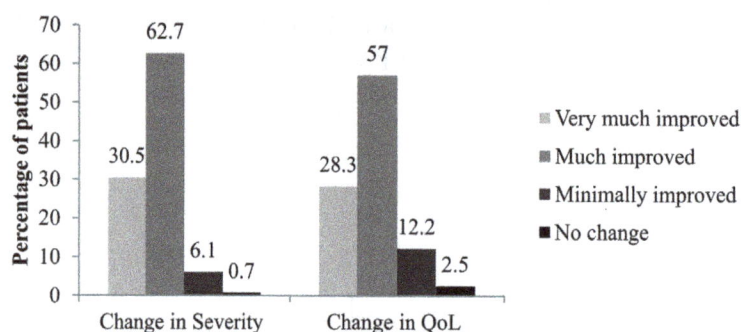

Figure 4. CGI per classifications of change in severity and change in QoL (intent-to-treat analysis set) CGI: Clinical Global Impression, QoL: Quality of Life.

Table 2. CGI-S classification at baseline and day 42 (intent-to-treat analysis set).

Severity	Baseline n (%)	Day 42 n (%)
Normal, not at all ill	0 (0.0)	58 (20.8)
Borderline mentally ill	2 (0.7)	114 (40.9)
Mildly ill	19 (6.5)	67 (24.0)
Moderately ill	140 (47.8)	30 (10.8)
Markedly ill	102 (34.8)	9 (3.2)
Severely ill	29 (9.9)	1 (0.4)
Most extremely ill	1 (0.3)	0 (0.0)

CGI-S: Clinical Global Impression Severity.

Table 3. Adverse events reported in >1% of patients (Safety analysis set) (order of frequency).

Adverse Drug Reaction (ADR)	n (%)
Patients with ≥1 ADR	72 (24.6)
Nausea	37 (12.6)
Somnolence	15 (5.1)
Headache	6 (2.0)
Vertigo	5 (1.7)
Asthenia	4 (1.4)
Constipation	4 (1.4)

due to ADRs during the study. Nausea in two patients, sleepiness and diarrhea in one patient each were the only severe ADRs. No clinically significant changes were observed in vital signs, body weight, BMI, pulse rate, DBP, and SBP.

4. Discussion

Prevalence of depression in Russian population is substantial, but studies dealing with the treatment needs in this population under routine settings are limited. Although, fluvoxamine is the preferred line of treatment for depression, studies examining its effectiveness under daily practice from Russia are scarce. This observational study established the efficacy of fluvoxamine-based treatment as evidenced by a significant improvement in HAMD-17 total scores and CGI scores. To the best of our knowledge, this is the first open-label observational study to examine the efficacy and safety of fluvoxamine-based treatment in Russian patients with depression under uncontrolled routine settings.

The high percentage of female patients with depression (72%) in this study is line with other published reports [24] [25] reporting high prevalence of depression in Russian females in comparison with the male population; similarly observed worldwide.

The efficacy results of this study are consistent with other studies using the same drug in populations from Europe and other regions [19] [26]-[28]. The observed 75% reduction in the HAMD-17 score with fluvoxamine treatment is similar to the clinically significant change of 71% recorded in another study [29].

Fluvoxamine in contrast to other anti-depressants is known to have an early onset of action, which is an important consideration as depressed patients are prone to harm themselves if not treated at an earlier stage. Early onset of action may also reduce the occurrence of treatment discontinuations, which may be due to lack of efficacy, one of the commonest factors seen in routine settings. Thus, decrease in HAMD-17 score as early as day 7 may explain why very few patients discontinued the treatment due to lack of efficacy [30]. These findings correlate with a double-blind study wherein fluvoxamine was reported to have a relatively faster onset of therapeutic action when compared with other SSRIs [19].

Similar to HAMD-17 total score, improvement was also noted in the CGI scores. A 46.67% reduction in the mean CGI-severity scores was recorded at the endpoint and a total of 20.8% patients were categorized as being "normal" and "not at all ill", as per the CGI-severity scale. Earlier studies have reported significantly more responders on the CGI-severity and a greater reduction of CGI-severity scores for fluvoxamine treatment when compared to other SSRIs at week 2, but not at week 4 or 6 [19]. As we only evaluated the CGI scores at baseline and week 6 (day 42), our study provides further evidence of a favorable response of fluvoxamine on CGI scores also at week 6.

Depression is associated with a poor quality of life [31]. This study showed improvement in quality of life of the patients over a 6-week treatment, which is in conformance with other studies [26] [32]. Improvements were also observed in quality of sleep, as measured by the HAMD-17 sleep sub-score and the results are in accordance with the previous studies [19] [33] where fluvoxamine treatment was shown to have a faster onset of action against depressive symptoms and better improvement in sleep quality as compared with other SSRIs.

Fluvoxamine treatment exhibited good safety and favorable tolerability profile in this study. Nausea and somnolence were the most commonly reported ADRs. These results are consistent with the previous studies [20] [34]-[36]. In this study, fluvoxamine treatment led to no remarkable changes in either body weight or BMI. These findings are highly encouraging in the treatment of depression as it enhances adherence and reduces non-compliance in patients requiring long-term treatment [20].

Although an open-label, uncontrolled study has its own limitations; the routine setting does provide a more realistic approximation of clinical practice when compared to a double-blind study. Limitation of the study was its short duration, which disallowed information about relapse and remission maintenance in patients with depression.

5. Conclusion

Treatment with fluvoxamine under routine settings showed marked improvement in Russian patients with depression as measured by HAMD-17 and CGI ratings and was thus efficacious as well as safe and well-tolerated. The lack of empirical evidence in the treatment of depression in primary care settings serves a major barrier in the management of depression. The routine setting of this study targets to fill this gap to some extent while validating and extending the safety and efficacy of fluvoxamine treatment for depression in the Russian population.

Acknowledgements

The authors thank Dr. Khushboo Nagdev and Dr. Shirin Ghodke (SIRO Clinpharm Pvt. Ltd.) for providing writing assistance. The authors also thank the study participants, without whom this study would not have been accomplished.

Conflict of Interest

This study was funded by Solvay Pharmaceuticals, Russia.

Disclosure

All authors met ICMJE criteria and all those who fulfilled those criteria were listed as authors. All authors had access to the study data and made the final decision about where to present these data.

References

[1] World Health Organization. (2012) Depression a Global Public Health Concern.
http://www.who.int/mental_health/management/depression/who_paper_depression_wfmh_2012.pdf

[2] Lépine, J.P. and Briley, M. (2011) The Increasing Burden of Depression. *Journal of Neuropsychiatric Disease and Treatment*, **7**, 3-7.

[3] Reddy, M.S. (2010) Depression: The Disorder and the Burden. *Indian Journal of Psychological Medicine*, **32**, 1-2. http://dx.doi.org/10.4103/0253-7176.70510

[4] Pakriev, S., Kovalev, J. and Mozhaev, M. (2009) Prevalence of Depression in a General Hospital in Izhevsk, Russia. *Nordic Journal of Psychiatry*, **63**, 469-474. http://dx.doi.org/10.3109/08039480903062950

[5] Bobak, M., Pikhart, H., Pajak, A., Kubinova, R., Malyutina, S., Sebakova, H., *et al.* (2006) Depressive Symptoms in Urban Population Samples in Russia, Poland and the Czech Republic. *The British Journal of Psychiatry*, **188**, 359-365. http://dx.doi.org/10.1192/bjp.188.4.359

[6] Nicholson, A., Pikhart, H., Pajak, A., Malyutina, S., Kubinova, R., Peasey, A., *et al.* (2008) Socio-economic Status over the Life-Course and Depressive Symptoms in Men and Women in Eastern Europe. *Journal of Affective Disorders*, **105**, 125-136. http://dx.doi.org/10.1016/j.jad.2007.04.026

[7] Patel, D. (2008) Depression is the Most Common Mental Disorder in Community Settings, and Is a Major Cause of Disability. *Occupational Medicine (London)*, **58**, 453. http://dx.doi.org/10.1093/occmed/kqn135

[8] Gurovich, I.Y., Schmukler, A.B., Storozhakova, Y.A., Kiryanova, E.M., Salnikova, L.I., Gazha, A.K., *et al.* (2013) Depressive Symptoms Diagnosis and Treatment of Schizophrenia and Schizophrenia Spectrum Disorders in Russian Clinical Practice. *Zhurnal Nevrologii i Psikhiatrii Imeni S.S. Korsakova*, **113**, 28-33.

[9] Smulevich, A.B., Drobizhev, M.A. and Ivanov, S.V. (2002) Schizophrenia and Schizophrenia Spectrum Disorders in General Hospital. *Zhurnal Nevrologii i Psikhiatrii Imeni S.S. Korsakova*, **102**, 9-13.

[10] Smulevich, A.V. (2003) Depression and Schizophrenia. *Zhurnal Nevrologii i Psikhiatrii Imeni S.S. Korsakova*, **103**, 4-13.

[11] Kozyrev, V.N., Smulevich, A.B., Drobizhev, M.I., Kraeva, G.K. and Kubrakov, M.A. (2003) Psychotropic Drugs Used in a Psychiatric Hospital (Pharmaco-Epidemiologic Aspects). *Zhurnal Nevrologii i Psikhiatrii Imeni S.S. Korsakova*, **103**, 25-32.

[12] Gartlehner, G., Hansen, R.A., Thieda, P., De Veaugh-Geiss, A.M., Gaynes, B.N., Krebs, E.E., *et al.* (2007) Comparative Effectiveness of Second-Generation Antidepressants in the Pharmacologic Treatment of Adult Depression. Agency for Healthcare Research and Quality, Rockville.
http://www.effectivehealthcare.ahrq.gov/repFiles/Antidepressants_Final_Report.pdf13

[13] von Wolff, A., Hölzel, L.P., Westphal, A., Härter, M. and Kriston, L. (2013) Selective Serotonin Reuptake Inhibitors and Tricyclic Antidepressants in the Acute Treatment of Chronic Depression and Dysthymia: A Systematic Review and Meta-Analysis. *Journal of Affective Disorders*, **144**, 7-15. http://dx.doi.org/10.1016/j.jad.2012.06.007

[14] National Institute for Health and Clinical Excellence (2009) Depression: The Treatment and Management of Depression in Adults (Update). National Clinical Practice Guideline 90.
http://www.nice.org.uk/nicemedia/pdf/CG90NICEguideline.pdf

[15] Hachisu, M. and Ichimaru, Y. (2000) Pharmacological and Clinical Aspects of Fluvoxamine (Depromel): The First Se-

lective Serotonin Reuptake Inhibitor Approved for Clinical Use Employed in Japan. *Folia Pharmacologica Japonica*, **115**, 271-279. http://dx.doi.org/10.1254/fpj.115.271

[16] Hrdina, P.D. (1991) Pharmacology of Serotonin Uptake Inhibitors: Focus on Fluvoxamine. *Journal of Psychiatry & Neuroscience*, **16**, 10-18.

[17] Fabre, L., Birkhimer, L.J., Zaborny, B.A., Wong, L.F. and Kapik, B.M. (1996) Fluvoxamine versus Imipramine and Placebo: A Double-Blind Comparison in Depressed Patients. *International Clinical Psychopharmacology*, **11**, 119-127.

[18] Kasper, S., Möller, H.J., Montgomery, S.A. and Zondag, E. (1995) Antidepressant Efficacy in Relation to Item Analysis and Severity of Depression: A Placebo-Controlled Trial of Fluvoxamine versus Imipramine. *International Clinical Psychopharmacology*, **9**, 3-12. http://dx.doi.org/10.1097/00004850-199501004-00001

[19] Dalery, J. and Honig, A. (2003) Fluvoxamine versus Fluoxetine in Major Depressive Episode: A Double-Blind Randomized Comparison. *Human Psychopharmacology*, **18**, 379-384. http://dx.doi.org/10.1002/hup.490

[20] Westenberg, H.G. and Sandner, C. (2006) Tolerability and Safety of Fluvoxamine and Other Antidepressants. *International Journal of Clinical Practice*, **60**, 482-491. http://dx.doi.org/10.1111/j.1368-5031.2006.00865.x

[21] Panteleeva, G.P., Abramova, L.I. and Korenev, A.N. (2000) Selective Serotonin Reuptake Inhibitors in the Therapy of Various Types of Endogenous Depressions. *Zhurnal nevrologii i psikhiatrii imeni S.S. Korsakova*, **100**, 36-41.

[22] Sheĭfer, M.S., Tsybina, M.I. and Davydenko, M.V. (2000) Fluvoxamine (Fevarin) in the Treatment of Depression. *Zhurnal nevrologii i psikhiatrii imeni S.S. Korsakova*, **100**, 64-67.

[23] Neznamov, G.G., Siuniakov, S.A., Teleshova, E.S., Dorofeeva, O.A., Chumakov, D.B. and Davydova, I.A. (2001) Therapeutic Action and Efficiency of Fevarin (Fluvoxamine) in Patients with Non-Psychotic Anxious and Apathic-Adynamic Depressions. *Zhurnal nevrologii i psikhiatrii imeni S.S. Korsakova*, **101**, 19-24.

[24] Averina, M., Nilssen, O., Brenn, T., Brox, J., Arkhipovsky, V.L. and Kalinin, A.G. (2005) Social and Lifestyle Determinants of Depression, Anxiety, Sleeping Disorders and Self-Evaluated Quality of Life in Russia—A Population-Based Study in Arkhangelsk. *Social Psychiatry and Psychiatric Epidemiology*, **40**, 511-518. http://dx.doi.org/10.1007/s00127-005-0918-x

[25] Gafarov, V.V., Panov, D.O., Gromova, E.A., Gagulin, I.V. and Gafarova, A.V. (2013) The Influence of Depression on Risk Development of Acute Cardiovascular Diseases in the Female Population Aged 25 - 64 in Russia. *International Journal of Circumpolar Health*, **72**. http://dx.doi.org/10.3402/ijch.v72i0.21223

[26] Sonawalla, S.B., Spillmann, M.K., Kolsky, A.R., Alpert, J.E., Nierenberg, A.A., Rosenbaum, J.F., et al. (1999) Efficacy of Fluvoxamine in the Treatment of Major Depression with Comorbid Anxiety Disorders. *The Journal of Clinical Psychiatry*, **60**, 580-583. http://dx.doi.org/10.4088/JCP.v60n0903

[27] Furuse, T. and Hashimoto, K. (2009) Fluvoxamine Monotherapy for Psychotic Depression: The Potential Role of Sigma-1 Receptors. *Annals of General Psychiatry*, **8**, 26. http://dx.doi.org/10.1186/1744-859x-8-26

[28] Kishimoto, A., Todani, A., Miura, J., Kitagaki, T. and Hashimoto, K. (2010) The Opposite Effects of Fluvoxamine and Sertraline in the Treatment of Psychotic Major Depression: A Case Report. *Annals of General Psychiatry*, **9**, 23. http://dx.doi.org/10.1186/1744-859x-9-23

[29] Zohar, J., Keegstra, H. and Barrelet, L. (2003) Fluvoxamine as Effective as Clomipramine against Symptoms of Severe Depression: Results from a Multicentre, Double-Blind Study. *Human Psychopharmacology*, **18**, 113-119. http://dx.doi.org/10.1002/hup.442

[30] Katoh, Y., Uchida, S., Kawai, M., Takei, N., Mori, N., Kawakami, J., et al. (2010) Onset of Clinical Effects and Plasma Concentration of Fluvoxamine in Japanese Patients. *Biological & Pharmaceutical Bulletin*, **33**, 1999-2002. http://dx.doi.org/10.1248/bpb.33.1999

[31] Rapaport, M.H., Clary, C., Fayyad, R. and Endicott, J. (2005) Quality-of-Life Impairment in Depressive and Anxiety Disorders. *American Journal of Psychiatry*, **162**, 1171-1178. http://dx.doi.org/10.1176/appi.ajp.162.6.1171

[32] Stein, M., Fyer, A., Davidson, J., Pollack, M. and Wiita, B. (1999) Fluvoxamine Treatment of Social Phobia (Social Anxiety Disorder): A Double-Blind, Placebo-Controlled Study. *American Journal of Psychiatry*, **156**, 756-760.

[33] Wilson, S.J., Bell, C., Coupland, N.J. and Nutt, D.J. (2000) Sleep Changes During Long-Term Treatment of Depression with Fluvoxamine—A Home-Based Study. *Psychopharmacology*, **149**, 360-365. http://dx.doi.org/10.1007/s002139900362

[34] Irons, J. (2005) Fluvoxamine in the Treatment of Anxiety Disorders. *Neuropsychiatric Disease and Treatment*, **1**, 289-299.

[35] Horii, A., Uno, A., Kitahara, T., Mitani, K., Masumura, C., Kizawa, K., et al. (2007) Effects of Fluvoxamine on Anxiety, Depression, and Subjective Handicaps of Chronic Dizziness Patients with or without Neuro-Otologic Diseases. *Journal of Vestibular Research*, **17**, 1-8.

[36] Omori, I.M., Watanabe, N., Nakagawa, A., Cipriani, A., Barbui, C., McGuire, H., *et al.* (2010) Fluvoxamine versus Other Anti-Depressive Agents for Depression. *Cochrane Database of Systematic Reviews*, **17**, Article ID: CD006114.
Malik, A.S., Boyko, O., Atkar, N. and Young, W.F. (2001) A Comparative Study of MR Imaging Profile of Titanium Pedicle Screws. *Acta Radiologica*, **42**, 291-293. http://dx.doi.org/10.1080/028418501127346846

24

Stealth Adapted Viruses: A Bridge between Molecular Virology and Clinical Psychiatry

W. John Martin

Institute of Progressive Medicine, South Pasadena, CA, USA
Email: wjohnmartin@ccid.org

Abstract

Cytopathic "stealth-adapted" viruses bypass the cellular immune defense mechanisms because of molecular deletion or mutation of critical antigen coding genes. They, therefore, do not provoke the inflammatory reaction typical of infections with the conventional viruses from which stealth adapted viruses are derived. Stealth adapted viruses establish persistent, systemic virus infections, which commonly involve the brain. The brain damage can cause major mood and cognitive disorders, fatigue, seizures and various manifestations of an impaired autonomic nervous system. Symptoms can also result from: 1) induced autoimmunity, 2) antibody formation against virus antigens, 3) virus-induced cellular damage to non-brain tissues and 4) induced heightened overall immune reactivity, such that normally unrecognized components of the virus begin to become targeted by the cellular immune system. This last mechanism is relevant to the reported neurological and psychiatric adverse effects of vaccination in certain individuals. It is also appropriate to consider the infectious component of stealth adapted virus infections since family members and others may be at risk for becoming infected.

Keywords

Stealth Adapted Viruses, Cytomegalovirus, African Green Monkey Simian Cytomegalovirus, SCMV, Encephalopathy, Polio Vaccine, Chronic Fatigue Syndrome, Autism, Schizophrenia, Alzheimer's Disease, Delusion, Schizovirus

1. Overview of Traditional Neurology and Psychiatry

Dysfunctional brain syndromes are traditionally viewed as comprising two distinct groupings of illnesses; neurological and psychiatric. Neurologists mainly address diseases that can be attributed to discrete anatomic lesions, with readily elicited physical signs pertaining to the affected region of the brain. Although the therapeutic options are usually limited, the causes of these illnesses have a rational basis in terms of defined neuro-anatomical lesions. As opposed to neurologists, psychiatrists and other mental health personnel, mostly address diseases lacking precise anatomic localization or biologic explanation. These diseases are expressed in terms of varying degrees of altered emotions, behaviors and cognitive processes; functions that are viewed as expressions of the "mind" rather than of the "organic brain". The availability of mind-altering drugs has helped shift the therapeutic emphasis for these diseases from simply trying to coerce the patient to change his or her ways (psychotherapy) to the somewhat more successful (if still empirical) psychopharmacological approach. The use of therapeutic drugs in psychiatry is predicated on the assumption that patients have an underlying disturbance in neural metabolism that can be at least partially restored pharmacologically. The etiology of the presumed "chemical imbalance" is rarely addressed and often assumed to be a result of an inappropriate behavioral adaptation to life stressors. This paper provides an alternative explanation for many psychiatric illnesses; one that is based on altered brain function resulting from infection with stealth adapted viruses.

2. Spatial Distribution of Normal Brain Function

The brain is unique among the body's organs in the spatial distribution of its many functions. Unlike other organs, damage to one area of the brain cannot be readily compensated for by heightened activities in other brain areas. Moreover, individual components of the brain participate in complex neural networks, which can subserve a variety of integrated functions. Even minimal damage to neurological tissue has the potential for profound symptomatic effects; compared to the effects of limited cellular damage occurring in extra-neural tissues. Not only is the brain tissue spatially complex, it is hampered by the inability of mature neuronal cells to replicate and to replace neurons damaged by either illness or normal senescence.

3. Assessment of Brain Function

The brain is responsible for motor, sensory, autonomic and cognitive functions. It also determines personality, mood, self-perception and social interactions. Assessment of gross deficits of sensory and motor functions is readily achieved in routine neurological examinations. Psychiatrists rarely, if ever, employ testing for more subtle sensory and motor changes, and for possible derangements of the autonomic nervous system. Many neurologists have also disregarded such tests as only providing inconsequential "soft signs". Complex assays, such as tilt-table testing for orthostatic hypotension can provide a quantitative measure of a specific autonomic function, but are unsuitable for everyday clinical practice. Neuroimaging techniques, such as computerized EEG, PET scans and functional MRI can also provide measures of brain activity but are also unsuitable for routine psychiatric practice. Furthermore, the etiological foundations for the minor imaging changes that have been seen in psychiatric patients are not yet established. Neuropsychiatric testing for minor personality disorders and for mild cognitive impairments requires an in-depth knowledge of the individual's pre-illness performance; information which is not generally available. One-time testing will, therefore, usually not reveal the early changes in personality or cognitive abilities that patients themselves or their friends may perceive.

4. Diagnostic Labeling of Psychiatric Illnesses

In spite of the shortcomings in assessments of many brain functions, psychiatrists have managed to categorize psychiatric illnesses into distinct clinical entities by grouping symptoms into a variety of syndromes [1]. These groupings obscure the fact that many symptoms are common to various disease categories. Moreover, the naming of an illness tends to overlook the considerable variability in symptoms, and especially in their relative severity between patients and even in a single patient over time. The lack of true diagnostic precision in reflected in such terms as "co-morbidity" and "borderline condition." The assumption that different syndromes have different underlying etiologies has also hampered efforts to find common causes of mental illnesses.

5. Etiology of Psychiatric Illnesses

In a similar way that diagnostic labels have tended to artificially sub-divide a spectrum of neuropsychiatric illnesses, the proponents of various etiologic theories have also tended to be exclusive rather than inclusive. The notion that organic brain illness is genetic, infectious, autoimmune or toxic, precludes the known interactions between all of these components. The aging process itself can slowly erode the limited functional reserves that may have survived an earlier insult. This can lead to a delay in the clinical expression of an illness until years after the initiating event has occurred. Of the four etiologic categories listed above, an infectious cause has the promise of being the most readily targeted for therapy, as well as having the added concern of being potentially transmissible between individuals. Chronic viral infection of the brain can present in many different ways depending simply on its localization to different regions of the brain and on the preexisting functional capacity levels prior to infection. Chronic infections can also render individuals susceptible to normally tolerated environmental factors and to other stressors of brain function [2].

6. Viruses and Psychiatric Illnesses

The digression of psychiatry from basic molecular biology is seen in the minimal attention currently given to the potential role of viral infections in psychiatric illnesses. Historically, such conditions as encephalitis lethargica, subacute sclerosing panencephalitis, multifocal leukoencephalopathy and general paresis of the insane were belatedly accepted as infectious [3]. The reality of AIDS dementia is also now unquestioned [4]. On the other hand, early attempts to detect viruses in patients with schizophrenia (schizoviruses) and other major psychiatric illnesses, failed to provide convincing and readily reproducible findings [5]. In spite of the availability of more sensitive technologies, such as the polymerase chain reaction (PCR), few psychiatrists are intellectually poised to consider viral infections as a likely cause of their patients' illnesses.

The prevailing model of a viral brain infection is that of herpes simplex virus (HSV) encephalitis. Typically, the patient will present with an acute onset (<2 weeks from the initial symptoms to severe illness); have progressively diminishing level of consciousness; show localizing signs, often to the temporal lobes, on clinical, radiologic and EEG examinations; and have numerous lymphoid cells in the cerebrospinal fluid (CSF) with increased protein levels [6]. Relatively mild meningitis/encephalitis-like illnesses are also commonly encountered in General Practice. If pursued vigorously, serological assays, changes in CSF, and virus cultures of feces will occasionally indicate an enteroviral infection [7]. The illnesses are considered to be short lasting without sequela. The notion of a persisting, sub-acute, non-inflammatory viral encephalopathy is rarely considered clinically or tested for using either viral cultures or molecular probe based assays.

7. Viral Pathogenesis

All viruses have the potential to mediate cellular changes by altering the normal metabolic balance within the cell through over utilization of the cell's energy resources [8] [9]. While this can eventually lead to cell death, an earlier cost can be the failure of the cell to perform all of its specialized functions [10]. Continued metabolic drain on the cell can lead to a loss of essential components such as adenosine triphosphate (ATP). A tipping point is reached when there is insufficient ATP to import magnesium into the cell; a required co-factor for ATP activity. Energy starved cells can show foamy vacuolization, swelling and intercellular fusion. Some viruses trigger a more active form of cellular death, called apoptosis, characterized by shrinkage and condensation of cellular components. Herpesviruses, especially HSV and human cytomegalovirus (hCMV), are especially cytotoxic when cultured with normal cells. So too are adenoviruses, influenza, polio and many enteroviruses. Certain human viruses, however, are essentially incapable of inducing a readily detectable cytopathic effect (CPE) in viral cultures on human cells. For example, rubella; hepatitis A, B, C and D; HTLV; Borna and Hantaan viruses are non-cytopathic on cultured cells. Moreover, primary clinical isolates of German measles and mumps viruses induce rather minimal CPE when directly cultured on human cells. For many of these non- or minimally-cytopathic viruses, the major in vivo tissue damage is a consequence of immune activation and lymphocyte killing of the infected cells [11].

8. Viral Immunity

The immune system can both reduce and enhance the extent of viral damage. Antibodies can provide an effective blockade preventing viruses from gaining access to normally permissive cells. In particular, antiviral antibodies can help prevent viruses passing through the blood to the brain. Cellular immunity can reduce viral load by destroying infected cells prior to the release of infectious viral particles. On the other hand, cellular immunity against viral antigens or against modified or inappropriately expressed cellular antigens can lead to immune damage of cells beyond that achieved by the virus itself.

Viruses have evolved various mechanisms to help evade the immune system. One such mechanism is the deletion of the genes coding for the major antigens recognized by the cellular immune system [12] [13]. This mechanism of bypassing the cellular immune defenses has been referred to as a "stealth adaptation."

9. Stealth Adapted Viruses

A corollary of the Clonal Selection Theory of Immunology [14] is that to be effectively recognized, a viral infected cell must present multiple copies of the antigen that is targeted by the responding antigen specific lymphocyte. This requirement restricts the number of different viral antigens, which can be presented to the cellular immune system. Even with large complex viruses, relatively few viral components are targeted for cellular immune defenses [15]. For certain viruses, e.g. hCMV, experimental studies suggested that the complete deletion of the three genes coding for the major viral components recognized by the cellular immune system, would likely yield defective, non-replicating, non-cytopathic viral sequences. The remaining sequences could, however, provide potential building blocks towards the evolution of a cytopathic, non-immunogenic "stealth adapted virus." Potentially, the downsized gene-depleted virus could, for example, form a synergy with a replicating non-cytopathic virus and/or incorporate certain cellular genes by recombination, to yield an atypically structured cytopathic virus. These concepts are embodied in the following definition of stealth adapted viruses:

"Molecularly heterogeneous grouping of atypically structured, cytopathic viruses that cause persistent systemic infection, often with neuropsychiatric manifestations, in the absence of significant anti-viral inflammation. Stealth adaptation is a generic, derivative process in which conventional viruses have lost or mutated the relatively few genes encoding the major antigens normally targeted by the cellular immune system. Stealth adapted viruses typically induce a vacuolating cytopathic effect (CPE) in a range of human and animal cells. The formation, progression, and/or host range of the CPE distinguish stealth adapted viruses from the CPE caused by conventional human cytopathic viruses, including herpesviruses, enteroviruses, and adenoviruses. Additional distinctions can be made on the basis of electron microscopy, serology, and molecular-based studies."

10. Origins and Replication of Stealth Adapted Viruses

Certain stealth viruses contain genetic sequences that are nearly identical to sequences found in African green monkey simian cytomegalovirus (SCMV) [13]. Other regions of these viruses are clearly different from SCMV. Other stealth adapted viruses contain genetic sequences or at least express serological markers related to common human herpesviruses, adenoviruses and enteroviruses. Similar to stealth adapted SCMV, evidence for various cellular genes, have been detected in the DNA and/or RNA fractions of several stealth adapted virus infected cultures. Electron microscopy has also revealed differences between stealth viral cultures in terms of the types and relative abundance of distinctive accumulations of variously structured, complex materials within cells showing the characteristic vacuolated CPE and in the tissue culture medium (unpublished data). An interesting observation is the apparent genetic instability and fragmentation of a stealth viral DNA genome [16]. A potential mechanism of stealth viral DNA replication is through the bridging of viral fragments with long RNA molecules. If so, this scaffolding effect could potentially be inhibited in the presence of short RNA molecules competing with the longer RNA molecule for binding to one of the fragments.

11. Relevance of the SCMV Origin of Certain Stealth Adapted Viruses

While stealth adapted viruses have presumably existed for eons, the increasing incidence of many current disease entities is consistent with the introduction of additional stealth adapted viruses through vaccines. Public health authorities have largely ignored the issue of SCMV as a possible contaminant of polio vaccines. This disregard occurred even though in 1972 a joint study by FDA and the vaccine manufacturer showed that all 11 monkey kidney cultures tested using sensitive indicator cell lines showed the presence of SCMV. Only 4 of these isolates would have been detected using the standard detection procedures, which remained in place despite of the above finding (correspondence of polio vaccine manufacturer).

A diverse array of animal cell lines has been used for the many human and animal vaccines that have been developed. It is not unreasonable to suggest that some of these vaccines may have generated stealth adapted viruses. It is also conceivable that vaccine viruses can contribute genetic elements to contaminating herpes and other viruses and that this could facilitate the emergence of replicating, non-immunogenic (stealth-adapted) viruses. Once within the human population, stealth adapted viruses can be passed via direct human-to-human contact as well as potentially by interspecies transmission.

12. Detection of Stealth Adapted Viruses

The most reliable method for detecting the diversity of stealth viruses is to co-culture the patient's blood with a variety of indicator cell types and observe the cultures for the induction of a transmissible CPE [17]. Typically, rhesus monkey kidney cells and a human fibroblast cell line such as MRC-5 cells are inoculated with the patient's frozen-thawed mononuclear cells and observed for 2 - 4 weeks. Frequent re-feeding of the cultures can help promote the development of the CPE. It is quite unusual (<10%) to observe a rapidly developing CPE in blood samples from randomly selected hospital outpatients. Conversely, it is unusual not to observe a strong positive CPE in cultures from patients with otherwise unexplained neurological or behavioral disorders.

The stealth virus CPE is best characterized by the formation of foci of enlarged, rounded cells, often with cell fusion (syncytia). Proliferation foci of affected cells can occasionally be seen. The actual appearance of the CPE differs between cultures and is best followed by repeated examination of individual cultures by the same observer. The CPE can be transferred to fresh cultures. Positive cultures can be further examined by staining cell smears or sectioned cell pellets using the patient's and other sera. Electron microscopic studies can also be performed. Cell derived DNA and RNA can also be used for molecular characterization. A series of PCR primer sets based on previously characterized stealth viruses can be used to screen for virus-derived DNA and RNA sequences. The primers can also be used to test for DNA and RNA dependent polymerases. Finally, the viral cultures can be used to test the effects of various anti-viral therapies.

As noted above, stealth viral infections are not necessarily confined to the brain and indeed blood samples are routinely used for stealth viral cultures. Other serological signs of viral infections can include unusually high levels of anti-herpesvirus antibodies. This may reflect the presence of the stealth virus or the two-way cross stimulation that can be seen between stealth adapted viruses and conventional herpesviruses. Broadly reactive herpesvirus primers can also be used in low stringency PCR based assays on DNA and RNA directly isolated from the patient's blood [17]. Other primer sets have been shown to cross react with several stealth virus isolates in low stringency PCR assays. Cloning and sequencing of the PCR products can be used to design more specific primer sets. The possible role of stealth adapted herpesviruses in secondary activation of parvo- and papovaviruses can also be assessed using serological and molecular probe based assays for these agents.

13. Stealth Adapted Viral Infection

Stealth viruses have been isolated from blood and CSF of patients with a spectrum of illnesses with neurological and neuropsychiatric manifestations [17]-[22]. The clinical diagnoses have included autism and attention deficit learning disorders in children, CFS, fibromyalgia, Gulf war syndrome and depression in adults, and dementia/Alzheimer's disease in the elderly. Severe acute encephalopathy and major psychotic reactions have also been associated with positive stealth adapted viral infections. The clinical diversity seen in stealth viral infected patients may relate to the predominant areas of the brain that are infected as well as the timing and intensity of the infection. Stealth viruses from humans have induced acute neurobehavioral diseases in experimental animals [23] accompanied by similar histological and electron microscopic changes as seen in brain biopsies of infected humans.

14. Histopathology

The predominant histological characteristic in both humans and in the animal model is the presence of occasional cells with distinctly vacuolated, lipid-rich cytoplasm and distorted abnormal nuclei [18] [22] [23]. The affected cells may show varying granules positive with periodic acid Schiff (PAS) stain. Deposited material can also accumulate around small blood vessels, possibly impairing gas exchange and nutrient delivery. The marked vacuolization seen in some biopsies is certainly suggestive of Creutzfeld Jacob prion disease [22].

Animal studies confirmed that the cellular changes were not confined to the brain but that signs of infection could be found in various organs throughout the body [23]. Nonetheless, the predominant clinical manifestations in the animals were neurobehavioral, consistent with the unique susceptibility of the brain to limited damage.

15. Clinical Manifestations of Illnesses Seen in Certain Stealth Adapted Virus Infected Patients

Numerous articles have described the protean clinical manifestations of major neuropsychiatric illnesses and conditions such as CFS and autism. This section is intended to highlight some of the clinical insights from extensive culturing of stealth adapted viruses from patients.

Stealth viral culture positive patients, whether presenting with a psychiatric or neurological illness, will not uncommonly report symptoms attributed to illnesses occurring elsewhere in the body. In some cases, such as in low back pain, the essence of the illness is a lowered pain threshold; more than the severity of the musculoskeletal changes. Similarly, pelvic pain can have a strong central nervous system component. Clinicians can err in over treating the localized area of pain without due regard to the underlying hypersensitivity of the patient's nervous system. The treated disease will likely recur or be replaced by an equally disabling painful condition occurring elsewhere in the body.

Various cardiovascular diseases, affecting the heart and/or peripheral circulation, can be ascribed to dysregulation by an impaired autonomic nervous system. Postural hypotension occurring in CFS patients is well described. An interesting illness encountered in some patients is erythromelalgia, in which inappropriate shunting of blood via opened arteriovenous connections compromises the capillary circulation with resulting pain [24].

The autonomic nervous system also controls aspects of gastrointestinal functioning and this can account for dysphagia and irritable bowel syndrome. It may also contribute to malabsorption, leaky gut syndrome and dysbiosis (abnormal gut flora). Bacteria sequences have been identified in some stealth adapted virus cultures [25]. This is consistent with some of these viruses being able to pass within bacteria. Indeed, atypical bacteria have been seen in fecal cultures of some CFS patients. Stealth adapted virus infection of the gut bacteria could, therefore, also contribute to dysbiosis.

Another diagnosis experienced by stealth adapted virus infected patients is delusional parasitosis [26]. Patients can produce pigmented particles with striking electrostatic properties, which the patients can easily mistake for living movements. When detected in the hair, the particles have also been misidentified as lice. The mother of a child reported severe mental deterioration requiring institutionalized care, after the anti-lice medication, Lindane, had been applied to her daughter's scalp and the house fogged with an insecticide.

A patient from whom strikingly positive cultures were repeatedly observed had numerous lipomas, which she said tended to come in episodes and slowly resolve. Her diagnosis was Dercum's disease, which is a condition largely unknown in conventional medicine [27]. This disease can be likened to periodic outbreaks of shingles. The difference is that instead of vesicular lesions developing in the skin, localized areas of excessive subcutaneous lipids are being produced; sometimes distributed within a single dermatome. Virus induced overproduction of intracellular lipids can explain liver steatosis seen in some stealth adapted virus infected patients. Using the same reasoning, intracellular lipids can inhibit glucose transport into cells, rendering cells somewhat insulin resistant. Obesity may result from the unsightly but possibly necessary disposal of lipids overproduced by virus infected parenchymal organs.

Virus infections can also provoke autoimmune reactions, especially to cellular DNA, as in systemic lupus erythematosus. Autoantibody production against mitochondrial phospholipids can lead to hypercoagulation, while antibodies to clotting factors can lead to excessive bleeding. Hashimoto's disease and Graves' disease can occur with auto-antibodies against thyroid antigens. Autoimmunity can also be directed to the nervous system, as can be seen with the extension of an apparent CFS to multiple sclerosis. Cases of limbic encephalopathy [28] can also be explained as an autoimmune response to neurotransmitters or to their receptors. Antibodies may also form against the virus, since many more virus antigens evoke humoral immunity than the relatively few antigens targeted by the cellular immune system. These antibodies can explain the vasculitis occurring in some stealth adapted virus culture positive patients [19]. The immune system itself can be directly damaged by virus infection leading to immune dysregulation.

An exception to the statement that limited localized damage is relatively less significant outside of the nervous system, is the occurrence of malignancy. Upon inquiry, breast cancer patients not uncommonly report on fatigue for years prior to the detection of their cancer and even after its removal. Multiple myeloma patients commonly have a prior history of neuropsychiatric illnesses. The consistent finding of positive cultures for stealth adapted viruses in multiple myeloma patients was confirmed in a double blind study [29]. Direct evidence for stealth adapted viruses was also obtained by using the PCR assay in patients with salivary tumors [30]. A patient with strikingly positive virus cultures had a glioblastoma, which is consistent with published evidence linking CMV to this tumor.

Virus infection of germ cells can potentially lead to genetic disorders in offspring. This has been noted in some patients with a genetic abnormality, not present as a somatic mutation in either of the parents. CMV is especially prone to infect the gonads and may induce genetic change in germ cell even prior to fertilization. This could account for the circumstances in which a de novo genetic disease occurs in children in whom one or more parent was stealth adapted virus infected.

16. Transmission of Stealth Adapted Virus Infections

The occurrence of family illnesses of presumptive infectious origin has been noted on several occasions. To cite one of these families: The mother openly declared she had CFS. She believed her husband also had the illness but was in denial since he was still required to work. The woman's mother was diagnosed with Parkinson's disease, while her son was diagnosed as schizophrenic. Within the family, they all recognized a basic similarity of their illnesses. Several other families with differing illnesses but all of presumptive infectious origin have been seen.

Community wide transmission of stealth adapted virus induced illnesses can easily explain many of the reported outbreaks of CFS-like illnesses. One such epidemic occurred in 1996 in the Mohave Valley area of Arizona and adjoining town of Needles, California [21]. The nation's blood and blood products supply is also an expected mode of transmission of stealth adapted viruses. Indeed, CDC was informed of positive stealth adapted virus cultures from 10% of blood donations collected in 2002 from the University of California Irvine.

Occupational exposure is also a potential risk factor, especially in individuals likely to come into close contact with others [31]. This group includes healthcare providers, schoolteachers, prison guards, etc. Avoiding becoming stealth adapted virus infected is of special concern to women anticipating pregnancy. A difficult issue, which also applies to conventional CMV infection, is the risk of daycare facilities and of pediatricians' medical offices in spreading infection to other children. Freshly infected children can expose their mother to the virus prior to or during her next pregnancy.

17. Summary

The specialization of medicine has focused attention on disorders that are essentially restricted to a single organ system. Multi-system diseases tend to fall outside the purview of most physicians and a balanced, comprehensive approach to their assessment is often lacking. The clinical evaluation of patients with a stealth viral induced encephalopathy should not be confined to disorders of brain function. Rather, the clinical evaluation should include seeking evidence for viral involvement of additional organs, as would be expected for a systemic virus infection. Efforts should also be undertaken to restrict the likely transmission of stealth adapted virus infections within families, certain occupations and whole communities.

References

[1]   American Psychiatric Association (2013) Diagnostic and Statistical Manual of Mental Disorders. 5th Edition (DSM-5), Amer Psychiatric Pub Inc., Arlington.

[2]   Noshpitz, J.D. and Coddington, R.D. (1990) Stressors and the Adjustment Disorders. John Wiley and Sons, New York.

[3]   Tselis, A. and Booss, J. (2003) Behavioral Consequences of Infections of the Central Nervous System: With Emphasis on Viral Infections. *Journal of the American Academy of Psychiatry and the Law*, **31**, 289-298.

[4]   Ances, B.M. and Ellis R.J. (2007) Dementia and Neurocognitive Disorders Due to HIV-1 Infection. *Seminars in Neurology*, **27**, 86-92. http://dx.doi.org/10.1055/s-2006-956759

[5]   Torrey, E.F. (1988) Stalking the Schizovirus. *Schizophrenia Bulletin*, **14**, 223-229. http://dx.doi.org/10.1093/schbul/14.2.223

[6]   Tyler, K.L. (2004) Herpes Simplex Virus Infections of the Central Nervous System: Encephalitis and Meningitis, including Mollaret's. *Herpes*, **11**, Suppl. 2, 57A-64A.

[7]   Rhoades, R.E., Tabor-Godwin, J.M., Tsueng, G. and Feuer, R. (2011) Enterovirus Infections of the Central Nervous System. *Virology*, **411**, 288-305. http://dx.doi.org/10.1016/j.virol.2010.12.014

[8]   White, D.O. and Fenner, F.J. (1994) Medical Virology. 4th Edition, Academic Press, San Diego.

[9] Carrasco, L. (1987) Mechanisms of Viral Toxicity in Animal Cells. CRC Press, Boca Raton.

[10] de la Torre, J.C., Borrow, P. and Oldstone, M.B. (1991) Viral Persistence and Disease: Cytopathology in the Absence of Cytolysis. *British Medical Bulletin*, **47**, 838-851.

[11] Zinkernagel, R.M. (1997) Immunology and Immunity Studied with Viruses. *Ciba Foundation Symposium*, **204**, 105-125.

[12] Martin, W.J. (1994) Stealth Viruses as Neuropathogens. College of American Pathologist's Publication. *CAP Today*, **8**, 67-70.

[13] Martin, W.J. (1999) Stealth Adaptation of an African Green Monkey Simian Cytomegalovirus. *Experimental and Molecular Pathology*, **66**, 3-7. http://dx.doi.org/10.1006/exmp.1999.2248

[14] Burnet, F.M. (1959) The Clonal Selection Theory of Acquired Immunity. Vanderbilt University Press, Nashville. http://dx.doi.org/10.5962/bhl.title.8281

[15] Wills, M.R., Carmichael, A.J., Mynard, K., Jin, X., Weekes, M.P., *et al.* (1996) The Human Cytotoxic T-Lymphocyte (CTL) Response to Cytomegalovirus Is Dominated by Structural Protein pp65: Frequency, Specificity, and T-Cell Receptor Usage of pp65-Specific CTL. *Journal of Virology*, **70**, 7569-7579.

[16] Martin, W.J. (1996) Genetic Instability and Fragmentation of a Stealth Viral Genome. *Pathobiology*, **64**, 9-17. http://dx.doi.org/10.1159/000164000

[17] Martin, W.J., Zeng, L.C., Ahmed, K. and Roy, M. (1994) Cytomegalovirus-Related Sequences in an Atypical Cytopathic Virus Repeatedly Isolated from a Patient with the Chronic Fatigue Syndrome. *American Journal of Pathology*, **145**, 441-452.

[18] Martin, W.J. (1996) Severe Stealth Virus Encephalopathy Following Chronic Fatigue Syndrome-Like Illness: Clinical and Histopathological Features. *Pathobiology*, **64**, 1-8. http://dx.doi.org/10.1159/000163999

[19] Martin, W.J. (1996) Stealth Viral Encephalopathy: Report of a Fatal Case Complicated by Cerebral Vasculitis. *Pathobiology*, **64**, 59-63. http://dx.doi.org/10.1159/000164009

[20] Martin, W.J. (1996) Simian Cytomegalovirus-Related Stealth Virus Isolated from the Cerebrospinal Fluid of a Patient with Bipolar Psychosis and Acute Encephalopathy. *Pathobiology*, **64**, 64-66. http://dx.doi.org/10.1159/000164010

[21] Martin, W.J. and Anderson, D. (1997) Stealth Virus Epidemic in the Mohave Valley. Initial Report of Viral Isolation. *Pathobiology*, **65**, 51-56. http://dx.doi.org/10.1159/000164103

[22] Martin, W.J. and Anderson, D. (1999) Stealth Virus Epidemic in the Mohave Valley: Severe Vacuolating Encephalopathy in a Child Presenting with a Behavioral Disorder. *Experimental and Molecular Pathology*, **66**, 19-30. http://dx.doi.org/10.1006/exmp.1999.2237

[23] Martin, W.J. and Glass, R.T. (1995) Acute Encephalopathy Induced in Cats with a Stealth Virus Isolated from a Patient with Chronic Fatigue Syndrome. *Pathobiology*, **63**, 115-118. http://dx.doi.org/10.1159/000163942

[24] Ljubojević, S., Lipozencić, J. and Pustisek, N. (2004) Erythromelalgia. *Acta Dermatovenerologica Croatica*, **12**, 99-105.

[25] Martin, W.J. (1999) Bacteria Related Sequences in a Simian Cytomegalovirus-Derived Stealth Virus Culture. *Experimental and Molecular Pathology*, **66**, 8-14. http://dx.doi.org/10.1006/exmp.1999.2239

[26] Martin, W.J. (2005) Alternative Cellular Energy Pigments Mistaken for Parasitic Skin Infestations. *Experimental and Molecular Pathology*, **78**, 212-214. http://dx.doi.org/10.1016/j.yexmp.2005.01.007

[27] Hansson, E., Svensson, H. and Brorson, H. (2012) Review of Dercum's Disease and Proposal of Diagnostic Criteria, Diagnostic Methods, Classification and Management. *Orphanet Journal of Rare Diseases*, **7**, 23. http://dx.doi.org/10.1186/1750-1172-7-23

[28] Ramanathan, S., Mohammad, S.S., Brilot, F. and Dale, R.C. (2014) Autoimmune Encephalitis: Recent Updates and Emerging Challenges. *Journal of Clinical Neuroscience*, **21**, 722-730.

[29] Durie, B.G., Collins, R.A. and Martin, W.J. (2000) Positive Stealth Virus Cultures in Myeloma Patients: A Possible Explanation for Neuropsychiatric Co-Morbidity. *Blood*, **96**, 29.

[30] Gollard, R.P., Mayr, A., Rice, D.A. and Martin, W.J. (1996) Herpesvirus-Related Sequences in Salivary Gland Tumors. *Journal of Experimental & Clinical Cancer Research*, **15**, 1-4.

[31] Joseph, S.A., Béliveau, C. and Gyorkos, T.W. (2006) Cytomegalovirus as an Occupational Risk in Daycare Educators. *Paediatrics & Child Health*, **11**, 401-407.

Abbreviation

SCMV—African green monkey simian cytomegalovirus,

hCMV—human cytomegalovirus,

CPE—cytopathic effect,

PCR—polymerase chain reaction,

CSF—cerebrospinal fluid.

25

Stress, Executive Function, Resilience and Quality of Life in Portuguese Subjects in Situations of Economic Insufficiency and Unemployment

Eduardo Gonçalves[1], Saul Neves de Jesus[2]

[1]Department of Psychiatry and Mental Health of Hospital Center of Algarve, Faro, Portugal
[2]Department of Psychology of Faculty of Social and Human Sciences of University of Algarve, Faro, Portugal
Email: eduar.goncalves@gmail.com

Abstract

The aim of this study is the investigation of the impact of stress of Portuguese subjects in situations of economic insufficiency and unemployment on executive function and quality of life and the coping strategies and resilience skills used. The sample consists of 41 participants. The psychometric instruments used are validated for Portuguese population, measure (perceived) stress, coping, material deprivation, resilience and quality of life, defined by World Health Organization. Executive function has been evaluated through performances at Stroop and Berg tasks. It has been concluded that, in this population, resilience skills and active coping strategies are positively correlated with quality of life. Quality of life is negatively correlated with material deprivation. Active coping strategies are supported by adequate executive function, which neurobiological substrate is dorso-lateral prefrontal cortex. Not active coping strategies correlate negatively with cognitive flexibility, suggesting the presence of a deficit at infero-lateral prefrontal cortex.

Keywords

Stress, Economic Insufficiency, Unemployment, Coping, Resilience, Quality of Life, Executive Function

1. Introduction (Theoretical Framework)

1.1. Stress, Coping, Emotion, Anxiety, Depression, Perceived Stress and Unifying (Heuristic) Model of Stress Process

Lazarus and Folkman (1984) [1] define the psychological stress as "a particular relation between the person and his/her involvement appraised by the person as taxing or excessive in relation to his/her resources, endangering his/her well-being." On this evaluation, and according to these authors, "cognitive appraisal can be more easily understood as the process of categorizing the stress encounter, and its various facets, with respect to their importance to the well-being". They identify two main categories of appraisal: the primary appraisal, which is an evaluation of what is at stake in the stressful encounter; the secondary appraisal, which is an evaluation of options and resources to handle the stressful meeting. Also they emphasize three major potential outcomes of the primary appraisal, which provide an initial classification of the implications for the adaptation to person's circumstances: they can be appraised as irrelevant to his/her well-being, if they not relate to the needs and objectives of the person; they can be appraised as benign and positive, if they are evaluated as reassuring or incrementing the person's well-being; or they can be appraised as stressful if the needs and objectives of the person are implicated in the situation in a way that exceeds the personal resources, being these appraisals which result in a reaction to stress, that mobilize the person to respond to the situation, evoked by stress, through coping. Lazarus and Folkman (1984) [1] also identified three subtypes of stressful appraisals, from which run a more accurate categorization of the nature of the conditions evocative of stress: damage (and loss); threat; challenge. Damage appraisals reflect situations in which a person has suffered some kind of prejudice (whether through injury, illness, loss of self-esteem or some other type of setback in his/her objectives and activities). Threat appraisals focus on the existing potential in the situation related with future obtaining of damage (and loss). Challenge appraisals are focused on the existing potential in the situation related with future obtaining of gain. The difference between stress-related damage or threats, on the one hand, and stress-related challenge, in the other, is in concordance with the distinction, advanced by Selye (1974) [2], between negative stress or distress and positive stress or eustress. The evaluation of control potential, existing within the individual, on the stressful transaction person-involvement, is mentioned, as an important form of secondary appraisal, by Lazarus and Folkman (1984) [1], who observe that challenge appraisals, rather than threat ones, are especially likely when the person has a sense of personal control over the transaction. Individuals sustain as important motivational commitments, including goals and personal values, which are identified as relevant antecedents of their primary appraisals. As for the situation, and also according to these authors, many formal properties of events, including their novelty, predictability, uncertainty, eminence, duration and ambiguity have been identified as potentially important for appraisal. For Lazarus and Folkman (1984) [1], coping consists of "cognitive and behavioral efforts, constantly changing, to manage specific external and/or internal demands that are assessed as exceeding the resources of the person". Moreover, they differentiate two basic functions corresponding to two different types of coping. Folkman and Lazarus (1980) [3] argue that problem focused coping refers to the "management or change of the transaction person-involvement, which is the source of stress," while emotion focused coping refers to "the regulation of stressful emotions" that arise in response to the problem. They also propose that problem focused coping includes more intra-personal strategies that would reduce the problem through motivational and cognitive changes, such as changing aspiration's level, developing new behavioral patterns, reducing investment's degree in the situation. Emotion focused coping is described as consisting primarily of a series of cognitive processes in order to reduce emotional distress, including avoidance, minimization, reevaluation of the situation in a more positive way, without really changing it (Lazarus & Folkman, 1984) [1]. Smith and Lazarus (1990) [4] argued that the knowledge of the emotional state of a person allows to gather more information about how that person is doing appraisals of his/her circumstances and the likelihood of behaving, than simply stating that the person is having a stressful experience. According to Lang (1995) [5], human experience can be characterized by two dimensions: valence and arousal (neuro-physiological activation). Valence refers to an evaluation continuum, that ranges from a state of displeasure (negative/unpleasant) to a state of pleasure (positive/pleasant), and arousal refers to an evaluation continuum that ranges from a state of calm to a state of maximum activation (excitation state of alert). While valence response guides the behavior by activating the motivational system (approach/appetitive behavior versus avoidance, withdrawal/aversive behavior), arousal corresponds to the magnitude of this response [5]. Negative emotions, in association with passive arousal, correspond to emotional/affective states of sadness, resignation, and, with greater intensity, to states of depression, evoked by damage (and loss) appraisals. Negative emotions, in association with active arousal, correspond to emotional/affective states of fear, and, with greater intensity, to anxiety states, evoked by threat appraisals. Positive emotions, in association with passive arousal, correspond to emotional/affective states of calm. Positive emotions, in association with active arousal, correspond to emotional/affective states of joy, and, with greater intensity, to excitement states. Anxiety disorders have repeatedly been associated with an increase in right prefrontal cortex and amygdala activity, abnormalities similar to those reported in depressed subjects [6]. Neuro-stimulation, in particular, high frequency (above 1 Hz) repetitive transcranial magnetic stimulation (rTMS) over left dorso-lateral prefrontal cortex treats depressive states [7]. Cohen *et al.* (1997) [8] have distinguished three perspectives to assess the role of stress in the risk for disease (environmental, biological and psychological perspectives). The environmental perspective focuses on the assessment of environmental events or experiences that are normatively (objectively) associated with substantial adaptation requirements. The biological perspective focuses on the activation of physiological systems, sympathetic-adrenal medullar system and hypothalamic-pituitary-adrenal axis, that are particularly sensitive to physical and psychological demands, and whose prolonged or repeated activation can put people at risk for the development of a variety of physical and psychiatric disorders. The psychological perspective on stress puts emphasis on the perception and evaluation of the potential threat posed by objective environmental experiences. When the demands of involvement are perceived as exceeding the competencies and strategies to cope with the situation, the individual is considered under stress and simultaneously experiences a negative emotional response. Psychological models of stress argue that the events only affect people who appraise them as stressful (perceived stress). Stress appraisals are determined, not only by the stimulus condition or the response variables but, by the person's interpretations of their relations with his/her involvement, that is, the perception of stress is a product of the meaning's interpretation of an event and the evaluation of the adequacy of personal coping resources. The primary appraisal depends on two classes of antecedent conditions: the perceived characteristics of the stimulus situation and the psychological structure of the individual. Some factors affecting primary appraisal of the stimulus situation include the potentiality of damaging confrontation, as well as the magnitude, intensity, duration and controllability of the stimulus. Individual factors affecting primary appraisal include beliefs about oneself and the involvement, the pattern and intensity of personal values and commitments, as well as personality dispositions [8] [9]. Cohen *et al.* (1997) [8] proposed a unifying model of environmental, psychological and biological perspectives on stress. When confronted with the environmental demands, the person appraises whether they represent a potential threat and if he/she has available skills to adaptively cope with those. Appraising coping resources as insufficient, one will realize his/her situation as stressful, and this stress evaluation results in negative emotional states. When very intense, these same states can directly contribute to the triggering of affective psychiatric disorders, and trigger behavioral or physiological responses that put a person at risk for physical and/or psychiatric disease/s. The model also provides for the possibility that environmental requirements may put the person at risk for disease, even when the evaluation does not result in stress perception nor negative emotional responses. In this model, they are identified two feedback loops, regarding the possibility that an affective state, associated with negative emotions (e.g., depression),can vies stress measurements, as well as the possibility of attribution of physiological activation to a stressor agent, when in fact this is determined by physical exercise or the action of toxic psychoactive substances. Thus, the perception of stress may influence the pathogenesis of physical illness, determining negative emotional states which directly affect physiological processes influencing behavior patterns or risk for disease [8].

1.2. Executive Function and Its Evaluation through Stroop and Berg Tasks

Executive function is a multifaceted neuropsychological construct that can be defined as forming, maintaining and shifting of mental sets, corresponding to the abilities to reason and generate goals and plans, maintain focus and motivation to follow through with goals and plans, and flexibly to alter goals and plans in response to changing contingencies. Set formation (*i.e.*, the generation of short- and long-term objectives), through planning and reasoning, with the use of neuro-cognitive processes of focusing attention, generativity, memory retrieval, working memory, sequencing, requires the integrity of dorso-lateral prefrontal cortex, whose injury determines the neuro-behavioral syndrome of disorganization. Set maintenance (*i.e.*, the execution of short- and long-term goals), through follow-through, with the use of neuro-cognitive processes of initiation, response selection (conflict resolution), selective attention, self-monitoring and vigilant attention, requires the integrity of the supero-median prefrontal cortex, whose injury determines the neuro-behavioral syndrome of apathy. Set maintenance, through social appropriateness and judgment, with the use of neuro-cognitive processes of inhibition and discrepancy detection, requires the integrity of the ventro-median prefrontal and orbito-frontal cortex, whose injury determines the neuro-behavioral syndrome of desinhibition. Set shifting (*i.e.*, the alteration in short- and long-term goals in response to changes in situations and contexts), through problem solving, with the use of the neuro-cognitive processes of discrepancy detection, cognitive flexibility, attention shifting, generativity, memory retrieval and working memory, requires the integrity of the dorso-lateral prefrontal cortex, whose injury determines the neuro-behavioral syndrome of perseverance. The experimental tasks used to test executive function can be divided into three main categories: cognitive control, working memory and emotional decision. Berg (Wisconsin sorting card test) and Stroop tasks evaluate cognitive control. Stroop tasks evaluate functions involved in set maintenance. Berg task evaluates functions involved in set formation and set shifting (cognitive flexibility). Tower of Hanoi/tower of London tasks evaluate working memory. Iowa gambling task requires participants to consider before a specific purpose, the relative contributions of rewards and punishments, and evaluates emotional decision [10]. Stroop tasks, which computerized version in Psycho Experiment Building Language (PEBL) is victoria Stroop task/test (VST), share the need to select cognitively one of several possible responses to a given stimulus (resolution of conflict/discrepancy), involving, among other functions, inhibition of a pre-potent response, and recruiting visuo-spatial executive components of language and processing speed [11]. Normal performance on Stroop tasks depends mainly on structural and functional integrity of dorso-lateral prefrontal cortex and anterior cingulate cortex [12]-[14]. There is an increase in Stroop interference effect in many psychopathological and neuro-psychiatric disorders, such as dementia and other neurodegenerative disorders (schizophrenia), attention deficit and depression [15]-[17]. Berg task (Wisconsin card sorting test), which computerized version is PEBL's Berg card sorting test (BCST) tests cognitive flexibility [10]. This task is used in the evaluation of patients with brain injury, neurodegenerative disease (including schizophrenia) and depression. Cognitive flexibility, *i.e.*, the mental ability to switch between thinking about two different concepts and think about several concepts at once, is a vital component of learning. Various cognitive components that functionally implement cognitive flexibility, such as recognition of the incorrectness of the environmental feedback stimulus, selection of new dimension through abstract thinking, *i.e.*, conceptual ability, learning how to learn (learning to learn/LTL), inner speech, response inhibition and updating working memory depend on structural and functional integrity of the infero-lateral prefrontal cortex (sub-region of dorso-lateral prefrontal cortex) and caudate nucleus [18] [19].

1.3. Economic Insufficiency (Poverty, Material Deprivation) and Unemployment

Poverty determines lack of opportunities, reduced accessibility to resources and a greater likelihood of life events with traumatogenic potential. By acting through stressors agents of socio-economic nature, such as the unemployment and the difficulty of access to housing, it is much more likely that poverty precede mental disorders, such as anxiety and depression, being an important risk factor for mental illnesss [20]. The relationship between poverty and mental illness is bidirectional, that is, poverty is a risk factor for certain mental illnesses, which, in turn, worsen the economic condition of the patient and their families. Some factors, such as education and employment, has a two-way relationship with poverty. The lack of employment results in financial difficulties, and poverty results in reduced opportunity to obtain gainful employment. Unemployed people and those who fail to obtain employment have more depressive symptoms than individuals who can get a job [21]. Limited resources resulting in reduced opportunity for education, which prevent access to most skilled jobs, increase individual vulnerability and insecurity and contribute to a persistently low social capital. The prevalence of common mental disorders is higher among individuals with low levels of education. Chronic poverty is often associated with low levels of family and community support, alcoholism, community insecurity and violent crime, family abuse and family desertion, particularly by men [20]. People in poverty reported higher levels of hopelessness, fatalism, lack of control over their circumstances, as well as a sense of life more oriented to the present than to the future and lower levels of life satisfaction and quality of life, aspects that perpetuate poverty, making it difficult to effectively change the socio-economic status of those who are in poverty situation. The personal debt is a particular source of stress. Working in poverty, represented by financial need and restrictive standards of living, correlates negatively with subjective well-being and is associated with increased risk for not meeting basic needs in mental health [22]. The sudden change of socio-economic status of an individual can result in acute and extreme distress, including suicidal ideation and attempts [23]. The chronically poor families do not provide a qualified involvement in child growth and development, and these children have worse cognitive performance and more behavioral problems compared to other children [24]. Adolescents in poverty are more prone to abuse alcohol and illegal drugs and to start an active sex life at an earlier age, as well as manifest greater mental health problems and lower levels of school performance [25]. Poverty generates less favorable family environment, with greater vulnerability of the parents to the debilitating effects of life events, as well as a decreased ability of them to provide consistent socio-family support [24] [25]. Poverty and material deprivation are associated, independently, to the risk for mental disorders in women, to add to the sources of stress usually related to women condition [26]. Studies of poverty and mental health have used a variety of indicators of poverty, including low financial income, material deprivation, unemployment and difficulties in obtaining housing. One of the most cited theoretical frameworks on the impact of unemployment on (physical and psychological) health is Jahoda's model of latent deprivation [27] [28]. This author believes that employment is beneficial from a financial point of view. As well, it provides subject's structure, meaningful activities, shared experiences, goals, social contact and opportunities for recognition and status. Morris, Cooke and Shaper (1994) [29] reported that men, who have suffered loss of employment (unemployment or retirement), are associated to twice the risk for early mortality, compared to men who are continuously employed, being this increase due to a variety of causes, including cancer and cardiovascular disease. Voss, Nylen, Floderus, Diderichsen and Terry (2004) [30] found that unemployment in men is associated with an increased risk of suicide and undetermined cause of death. Cohen *et al.* (2007) [31] found that unemployed individuals had less cytotoxic activity of their natural killer cell, and that their immune and inflammatory function recovered quickly when they returned to be employed. Janicki-Deverts, Cohen, Matthews and Cullen (2008) [32] found that an unemployment history is associated with increased C-reactive protein levels, an inflammatory marker of early expression in the evolution of cardiovascular disease. Lindstrom (2005) [33] and Brown *et al.* (2003) [34] also reported increased risk for psychological distress in unemployed people. Maier *et al.* (2006) [35] studied the impact of unemployment, over time, on the capacity for physical work. Unemployment is associated with a decrease in opportunities for physical activity and with increased psychological/distress suffering. Chronic stress is the main pathway through which unemployment exerts its negative impact on health.

1.4. Quality of Life and Resilience

The working group of world health organization on quality of life [36] defined quality of life as "the individual's perception of his/her position in life, in the context of culture and values system in which he/she lives, and in relation to his/her objectives, expectations, standards and concerns". The recognition of the multidimensional nature of the construct is reflected in the structure of the evaluation instruments, including the brief version of the scale of quality of life (WHOQOL BREF), based on physical, psychological, social and environmental domains. Wagnild (2010) [37] shown that resilience protects against negative emotions and thus has the potential to reduce its pathophysiological effects. The resilience scale she proposed, resilience state scale [38] [39], includes four factors: perseverance; meaningful life (purpose); equanimity; existential aloneness (coming home to oneself) and self-reliance. Perseverance refers to the enthusiastic persistence in finding solutions to problems, overcoming adversity, and the will to continue to rebuild life, with an attitude of self-confidence. The meaning of life refers to the awareness that one has something meaningful to live, to the notion that life has a meaning (a reason) in which the individual focuses, avoiding being obsessed with disputes that can't be solved, involving determination and satisfaction with the achievement of defined goals. Equanimity depends on a balanced and focused perspective on the purposes of life, with the capacity to accept the variety of experiences (even adverse) calmly and enthusiastically and the ability to exercise self-esteem. Existential aloneness and self-reliance refer to the awareness that each person's life path is unique and faced in solitude, getting the person confident on his/her ability to depend essentially in him/herself.

2. Empirical Study

2.1. Methods

This research focused on the impact of unemployment and/or economic insufficiency/poverty (material deprivation) on quality of life, as defined by world health organization. Participants in this study gave written informed, free consent. This study has been developed in concordance with the principles contained in Helsinki Declaration. It is a descriptive, quantitative, correlational, not experimental study. It has been used Pearson correlation coefficient r. It has been used a convenience sample. Dependent variables comprise the dimensions relating to coping, resilience, quality of life and executive function. Independent variables respect stress associated with situations of unemployment and/or economic insufficiency/poverty (material deprivation). The psychometric scales have been validated for the Portuguese population, and executive function has been evaluated through computerized Stroop and Berg tasks.

2.2. Participants

The sample consists of 41 participants, residents in the Portuguese city of Olhão, and 61% are female. The age presents a mean value of 37.2 years, with a dispersion of values of 25%. As for the time of unemployment, 34% of the participants were employed less than 2 years, 22% between 2 and 5 years, 20% between 5 and 10 years and 24% over 10 years. In the sample, 10% of the participants have been unemployed for three months, 20% for 6 months, 35% for one year, 32% for over two years and one participant was always unemployed. As for the annual financial income, 61% of participants are from the income tax level (AT/IRS) [40] of 11.5% (*i.e.*, have annual income below 4898 euros), 12% are ranking at level 14.0% (*i.e.*, have annual income between 4898 and 7410 euros) and 27% are in the level of 24.5% (that is, have annual incomes between 7410 and 18,375 euros). In the sample, 51% of the participants live accompanied, and 59% have dependent children (financially in charge). As for the monthly financial income, 24% of respondents say they do not have an individual income higher than 421 euros, 32% are currently receiving unemployment benefits. In this study, 98% of respondents say that, with unemployment, their financial situation has worsened, and 95% say they live in a country of risk (for poverty).As for scholarship, 98% of participants have basic or mean (not superior) academic formation. As for health habits, 81% of the respondents claim that their daily diet is balanced in proteins, sugars, fats, vitamins, minerals (including salt) and water, 27% regularly practice exercise, 34% consume drinks containing alcohol, and 51% drink coffee and/or smoke tobacco (nicotine). In this study, 15% of participants suffer from chronic physical diseases.

2.3. Material

2.3.1. Coping
Coping scale brief COPE [41] [42] is a dichotomous scale with two possible answers (from "0" to "1") between "no" and "yes." It consists of 28 items, which are organized into 14 dimensions: active coping (dimension 1); planning (dimension 2); use of instrumental support (dimension 3); use of social emotional support (dimension 4); religion (dimension 5); positive reinterpretation (dimension 6); self-blame (dimension 7); acceptance (dimension 8); expression of feelings (dimension 9); denial (dimension 10); self-distraction (dimension 11); behavioral divestment (dimension 12); use of substances (dimension 13); humor (dimension 14). For each of the dimensions, the values were determined by calculating the sum of the items that constitute them. The minimum possible value is 0 and the maximum possible value is 28, and for each dimension, the minimum value is 0 and the maximum value is 2.

2.3.2. Resilient Coping
Brief resilient coping scale [43] [44] is an ordinal Likert scale with five possible answers ("1" to "5") between "almost never" and "almost always." It consists of four items, which are organized in a single dimension. Their values were determined by calculating the sum of the items that constitute them. The minimum possible value is 4 and the maximum possible value is 20.

2.3.3. Resilience
Resilience state scale [38] [39] is an ordinal Likert scale with seven response alternatives ("1" to "7") between "totally disagree" and "totally agree". It consists of 23 items, which are organized in a single dimension. Their values were determined by calculating the sum of the items that constitute them. The minimum value is 23 and the maximum value is 161.

2.3.4. Perceived Stress
Perceived stress scale [45] [46] is an ordinal Likert scale with five possible answers ("0" to "4") between "never" and "often". It consists of 10 items, which are organized in a single dimension, and the scale of the items 4, 5, 7

and 8 (indicated with R) is recoded conversely, since the formulation is held in the negative. Their values were determined by calculating the sum of the items that constitute them. The minimum value is 0 and the maximum value is 40.

2.3.5. Life Experiences Survey

Life experiences survey [47] [48] is an ordinal Likert scale with seven possible answers ("1" to "7") between "very negative" and "very positive". It consists of 60 items. Their values were determined by calculating the frequency with which each experience occurs and the frequency of the sample elements who consider it negative and also of those who consider it positive.

2.3.6. Material Deprivation

Material deprivation scale [49] is a dichotomous scale with two possible answers (from "0" to "1") between "no" and "yes." It consists of nine items which are organized in a single dimension. Items are: capacity to ensure the immediate payment of an unexpected expense of 421 euros (that is, close to the monthly value of the current poverty line) without resorting to loan (item 1); no ability to pay a week's holiday per year away from home, supporting the cost of accommodation and travel for all household members (item 2); delay, motivated by economic difficulties, in some of the regular payments for rent, current credit, benefits or costs of primary residence, or other expenses not related to the principal residence (item 3); no financial capacity to have a meal with meat or fish (or vegetarian equivalent) at least each two days (item 4); no financial capacity to keep home adequately warm (item 5); without availability of washing machine due to economic difficulties (item 6); no color television availability due to economic difficulties (item 7); no landline or mobile phone availability due to economic difficulties (item 8); no car availability (light passenger or mixed) due to economic difficulties (item 9). Their values were determined by calculating the sum of the items that constitute them. The minimum value is 0 and the maximum value is 9.

2.3.7. Quality of Life

Short/brief version of the scale of quality of life/WHOQOL BREF [36] [50] is an ordinal Likert scale with five possible answers ("1" to "5"). It consists of 26 items, which are organized into a general index and four domains. For items marked with an "R", the scale is recoded in reverse because its formulation is held in the negative. For each dimension, its values were determined by calculating the sum of the items that constitute them. For the general index, the minimum value is 2 and the maximum value is 10; for domain 1 (physical), the minimum possible value is 7 and the maximum possible value is 35; for domain 2 (psychological), the minimum possible value is 6 and the maximum possible value is 30; for domain 3 (social), the minimum possible value is 3 and the maximum possible value is 15; for domain 4 (environmental), the minimum possible value is 8 and the maximum possible value is 40. The values of the scores obtained for the various domains were then processed on a scale of 0 to 100.

2.3.8. Victoria Stroop Task

In victoria Stroop task/VST [51] [52], it have been used the values of the efficiencies of color/dot (C/D) and color/word (C/W).

2.3.9. Berg Card Sorting Test

In Berg card sorting test/BCST [53]-[55], it has been used the parameter values of perseverative errors, learning to learn (LTL) and correct answers.

2.4. Results

For brief COPE scale, Cronbach's alpha value is 0.851, and the mean value is 10.8. The coping strategy that occurs more frequently is active coping, followed by positive reinterpretation and planning. For brief resilient coping scale, Cronbach's alpha value is 0.717, with a mean value of 13.4 (higher than the midpoint of measurement scale, which is 12) and most of the values are located between 10 and 16. For resilience state scale, Cronbach's alpha value is 0.904, with a mean value of 129.8 (above the midpoint of measurement scale, which is 92) and most of the values located between 110 and 150. For perceived stress scale, Cronbach's alpha value is 0.854, with a mean value of 18.27 (below the midpoint of the measurement scale, which is 20) and most of the values located between 15 and 25. For life experiences survey, Cronbach's alpha value is 0.929, and the event considered negative with higher occurrence is "great change in their economic level" (item 19, which corresponds to 56%), followed by "change in sleep habits" (item 4, which corresponds to 39%), "change in employment status" (item 13, which corresponds to 35%) and "to be fired from job" (item 32, which corresponds to 34%). The event considered positive with higher occurrence is "great change in the amount and how to occupy leisure time"(item 29, which corresponds to 51%), followed by "great change in social activities" (item 36, which corresponds to 39%) and "great change of proximity of family members" (item 20, which corresponds to 29%). For material deprivation scale, Cronbach's alpha value is 0.763, with a mean value of 3.20 (lower than the midpoint of measurement scale, which is 4.50), and most of the values located between 0 and 4. For quality of life scale (WHOQOL BREF), Cronbach's alpha value is 0.647. For domain 1 (physical), Cronbach's alpha value is 0.823; for domain 2 (psychological), Cronbach's alpha value is 0.749; for domain 3 (social), Cronbach's alpha value is 0.759; for domain 4 (environmental), Cronbach's alpha value is 0.736. All mean values are higher than the midpoint, although most related with social domain, followed by the physical and psychological domains. Respecting the efficiency of C/D of VST, the mean value is 1.04, with the majority of the values located between 0.50 and 1.25. Respecting the efficiency of C/W of VST, the mean value is 1.31, with the majority of the values located between 0.75 and 1.75. Perseverative errors of BCST have a mean value of 15.0, with a dispersion of values of 75% (the distribution of values of perseverative errors mainly takes place between 0 and 15). Correct answers of BCST have a mean value of 71.4, with a dispersion of values of 22% (the distribution of values of correct responses mainly takes place between 50 and 90). Learning to learn (LTL) of BCST has a mean value of −0.02, with a dispersion of values of 31.297% values (the distribution of values of LTL occurs mainly between −5 and 5).The correlation analysis between variables shows that there are statistically significant positive correlations between:the efficiency of C/D of VST and the overall value of brief COPE, $r = 0.333$, $p < 0.05$; the efficiency of C/D of VST and dimension 1 (active coping) of brief COPE, $r = 0.351$, $p < 0.05$; the efficiency of C/W of VST and the overall value of brief COPE, $r = 0.355$, $p < 0.05$; the efficiency of C/W of VST and dimension 1 (active coping) of brief COPE, $r = 0.452$, $p < 0.01$; the efficiency of C/D of VST and domain 3 (social) of WHOQOL BREF, $r = 0.313$, $p < 0.05$; the life event "to borrow some money" (item 31 of life experiences survey) and the overall value of perceived stress scale, $r = 0.692$, $p = 0.013$; the brief resilient coping scale and the domain 2 (psychological) of WHOQOL BREF, $r = 0.512$, $p < 0.01$; the brief resilient coping scale and the domain 3 (social) of WHOQOL BREF, $r = 0.368$, $p < 0.05$; the resilience state scale and the domain 2 (psychological) of WHOQOL BREF, $r = 0.677$, $p < 0.01$; the resilience state scale and the domain 3 (social) of WHOQOL BREF, $r = 0.375$, $p < 0.05$; the resilience state scale and the domain 4 (environmental) of WHOQOL BREF, $r = 0.396$, $p < 0.01$. There are statistically significant negative correlations between: LTL of BCST and dimension 7 (self-blame) of brief COPE, $r = −0.437$, $p < 0.05$; material deprivation and the general value of WHOQOL BREF, $r = −0.322$, $p = 0.040$; the perceived stress scale and the resilience state scale, $r = −0.539$, $p < 0.01$; the perceived stress scale and brief resilient coping scale, $r = −0.373$, $p = 0.016$.

2.5. Discussion and Conclusion

This research focused on the impact of the economic insufficiency (poverty, material deprivation) and unemployment in quality of life, as defined by World Health Organization. As for the annual financial income, 61% of participants are from the income tax level (AT/IRS) [40] of 11.5% (*i.e.*, have annual income below 4898 euros), 12% are ranking at level 14.0% (*i.e.*, have annual income between 4898 and 7410 euros) and 27% are in the level of 24.5% (that is, have annual incomes between 7410 and 18,375 euros). In the sample, 51% of the participants live accompanied, and 59% have dependent children (financially in charge). As for the monthly financial income, 24% of respondents say they do not have an individual income higher than 421 euros, 32% are currently receiving unemployment benefits. In this study, 98% of respondents say that, with unemployment, their financial situation has worsened, and 95% say they live in a country of risk (for poverty). Material deprivation has a mean value of 3.20. There is a negative correlation between material deprivation and quality of life. As for the time of unemployment, 34% of the participants were employed less than 2 years, 22% between 2 and 5 years, 20% between 5 and 10 years and 24% over 10 years. In the sample, 10% of the participants have been unemployed for three months, 20% for 6 months, 35% for one year, 32% for over two years and one participant was always unemployed. As for scholarship, 98% of participants have basic or mean (not superior) academic formation. For life experiences survey, Cronbach's alpha value is 0.929, and the event considered negative with higher occurrence is "great change in their economic level" (item 19, which corresponds to 56%), followed by "change in sleep habits" (item 4, which corresponds to 39%), "change in employment status" (item 13, which corresponds to 35%) and "to be fired from job" (item 32, which corresponds to 34%). The event considered positive with higher occurrence is "great change in the amount and how to occupy leisure time" (item 29, which corresponds to 51%), followed by "great change in social activities" (item 36, which corresponds to 39%) and "great change of proximity of family members" (item 20, which corresponds to 29%). There is a positive correlation between perceived stress and life event "to borrow some money" (item 31 of life experiences survey). By acting through stressors agents of socio-economic nature, such as unemployment and the difficulty of access to housing, it is much more likely that poverty precedes mental disorders such as anxiety and depression, as well as it constitutes an important risk factor for mental illness [20]. The personal debt is a particular source of stress. Working in poverty, represented by financial need and restrictive standards of living, correlates negatively with subjective well-being, and is associated with increased risk for not meeting basic needs in mental health [22]. Poverty and material deprivation are associated, independently, concerning risk of mental disorders in women, to add to the sources of stress usually related to women condition [26]. Some factors, such as education and employment, has a two-way relationship with poverty. The lack of employment results in financial difficulties and poverty results in reduced opportunity to obtain gainful employment. Unemployed people and those who fail to obtain employment have more depressive symptoms than individuals who can get a job [21]. Morris, Cooke and Shaper (1994) [29] reported that the men, who have suffered job loss (due to unemployment or retirement), is associated with a risk two times higher of (early) mortality, compared to men who are (continuously) employed, this increase being due to a variety of causes, including cancer and cardiovascular disease. Voss, Nylen, Floderus, Diderichsen and Terry (2004) [30] found that unemployment in men is associated with an increased risk of suicide and undetermined cause of death. Lindstrom (2005) [33] and Brown et al. (2003) [34] also reported increased risk of psychological distress in unemployed people. The prevalence of common mental disorders is higher among individuals with low levels of education. In this work, it is found negative correlations between: perceived stress and resilience; perceived stress and resilient coping. There are positive correlations between: resilient coping and quality of life; resilience and quality of life. The perception of stress may influence the pathogenesis of physical illness, determining negative emotional states which directly affect physiological processes influencing behavior patterns or risk for disease [8]. Wagnild (2010) [37] has shown that the resilience protects against negative emotions and thus has the potential to reduce their pathophysiological effects. In this study, there are positive correlations between: performance in the Stroop task, which assesses executive function, and quality of life; Stroop task and active coping (dimension 1) of brief COPE. There is a negative correlation between the performance in Berg task, which assesses cognitive flexibility (performance in the parameter "learning to learn/LTL"), and self-blame (dimension 7 of brief COPE). The adequate performance in Stroop tasks depends mainly on structural and functional integrity of the dorso-lateral prefrontal cortex and anterior cingulate gyrus. The dorsolateral prefrontal cortex is the neuro-biological correlate of working memory [12]-[14]. Berg task is a neuropsychological task that evaluates cognitive flexibility [11] [12]. Various cognitive components that functionally implement cognitive flexibility, such as recognition of the incorrectness of the environmental feedback stimulus, selection of new dimension through abstract thinking, i.e., conceptual ability, learning how to learn (learning to learn/LTL), inner speech, response inhibition and updating working memory depend on structural and functional integrity of the infero-lateral prefrontal cortex, sub-region of dorso-lateral prefrontal cortex [17], and caudate nucleus [18] [19]. This work allowed to highlight that quality of life is positively correlated with resilience skills and active coping strategies. This type of coping is supported by a suitable executive function, as demonstrated in this study. Responsible for the use of active coping strategies is an adequate structural and functional integrity of prefrontal cortex, brain region which is a predominant target of the pathophysiological impact of (chronic) stress. Participants who predominantly use not active coping strategies (self-blame) have less adequate performances in Berg task. The use of not active coping strategies is associated with decreased cognitive flexibility, and suggests dysfunction of infero-lateral prefrontal cortex, in this population.

References

[1]   Lazarus, R S. and Folkman, S. (1984) Stress, Appraisal, and Coping. Springer, New York.

[2]   Selye, H. (1974) Stress without Distress. J. B. Lippincott, Philadelphia.

[3]   Folkman, S. and Lazarus, RS. (1980) An Analysis of Coping in a Middle Aged Community Sample. *Journal of Health and Social Behavior*, **21**, 219-239. http://dx.doi.org/10.2307/2136617

[4]   Smith, C.A. and Lazarus, R.S. (1990) Emotion and Adaptation. In: Pervin, L.A., Ed., *Handbook of Personality: Theory and Research*, Guilford, New York, 609-637.

[5]   Lang, P.J. (1995) The Emotion Probe: Studies of Motivation and Attention. *American Psychologist*, **50**, 372-385. http://dx.doi.org/10.1037/0003-066X.50.5.372

[6]   Drevets, W.C., Bogers, W. and Raichle, M.E. (2002) Functional Anatomical Correlates of Antidepressant Drug Treatment Assessed Using PET Measures of Regional Glucose Metabolism. *European Neuropsychopharmacology*, **12**, 527-544. http://dx.doi.org/10.1016/S0924-977X(02)00102-5

[7]   George, M.S., Lisanby, S.H. and Sackeim, H.A. (1999) Transcranial Magnetic Stimulation—Applications in Neuropsychiatry. *Archives of General Psychiatry*, **56**, 300-311. http://dx.doi.org/10.1001/archpsyc.56.4.300

[8]   Cohen, S., Kessler, R.C. and Underwood Gordon, L. (1997) Measuring Stress: A Guide for Health and Social Scientists. Oxford, New York.

[9]   Cohen, S., Evans, G.W., Krantz, D.S. and Stokols, D. (1986) Behavior, Health and Environmental Stress. Plenum Press, New York. http://dx.doi.org/10.1007/978-1-4757-9380-2

[10]   Suchy, Y. (2009) Executive Functioning: Overview, Assessment, and Research Issues for non-Neuropsychologists. *Annals of Behavioral Medicine*, **37**, 106-116. http://dx.doi.org/10.1007/s12160-009-9097-4

[11]   Golden, C.J. (1978) Stroop Color and Word Test: A Manual for Clinical and Experimental Uses. Skoelting, Chicago.

[12]   Fuster, J.N.M. (2000) The Prefrontal Cortex of the Primate: A Synopsis. *Psychobiology*, **28**, 125-131.

[13]   Stuss, D.T., Alexander, M.P., Floden, D., *et al.* (2002) Fractionation and Localization of Distinct Frontal Lobe Processes: Evidence from Focal Lesions in Humans. Oxford University Press, London.

[14]   Lezak, M.D., Howieson, D.B. and Loring, D.W. (2004) Neuropsychological Assessment. Oxford University Press, New York.

[15]   Pujol, J., Vendrell, P., Deus, J., *et al.* (2001) The Effect of Medial Frontal and Posterior Parietal Demyelinating Lesions on Stroop Interference. *Neuroimage*, **13**, 68-75. http://dx.doi.org/10.1006/nimg.2000.0662

[16]   Bush, G., Frazier, J.A., Rauch, S.L., *et al.* (1999) Anterior Cingulate Cortex Dysfunction in Attention-Deficit/ Hyperactivity Disorder Revealed by fMRI and the Counting Stroop. *Biological Psychiatry*, **45**, 1542-1552. http://dx.doi.org/10.1016/S0006-3223(99)00083-9

[17]   Kaufmann, L., Ischebeck, A., Weiss, E., *et al.* (2008) An fMRI Study of the Numerical Stroop Task in Individuals with and without Minimal Cognitive Impairment. *Cortex*, **44**, 1248-1255. http://dx.doi.org/10.1016/j.cortex.2007.11.009

[18]   Monchi, O., Petrides, M., Petre, V., Worsley, K. and Dagher, A. (2001) Wisconsin Card Sorting Revisited: Distinct Neural Circuits Participating in Different Stages of the Task Identified by Event-Related Functional Magnetic Resonance Imaging. *The Journal of Neuroscience*, **21**, 7733-7741. http://unf-montreal.ca/oury/Site/publications/J_Neurosci_2001.pdf

[19]   Frank, M.J., Loughry, B. and O'Reilly, R.C. (2001) Interactions between Frontal Cortex and Basal Ganglia in Working Memory: A Computational Model. *Cognitive, Affective, & Behavioral Neuroscience*, **1**, 137-160. http://dx.doi.org/10.3758/CABN.1.2.137

[20]   Patel, V. and Kleinman, A. (2003) Poverty and Common Mental Disorders in Developing Countries. *Bulletin of the World Health Organization*, **81**, 609-615.

[21]   Simon, G.E., Revicki, D., Heiligenstein, J., *et al.* (2000) Recovery from Depression, Work Productivity, and Health Care Costs among Primary Care Patients. *General Hospital Psychiatry*, **22**, 153-162. http://dx.doi.org/10.1016/S0163-8343(00)00072-4

[22]   Vetter, S., Endrass, J., Schweizer, I., *et al.* (2006) The Effects of Economic Deprivation on Psychological Well-Being among the Working Population of Switzerland. *BMC Public Health*, **6**, 223. http://dx.doi.org/10.1186/1471-2458-6-223

[23]   Elder, G.H. and Caspi, A. (1988) Economic Stress in Lives: Developmental Perspectives. *Journal of Social Issues*, **44**, 25-45. http://dx.doi.org/10.1111/j.1540-4560.1988.tb02090.x

[24]   National Institute of Child Health and Human Development, NICHD (2006) Duration and Developmental Timing of Poverty and Children's Cognitive and Social Development from Birth through Third Grade. *Child Development*, **76**, 795-810.

[25]   Goosby, B.J. (2006) Poverty and Adolescent Mental Health: The Role of Maternal Psychological Resources. *Proceedings of the Annual Meetings of the Population Association of America*, Los Angeles, 30 March-1 April 2006. http://paa2006.princeton.edu/papers/60518

[26] Patel, V., Kirkwood, B.R., Pednekar, S., Weiss, H. and Mabey, D. (2006) Risk Factors for Common Mental Disorders in Women Population-Based Longitudinal Study. *The British Journal of Psychiatry*, **189**, 547-555. http://dx.doi.org/10.1192/bjp.bp.106.022558

[27] Ezzy, D. (1993) Unemployment and Mental Health: A Critical Review. *Social Science and Medicine*, **37**, 41-52. http://dx.doi.org/10.1016/0277-9536(93)90316-V

[28] Janlert, U. and Hammarstrom, A. (2009) Which Model Is Best? Explanatory Models of the Relationship between Unemployment and Health. *BMC Public Health*, **9**, 235. http://dx.doi.org/10.1186/1471-2458-9-235

[29] Morris, J.K., Cook, D.G. and Shaper, A.G. (1994) Loss of Employment and Mortality. *BMJ*, **308**, 1135-1139. http://dx.doi.org/10.1136/bmj.308.6937.1135

[30] Voss, M., Nylen, L., Floderus, B., Diderichsen, F. and Terry, P.D. (2004) Unemployment and Early Cause-Specific Mortality: A Study Based on the Swedish Twin Registry. *American Journal of Public Health*, **94**, 2155-2161. http://dx.doi.org/10.2105/AJPH.94.12.2155

[31] Cohen, F., Kemeny, M.E., Zegans, L.S., *et al.* (2007) Immune Function Declines with Unemployment and Recovers after Stressor Termination. *Psychosomatic Medicine*, **69**, 225-234. http://dx.doi.org/10.1097/PSY.0b013e31803139a6

[32] Janicki-Deverts, D., Cohen, S., Matthews, K.A. and Cullen, M.R. (2008) History of Unemployment Predicts Future Elevations in C-Reactive Protein among Male Participants in the Coronary Artery Risk Development in Young Adults (CARDIA) Study. *Annuals of Behavioral Medicine*, **36**, 176-185. http://dx.doi.org/10.1007/s12160-008-9056-5

[33] Lindstrom, M. (2005) Psychosocial Work Conditions, Unemployment and Selfreported Psychological Health: A Population-Based Study. *Occupational Medicine*, **55**, 568-571. http://dx.doi.org/10.1093/occmed/kqi122

[34] Brown, D.W., Balluz, L.S., Ford, E.S., *et al.* (2003) Associations between Short- and Long-Term Unemployment and Frequent Mental Distress among a National Sample of Men and Women. *Journal of Occupational and Environmental Medicine*, **45**, 11569-1166. http://dx.doi.org/10.1097/01.jom.0000094994.09655.0f

[35] Maier, R., Egger, A., Barth, A., *et al.* (2006) Effects of Short- and Long-Term Unemployment on Physical Work Capacity and on Serum Cortisol. *International Archives of Occupational and Environmental Health*, **79**, 193-198. http://dx.doi.org/10.1007/s00420-005-0052-9

[36] WHOQOL Group (1994) The Development of the World Health Organization Quality of Life Assessment Instrument (The WHOQOL). In: *Quality of Life Assessment: International Perspectives*, Springer Verlag, Berlin, Heidelberg, 41-57.

[37] Wagnild, G.M. (2010) Discovering Your Resilience Core. Resiliencescale.com. http://resiliencescale.net/papers.html

[38] Wagnild, G.M. and Young, H.M. (1993) Development and Psychometric Evaluation of the Resilience Scale. *Journal of Nursing Measurement*, **1**, 165-178.

[39] de Carvalho Ng, C.A.F. and Pereira, I.D. (2012) Adaptação da "Theresiliencescale" para a população adulta portuguesa. *Psicologia USP*, **23**, 417-433. http://dx.doi.org/10.1590/S0103-65642012005000008 http://www.revistas.usp.br/psicousp/article/viewFile/42178/45851

[40] Autoridade Tributária e Aduaneira do Ministério das Finanças do Governo de Portugal (AT) (2012) Modelo 3 de Imposto sobre o Rendimento das Pessoas Singulares(IRS). http://info.portaldasfinancas.gov.pt/NR/rdonlyres/8687C530-4D05-4CB6-ABFA-0697CC4C180F/0/IRS_2012_internet.pdf

[41] Ribeiro, J.L.P. and Rodrigues, A.P. (2004) Questões acerca do coping: A propósito do estudo de adaptação do Brief Cope. *Psicologia, Saúde & Doenças*, **5**, 3-15. http://hdl.handle.net/10400.12/1054

[42] Carver, C.S. (1997) You Want to Measure Coping but Your Protocol's Too Long: Consider the Brief COPE. *International Journal of Behavioral Medicine*, **4**, 92-100. http://dx.doi.org/10.1207/s15327558ijbm0401_6

[43] Ribeiro, J.L. and Morais, R. (2010) Adaptação portuguesa da escala breve de coping resiliente. *Psicologia, Saúde & Doenças*, **11**, 5-13.

[44] Sinclair, V.G. and Wallston, K.A. (2004) The Development and Psychometric Evaluation of the Brief Resilient Coping Scale. *Assessment*, **11**, 94-101. http://dx.doi.org/10.1177/1073191103258144

[45] Pais Ribeiro, J. and Marques, T. (2009) A avaliação do stresse: A propósito de um estudo de adaptação da escala de percepção de stresse. *Psicologia, Saúde & Doenças*, **10**, 237-248. http://hdl.handle.net/10400.12/1091

[46] Cohen, S., Kamarck, T. and Mermelstein, R. (1983) A Global Measure of Perceived Stress. *Journal of Health and Social Behavior*, **24**, 385-396. http://www.jstor.org/stable/2136404 http://dx.doi.org/10.2307/2136404

[47] Silva, I., Pais-Ribeiro, J., Cardoso, H. and Ramos, H. (2003) Contributo para a adaptação da Life Experiences Survey

(LES) à população diabética portuguesa. *Revista Portuguesa de Saúde Pública*, **21**, 49-60. https://cms.ensp.unl.pt/www.ensp.unl.pt/dispositivos-de-apoio/cdi/cdi/sector-de-publicacoes/revista/2000-2008/pdfs/2-05-2003.pdf

[48] Sarason, I., Johnson, J. and Siegel, J. (1978) Assessing the Impact of Life Changes: Development of the Life Experiences Survey. *Journal of Consulting and Clinical Psychology*, **46**, 932-946. http://dx.doi.org/10.1037/0022-006x.46.5.932

[49] Instituto Nacional de Estatística (2010) Sobre a pobreza, as desigualdades e a privação material em Portugal (On-poverty, Inequality, and Material Deprivation in Portugal). INE, Lisboa.

[50] Vaz-Serra, A., Canavarro, M.C. and Simões, M.R. (2006) Estudos psicométricos do instrumento de avaliação da qualidade de vida da Organização Mundial de Saúde (WHOQOL-Bref) para Português de Portugal. *Psiquiatria Clínica*, **27**, 41-49. http://hdl.handle.net/10849/181

[51] Mueller, S. (2010) The Stroop Test (Web Log Post). PEBL Blog. http://peblblog.blogspot.com/2010/05/stroop-test.html

[52] Troyer, A.K., Leach, L. and Strauss, E. (2006) Aging and Response Inhibition: Normative Data for the Victoria Stroop Test. *Aging, Neuropsychology & Cognition*, **13**, 20-35. http://dx.doi.org/10.1080/138255890968187

[53] Berg, E.A. (1948) A Simple Objective Technique for Measuring Flexibility in Thinking. *The Journal of General Psychology*, **39**, 15-22. http://dx.doi.org/10.1080/00221309.1948.9918159

[54] Piper, B. (2012) Video of the Berg (Wisconsin) Card Sorting Task (Web Log Post). PEBL Blog. http://peblblog.blogspot.pt/2012/07/video-of-berg-wisconsin-card-sorting.html

[55] Fox, C.J., Mueller, S.T., Gray, H.M., Raber, J. and Piper, B.J. (2013) Evaluation of a Short-Form of the Berg Card Sorting Test. *PLoS ONE*, **8**, 1-4. http://dx.doi.org/10.1371/journal.pone.0063885

26

Mental Health Literacy and the Belief in the Supernatural

Leslie Lim[1], Justine Goh[1], Yiong-Huak Chan[2], Shi-Hui Poon[1]

[1]Department of Psychiatry, Singapore General Hospital, Republic of Singapore
[2]National University Health System, National University of Singapore, Republic of Singapore
Email: leslie.lim.e.c@sgh.com.sg

Abstract

Objective: Mental health literacy affects treatment seeking. We compare literacy levels of psychiatric outpatients and a control group of outpatients seeking treatment for non-psychiatric disorders in the same hospital. We hypothesized higher levels of mental health literacy among psychiatric patients than controls, with younger age and higher educational levels associated with better literacy. We also hypothesized that there would be an inverse relationship between educational level and the belief in the supernatural causality of mental disorders. Methods: Literacy was estimated by showing psychiatric outpatients and a control group of non-psychiatric patients vignettes depicting a case of major depression and a case of generalised anxiety disorder. Their opinions regarding diagnosis, etiology, treatment, and attitudes towards mental health services were ascertained by structured questionnaires. Results: Psychiatric patients did not demonstrate superior mental health literacy compared to controls, with the exception of knowing where to obtain a psychiatric referral. Lower age and higher education levels of psychiatric patients were associated with better literacy. The higher the education level is, the less likely to attribute the causality of mental disorders to supernatural elements. Conclusion: This study highlights the need for a program of psycho-education targeting patients, their relatives, and the public.

Keywords

Mental Health Literacy, Age, Education Level, Belief in the Supernatural

1. Introduction

Low rates of help seeking among persons with mental disorders have been widely reported [1]-[4]. One of the reasons cited for this phenomenon is poor understanding of mental disorders, their etiology, symptoms, treatment, and prevention. Such knowledge is also termed "mental health literacy" [5]. There is growing evidence that poor mental health literacy (MHL) negatively impacts help-seeking behaviors and influences decisions regarding treatment and compliance [6]-[10].

Cultural factors also play a role in determining treatment preferences. For instance, the prevalent belief among people in Southeast Asia is to attribute mental illness causation to demonic spirits and supernatural elements [11]-[13]. Not surprisingly, some have preferred to consult traditional healers rather than seeking professional help from mental health services [1] [11] [13].

Most literacy research has assessed the general population. A notable exception was the study by Goldney *et al.* [14] who utilised a case vignette describing depression to measure literacy in depressed patients. They found that depressed subjects' knowledge about depression was similar to that of non-depressed persons, despite the apparent familiarity of patients with the nature of the disorder and its treatment. In contrast, Furnham and Blythe, while not using the vignette method, found that lay persons without schizophrenia were able to display a higher degree of literacy if they had prior interactions with schizophrenia patients [15].

Our present study seeks to measure and compare the mental health literacy of patients undergoing psychiatric outpatient treatment to that of a control group of patients seeking treatment for non-psychiatric disorders in the same hospital. We hypothesized higher levels of mental health literacy among psychiatric patients compared to controls and that literacy would be positively associated with younger age and higher educational levels. We also hypothesized that there would be an inverse relationship between educational level and the belief in the supernatural causality of mental disorders.

2. Methods

2.1. Participants and Procedure

The study was conducted in the psychiatric outpatient clinic of a large general hospital in Singapore, a city state with a population of over 5 million. Over a period from 1 November 2014 to 31 March 2015, patients with anxiety and depressive disorders were interviewed by a trained research coordinator, who had access to their clinic records. We included patients between the ages of 21 to 75 years, who were able to understand written English or Mandarin, and who consented to participate in the study. Patients with organic mental conditions such as delirium or dementia, and psychosis were excluded. Control participants consisted of patients from other disciplines attending outpatient treatment from the same general hospital. Patients were approached with the approval of their respective hospital consultants, and subsequently interviewed if they were agreeable to participate in the study. The study was approved by the hospital's Institutional Review Board.

2.2. Materials

Participants were presented with two vignettes describing cases meeting Diagnostic and Statistical Manual of Mental Disorders, Fourth Edition, Text Revision (DSM-IV-TR) diagnostic criteria [16] for Major Depressive Disorder (MDD) and Generalised Anxiety Disorder (GAD) respectively. We used a structured questionnaire with a multiple choice response format. To assess recognition of MDD and GAD in the vignettes, participants were asked what type of illness they felt the subject in the vignette was suffering from (e.g. "physical illness/ mental illness/spiritual condition/none of the above/don't know") and if they recognized a mental illness, what they thought the diagnosis was (e.g. "Acute stress disorder/Major Depression/Generalised Anxiety Disorder/ Panic Disorder/Obsessive-Compulsive Disorder/Schizophrenia/Others").

Knowledge of interventions and treatments available was also tested by asking participants whether they felt certain interventions were needed to help resolve the problem, with interventions including "Physical exercise", "Diet", "Psychotherapy", "Medication", "Vitamins", and "Exorcism". We also enquired whether they held beliefs regarding the possible supernatural causation of mental disorders.

2.3. Psychiatric Assessments

We used the Mini-International Neuropsychiatric Interview (MINI) [17] to assess for any psychiatric morbidity in the controls and to confirm that the group of psychiatric patients and controls did not meet our exclusion criteria.

2.4. Statistical Analysis

Data were analysed using the Statistical Package for the Social Sciences (SPSS) 22.0 program. Pearson's chi-squared tests were conducted to identify any significant differences in demographic variables between the psychiatric patients and the control participants. One-way Analyses of Covariance (ANCOVA) were conducted to determine whether there was any significant difference in the mental health literacy scores of the psychiatric patients and control participants, while controlling for certain demographic variables. Significance was set at $p < 0.05$.

3. Results

A total of 131 patients, comprising 70 with psychiatric illness (mainly anxiety and depression) and 61 control subjects, were recruited into the study. **Table 1** shows the characteristics of the sample. The mean age of the psychiatric patients was 51.6 years (SD = 13.5) and the controls 44.8 years (SD = 12.5). The differences in ages was significant according to a one-way Analysis of Variance (ANOVA), $F(1,129) = 8.896, p = 0.003$. There was also a significantly smaller percentage of psychiatric patients than control participants who were actively employed, $\chi^2 (5, n = 131) = 14.71, p = 0.012$.

Each correct answer was given one mark. The scores for each component of mental health literacy were tallied. This yielded subtotals, from which the total composite score was obtained by addition of subtotal scores. Please refer to **Table 2** which shows the component items and their maximum scores.

Table 1. Characteristics of the patients.

	Psychiatric patients		Non-psychiatric patients		p-value
	Number (N = 70)	Percentage (%)	Number (N = 61)	Percentage (%)	
Gender					0.964
Male	37	52.9	32	52.5	
Ethnicity					0.931
Chinese	62	88.6	51	83.6	
Non-Chinese	8	11.4	10	16.4	
Education Level					0.305
Primary to Secondary	38	54.3	26	42.6	
Junior college/Polytechnic	12	17.1	18	29.5	
Tertiary (University)	20	28.6	17	27.9	
Employment Status					0.012
Employed	38	54.3	47	77.0	
Unemployed	7	10.0	0	0	
Not in labour force	25	35.7	14	23.0	
Marital Status					0.172
Never married	19	27.1	15	24.6	
Married	41	58.6	42	68.9	
Divorced or separated	5	7.1	4	6.6	
Widowed	5	7.1	0	0	
Religion					0.483
Christianity	24	34.3	20	32.8	
Muslim	2	2.9	6	9.8	
Buddhist or Taoist	25	35.7	23	37.7	
Hindu	2	2.9	1	1.6	
No religion	17	24.3	11	18.0	

Table 2. A description of the sub-score items.

Composite score items (each correct answer was awarded one point)	Maximum score (points)
Vignette Identification (MDD) Perceived type of illness Name of disorder if perceived to be mental illness	2
Vignette Identification (GAD) Perceived type of illness Name of disorder if perceived to be mental illness	2
Description of persons with mental illness Perceived descriptors of people with mental illness	7
Purpose of psychiatric medication Perceived purpose of psychiatric medication	4
Side effects of psychiatric medication Perceived side effects of psychiatric medication	4
Where to obtain a psychiatric referral Perceived sources of psychiatric referral	3
Total score *Sum total of composite scores for:* *Vignette Identification (MDD)* *Vignette Identification (GAD)* *Description of persons with mental illness* *Purpose of psychiatric medication* *Side effects of psychiatric medication* *Where to obtain a psychiatric referral*	22

An ANOVA showed no significant differences in the sub-scores of mental health literacy between psychiatric patients and controls (all $p > 0.05$). Since the ages and employment statuses of the control participants were found to be significantly different from that of the psychiatric patients, an ANCOVA was conducted to control for these two demographic variables, which were entered as covariates. Results of the ANCOVA showed no significant differences in all the sub-scores of mental health literacy between the psychiatric patients and control participants, with the only exception being knowledge of where to obtain a psychiatric referral, where psychiatric patients scored higher than the control group, $F(1, 122) = 7.25, p = 0.008$.

There were no significant differences between the total composite scores of the psychiatric patients and control participants, $F(1, 122) = 1.66, p = 0.200$.

However, simple linear regression analyses suggested an inverse relationship between age and total composite scores, which was significant for the psychiatric group ($p = 0.046$), but not significant for controls ($p = 0.984$). Additionally, there was a significant negative association between education level and belief in supernatural causes of both depression, $\chi^2 (12, n = 70) = 40.47, p < 0.001$, and GAD, $\chi^2 (12, n = 70) = 40.17, p < 0.001$, with the better educated less likely to subscribe to supernatural attributions. This negative association, however, was only statistically significant for the psychiatric patients, but not the controls.

When shown vignettes depicting anxiety and depression, the older psychiatric patients were not more likely to attribute the features of depression ($p = 0.748$), and anxiety ($p = 0.559$) to supernatural factors than the controls. There was no association between supernatural attributions of depression ($p = 0.559$) and anxiety ($p = 0.085$) and the total composite score of mental health literacy among the psychiatric patients.

Table 3 shows the results of the ANCOVA.

A one-way Analyses of Variance (ANOVA) to examine the relationships between demographic variables and the total composite score revealed that among psychiatric patients, scores differed significantly between different levels of education, $F(3, 66) = 5.041, p = 0.003$. A Bonferroni post-hoc test revealed that those attaining Junior College/Polytechnic education (11.5 ± 2.4 points, $p = 0.042$) and University level (11.1 ± 4.0 points, $p = 0.049$) had significantly higher total mental health literacy scores than those with Primary education (7.3 ± 3.4 points). Thus, the better educated had a better grasp of MHL.

Table 3. Means of each Sub-Score.

Sub-scores	Psychiatric patients (N = 70)		Non-psychiatric patients (N = 61)	
	Mean	S.D.	Mean	S.D.
Vignette Identification (MDD)	1.22	0.17	1.09	0.19
Vignette Identification (GAD)	1.27	0.14	1.13	0.17
Description of persons with mental illness	1.19	0.27	1.22	0.31
Purpose of psychiatric medication	2.11	0.25	2.03	0.29
Side effects of psychiatric medication	1.74	0.31	1.67	0.36
Where to obtain a psychiatric referral*	2.00	0.16	1.59	0.19
Total composite score	9.53	0.67	8.72	0.78

*$F(1, 122) = 7.25, p = 0.008$.

4. Discussion

Our study is unique in that it assesses psychiatric patients' ability to recognise features of common psychiatric conditions, whereas previous researchers only assessed such knowledge from members of the general population. An unexpected finding was that psychiatric patients did not demonstrate better literacy levels compared to non-psychiatric controls. This concurs with the findings of Goldney *et al.* [14] but is contrary to our hypothesis that psychiatric patients would display better literacy compared to non-psychiatric patients.

A recent study on breast cancer patients in this country has revealed poor mental health literacy levels in that less than half were able to identify anxiety and depressive features in vignettes shown to the patients [18]. However, the authors did not utilise a comparison group. In that study, patients indicated that they would turn to close family members for help with psychosocial distress, rather than seek consultation with mental health specialists. Over one half cited reasons such as fear and embarrassment for their disinclination to obtain help from mental health services [18].

This confirms the widespread notion of stigma being one of the barriers to help-seeking. In the case of those already receiving professional help, improved mental health literacy is an added advantage towards treatment adherence in the face of on-going negative public sentiments toward receiving psychiatric help.

Most studies from the West have revealed that between 35% - 68% respondents correctly identified the diagnosis in a vignette depicting a psychiatric condition [8] [19] [20]. When shown features of MDD, slightly over a third (about 35%) of our patients gave the correct diagnosis, a quarter (25%) thought there was no mental illness, and over a fifth (21%) thought the diagnosis was an anxiety disorder. In the case of the GAD vignette, the results were fairly similar. Some 30% correctly identified the disorder, 14% thought there was no mental illness, while another 14% thought the vignette depicted a case of "stress". Those who failed to identify any mental illness or who dismissed an anxiety disorder as merely a case of "stress" might not see the need to seek psychiatric help. Some hold the belief that psychiatrists only treat the severely mentally ill, and consider "stress" not worthy of psychiatric attention. These would most likely turn to traditional healers or to close family members for help and support should they experience psychiatric symptoms.

Whether the correct identification would translate into professional help-seeking is not clear, with some authors of a literature review suggesting that increased health literacy does not necessarily lead to increased medication adherence [20]. One reason could be stigma as mentioned earlier, while another reason could be public misperception over the safety and efficacy of psychotropic medications [21] [22].

It was possible that those who identified no psychiatric diagnosis in the vignettes were influenced by cultural factors. For instance, in Southeast Asia, there is a strong belief in the role of supernatural agents (from witchcraft and black magic to evil spirits and divine anger) in bringing about mental disorders [11]-[13]. In fact, there was a trend, just short of significance ($p = 0.056$), for psychiatric patients to attribute the causality of the depressive condition to supernatural factors in contrast to the controls (see **Table 4**). The reasons for this are unclear. One possible explanation is that in families of psychiatric patients, in the absence of physical pathology, family members tend to attribute these symptoms to a spiritual affliction and advise consultation with traditional healers, thus influencing patients into making similar assumptions, as they had been culturally accustomed to believe.

Table 4. Belief in supernatural causality of depression and anxiety.

	Psychiatric patients		Non-psychiatric patients		
	Number ($N = 70$)	Percentage (%)	Number ($N = 61$)	Percentage (%)	p-value
Belief in supernatural causality of depression					0.056
Don't know	12	17.1	4	6.5	
Disagree	55	78.6	57	93.4	
Agree	3	4.3	0	0	
Belief in supernatural causality of anxiety					0.760
Don't know	9	5.7	6	9.8	
Disagree	58	82.9	54	88.5	
Agree	3	4.3	1	1.6	

However, for the control subjects, most of whom do not have psychiatric symptomatology and are clearly suffering from physical conditions, the question of supernatural causality would not have not arisen. Hence, the controls are less likely to attribute the depressive condition to the supernatural.

Our findings also suggest that while older psychiatric patients tended to have lower mental health literacy scores, age was not a determinant to supernatural attributions. Such beliefs are more likely held by those with less education. Another interesting finding was that belief in the supernatural did not seem to affect composite literacy scores. This suggests that good literacy is not mutually exclusive to cultural belief systems, in that they can co-exist in parallel in the same patient. Those with high literacy scores may still ascribe mental illness to spiritual factors.

Conversely, the higher the education level the less inclined to believe in supernatural explanations of illness etiology. Instead, the more highly educated showed better literacy levels, thus confirming our hypothesis. This contrasts with the control group where there was no association between education level and literacy. A possible explanation is that psychiatric patients had a vested interest in understanding more about their conditions than controls, and among the better educated, familiarity and ease of access to on-line information might have contributed to improved literacy levels.

An added clinical utility of mental health literacy is the ability to advise others suspected of having a psychiatric illness to seek the appropriate help, or what has been referred to as "psychiatric first-aid" [2]. Here, the patients' knowledge of where to obtain psychiatric help may be of benefit not only to themselves, but also to those they might be called upon to advise in the future.

There are certain strengths and limitations to our study worth mentioning. We have assessed the health literacy of a group of psychiatric outpatients and compared their responses with those from a control group of non-psychiatric outpatients. To the best of our knowledge, the study of mental health literacy in patients and comparisons with a control group has seldom been performed in mental health literacy research. Owing to a modest sample size, our study may have been slightly underpowered; hence, certain observed differences between the two groups have only emerged as trends. We did not attempt to match the socio-demographic characteristics of both groups. This has yielded groups with different ages and employment statuses. In order to overcome this problem, we have applied the appropriate statistical tests to take into account these differences. The generalizability of our findings could be limited by the demographic characteristics—in particular, age, ethnicity, and education status of the cohort, and that it was based upon a single hospital study. Notwithstanding our limitations, we have managed to test and to confirm some of our hypotheses.

The finding that the level of psychiatric patients' mental health literacy was no better than that of the controls is a cause for great concern. This underlines the urgent need for a concerted program of psycho-education to patients, their relatives, and to the general public. Since the lesser educated and the older participants achieved the lowest scores on MHL, the program should, perhaps, target this group, as a start. Although some have found that increased literacy did not translate into treatment adherence [20], there are a number of reasons for regarding these findings with some caution. Firstly, the latter was a European study whose findings might not be generalizable to a Southeast Asian setting. Secondly, the association between literacy and treatment adherence has never been tested in this country. Therefore, we cannot assume that this intervention will result in failure even before it is started. Thirdly, we will certainly not expect treatment adherence or attitudes to treatment to spontaneously improve in the absence of any educational program being implemented. Conversely, should such a program be conducted, it will at least allow future research to assess its effects on literacy, attitudes, and help-seeking behavior.

Acknowledgements

The authors wish to thank Dr. Sharon Cohan Sung for valuable comments on an earlier draft of the manuscript. We gratefully acknowledge the Lee Foundation for sponsoring this study.

References

[1]   Ng, T.P., Fones, C.S.L. and Kua, E.H. (2003) Preference, Need and Utilization of Mental Health Services, Singapore National Mental Health Survey. *Australian and New Zealand Journal of Psychiatry*, **37**, 613-619.

[2]   Jorm, A.F., Kitchener, B.A. and Mugford, S.K. (2004) Experiences in Applying Skills Learned in a Mental Health First Aid Training Course: A Qualitative Study of Participants' Stories. The WHO World Mental Health Survey Consortium: Prevalence, severity, and Unmet Need for Treatment of Mental Disorders in the World Health Organization World Mental Health Surveys. *JAMA*, **291**, 2581-2590.

[3]   Zachrisson, H.D., Rödje, K. and Mykletun, A. (2006) Utilization of health Services in Relation to Mental Health Problems in Adolescents: A Population Based Survey.*BMC Public Health*, **6**, 34. http://dx.doi.org/10.4103/0253-7176.70510

[4]   Topuzoğlu, A., Binba, T., Ulaş, H., Elbi, H,, Aksu T. F., Zağlı, N. and Alptekin, K. (2015) The Epidemiology of Major Depressive Disorder and Subthreshold Depression in Izmir, Turkey: Prevalence, Socioeconomic Differences, Impairment and Help-Seeking. *Journal of Affective Disorders*, **181**, 78-86. http://dx.doi.org/10.3109/08039480903062950

[5]   Jorm, A.F., Korten, A.E., Jacomb, R.A., *et al.* (1997) Mental Health Literacy: A Survey of the Public's Ability to Recognise Mental Disorders and Their Beliefs about the Effectiveness of Treatment. *Medical Journal of Australia*, **166**, 182-186. http://dx.doi.org/10.1192/bjp.188.4.359

[6]   Angermeyer, M.C. and Dietrich, S. (2006) Public Beliefs about and Attitudes towards People with Mental Illness: A Review of Population Studies. *Acta Psychiatrica Scandinavica*, **113**, 163-179. http://dx.doi.org/10.1016/j.jad.2007.04.026

[7]   Angermeyer, M.C., Matschinger, H. and Riedel-Heller, S.G. (1999) Whom to Ask for Help in a Case of a Mental Disorder? Preferences of the Lay Public. *Social Psychiatry and Psychiatric Epidemiology*, **34**, 202-210. http://dx.doi.org/10.1093/occmed/kqn135

[8]   Lauber, C., Nordt, C., Falcato, L. and Rössler, W. (2003) Do People Recognise Mental illness? Factors Influencing Mental Health Literacy. *European Archives of Psychiatry and Clinical Neuroscience*, **253**, 248-251.

[9]   Rüsch, N., Evans-Lacko, S.E., Henderson, C., Flach, C. and Thornicroft, G. (2011) Knowledge and Attitudes as Predictors of Intentions to Seek Help for, and Disclose, a Mental Illness. *Psychiatric Services*, **62**, 675-678.

[10] Ten Have, M., de Graaf, R., Vilagut, G., Kovess, V., Alonso, J., *et al.* (2010) Are Attitudes towards Mental Health Help-Seeking Associated with Service Use? Results from the European Study of Epidemiology of Mental Disorders. *Social Psychiatry and Psychiatric Epidemiology*, **45**, 153-163.

[11] Ng, B.Y. (2001) Till the Break of Day: A History of Mental Health Services in Singapore, 1841-1993. Singapore University Press, Singapore.

[12] Kua, E.H., Chew, P.H. and Ko, S.M. (1993) Spirit Possession and Healing among Chinese Psychiatric Patients. *Acta Psychiatrica Scandinavica*, **88**, 447-450. http://dx.doi.org/10.1111/j.1600-0447.1993.tb03489.x

[13] Razali, S.M., Khan, U.A. and Hasanah, C.I. (1996) Belief in Supernatural Causes of Mental Illness among Malay Patients: Impact on Treatment. *Acta Psychiatrica Scandinavica*, **94**, 229-233. http://dx.doi.org/10.1111/j.1600-0447.1996.tb09854.x

[14] Goldney, R.D., Fisher, L.J., Wilson, D.H. and Cheok, F. (2002) Mental Health Literacy of Those with Major Depression and Suicidal Ideation: An Impediment to Help Seeking. *Suicide and Life-Threatening Behavior*, **32**, 394-403. http://dx.doi.org/10.1521/suli.32.4.394.22343

[15] Furnham, A. and Blythe, C. (2012) Schizophrenia Literacy: The Effect of Direct Experience with the Illness. *Psychiatry Research*, **198**, 18-23. http://dx.doi.org/10.1016/j.psychres.2011.12.025

[16] American Psychiatric Association (2000) Diagnostic and Statistical Manual of Mental Disorders. Fourth Edition, Text Revision, American Psychiatric Association, Washington DC. http://dx.doi.org/10.1176/appi.books.9780890423349

[17] Lecrubier, Y., Sheehan, D.V., Weiller, E., Amorim, P., Bonora, I., Sheehan, K.H., *et al.* (1997) The Mini International

Neuropsychiatric Interview (MINI). A Short Diagnostic Structured Interview: Reliability and Validity According to the CIDI. *European Psychiatry*, **12**, 224-231. http://dx.doi.org/10.1016/S0924-9338(97)83296-8

[18] Cheung, Y.T., Ong, Y.Y., Ng, T., Tan, Y.P., Fan, G., Chan, C.W., *et al.* (2015) Assessment of Mental Health Literacy in Patients with Breast Cancer. *Journal of Oncology Pharmacy Practice*, In Press. http://dx.doi.org/10.1177/1078155215587541

[19] Deen, T.L. and Bridges, A.J. (2011) Depression Literacy: Rates and Relation to Perceived Need and Mental Health service Utilization in a Rural American Sample. *Rural Remote Health*, **11**, 1803.

[20] Palazzo, M.C., Dell'Osso, B., Altamura, A.C., Stein, D.J. and Baldwin, D.S. (2014) Health Literacy and the Pharmacological Treatment of Anxiety Disorders: A Systematic Review. *Human Psychopharmacology: Clinical and Experimental*, **29**, 211-215. http://dx.doi.org/10.1002/hup.2397

[21] Angermeyer, M.C. and Matschinger, H. (2004) Public Attitudes towards Psychotropic Drugs: Have There Been any Changes in Recent Years? *Pharmacopsychiatry*, **37**, 152-156. http://dx.doi.org/10.1055/s-2004-827169

[22] Priest, R.G., Vize, C., Roberts, A., *et al.* (1996) Lay People's Attitudes to Treatment Campaign Just before Its Launch. *British Medical Journal*, **313**, 858-859. http://dx.doi.org/10.1136/bmj.313.7061.858

27

Meige Syndrome: An Eternal Diagnostic Confusion

Amit Chauhan[1], Shravani Chauhan[2*]

[1]Department of Orthopedics, Park Hospital, Gurgaon, Haryana, India
[2]Department of Psychiatry, VIMHANS, New Delhi, India
Email: *shrav1980@gmail.com

Abstract

Meige syndrome is an idiopathic dystonia characterized by combination of blepharospasm and involuntary movements of the lower facial and/or masticatory (jaw) muscles. The condition is rare and has a variety of clinical presentations which often lead to its misdiagnosis. We report a case of Meige syndrome repeatedly misdiagnosed and treated unsuccessfully as conversion disorder.

Keywords

Meige Syndrome, Orofacial Dystonia, Diagnostic Confusion

1. Introduction

Meige syndrome is an idiopathic dystonia characterized by symmetrical blepharospasm and oromandibular dystonia [1]. It is used synonymously with Brueghel's syndrome or segmental craniocervical dystonia. Although the causes of this syndrome are unknown, it has been reported to be induced by certain kinds of drugs such as antipsychotic drugs and dopamine agonists, cerebellar degeneration, basal ganglia dysfunction, and brain tumors [2]. The condition is rare and has clinical presentations like abnormal blinking, squinting/eyes closing during speech, trismus, clenching or grinding of teeth, lip tightening and pursing, deviation or protrusion of the tongue and drawing back of corners of the mouth. In some patients, dystonic spasms may be provoked by certain activities, such as talking, chewing, or biting. The variety of symptoms and low prevalence of the syndrome often leads to its misdiagnosis in psychiatry, ophthalmology and neurology. We report a case of Meige syndrome repeatedly misdiagnosed and treated as conversion disorder.

---

*Corresponding author.

2. Case Report

Mrs S., a 60-year-old lady, presented in orthopedic outpatient department with 3-year complaint of tightening of oral, facial and neck muscles along with neck pain for last 3 months. After initial assessment for cervical spondylosis, the orthopedician referred her to psychiatry for evaluation of the abnormal facial grimacing movements. On detailed history taking, patient revealed that symptoms started acutely 3 years back with repeated blinking of eyes. There were no apparent precipitating factors, no history of medication intake with negative family history of neurological and psychiatric illness and no comorbid medical illness. She was initially shown to an ophthalmologist who did not prescribe any specific medication. Two to three months after onset of increased eye blinking, patient started having painless tightening of neck muscles and subsequent upward deviation of face and neck, not relieved by massage or rest. This was followed by difficulty in opening her mouth (trismus) along with clenching and grinding of teeth (bruxism) whenever she tried to speak. Within six months, patient started having difficulty in opening her mouth to eat food along with protrusion of tongue and increased frequency of neck muscle tightening leading to bizarre grimacing of the face. She was referred to a psychiatrist, who diagnosed her as conversion disorder and prescribed amitriptylline (50 mg/day), haloperidol (10 mg/day) and trihexyphenidyl (4 mg/day). Two months after medication, there was no improvement so she was referred for neurological opinion. Routine blood tests and imaging (CT scan) were normal. Patient was confirmed as a case of conversion disorder and prescribed fluoxetine (20 mg/day), olanzapine (10 mg/day) and trihexyphenidyl (4 mg/day). She took above medication for few months and subsequently discontinued as symptoms worsened. Disappointed with treatment outcome, patient stopped taking medication for next one year during which her symptoms continued.

For last three months, patient started feeling pain in her neck during movement, especially during neck flexion. For this reason, she consulted an orthopedic surgeon, who referred her to psychiatric outpatient department. On clinical examination, patient presented with uncontrollable closing of eyes (blepharospasm), upward deviation of neck, grimacing of face, trismus and bruxism along with inability to speak properly due to neck muscle spasm. After thorough neurological and psychiatric check up, a diagnosis of idiopathic craniocervical dystonia/ Meige syndrome was made and patient started on baclofen, a GABA-agonist drug. The drug was started at 20 mg/day, increased by 10 mg every three days reaching a maximum dose of 60 mg/day. There was gradual improvement in trismus, bruxism and dysarthria, though blepharospasm showed minimal improvement. After three months of follow up, patient reported improved quality of life but continued to have eye symptoms and occasional neck and jaw spasms.

3. Discussion

Historically, Dr. Horatio Wood, a Philadelphia neurologist, first drew attention to blepharospasm and other cranial dystonias in 1887 [3]. In 1910, Dr. Henri Meige, a French neurologist, described ten patients with involuntary closure of the eyelids [1]. More than half a century later, an American neurologist, George Paulson, reported three patients with blepharospasm and oromandibular dystonia and emphasized the probability of a common pathophysiological basis [4]. Though studied for a long time, the cause of Meige syndrome still remains elusive and treatment remains debatable. Basal ganglion dysfunction has been postulated with involvement of dopamine receptors [5]. In the nigro-striatal pathway, one of the retrograde loops in the feed-back control of dopamine synthesis by nigral neurons is dependent on GABA. Increasing GABA activity through GABA agonists that cross the blood-brain barrier could result in a decreased dopaminergic action in the nigro-striatal pathway and, thus, ameliorate the dystonic symptoms which might have been produced by its increased function [5]. Baclofen, a GABA agonist, has been tried in dystonias for the above reason and has shown variable results. Other medical treatments like anti cholinergics, botulinum toxin injections and benzodiazepines usually present disappointing results. Surgical treatments include bilateral deep brain stimulation of the globus pallidus internus which has become a first choice treatment for drug refractory, primary, segmental, or generalized dystonias [6].

The authors report no proprietary or commercial interest in any product mentioned or concept discussed in this article.

References

[1]   Meige, H. (1910) Les convulsions de la face, une forme clinique deconvulsion faciale, bilatérale et médiane. *Revista de*

Neurología, **20**, 437-443.

[2]   Hayashi, T., Furutani, M., Taniyama, J., *et al.* (1998) Neuroleptic Induced Meige's Syndrome Following Akathisia: Pharmacologic Characteristics. *Psychiatry and Clinical Neurosciences*, **52**, 445-448. http://dx.doi.org/10.1046/j.1440-1819.1998.00408.x

[3]   Wood, H.C. (1887) Nervous Diseases and Their Diagnosis: A Treatise upon the Phenomena Produced by Diseases of the Nervous System. JB Lippincott, Philadelphia, 1937.

[4]   Paulson, G.W. (1972) Meige's Syndrome. Dyskinesia of the Eyelids and Facial Muscles. *Geriatrics*, **8**, 69-73.

[5]   De Andrade, L.A. and Bertolucci, P.H. (1985) Treatment of Meige Disease with a GABA Receptor Agonist. *Arquivos de Neuro-Psiquiatria*, **43**, 260-266. http://dx.doi.org/10.1590/S0004-282X1985000300004

[6]   Reese, R., Gruber, D., Schoenecker, T., *et al.* (2011) Long-Term Clinical Outcome in Meige Syndrome Treated with Internal Pallidum Deep Brain Stimulation. *Movement Disorders*, **26**, 691-698. http://dx.doi.org/10.1002/mds.23549

28

Mental and Cardiovascular Health of Portuguese Subjects in a Situation of Economic Insufficiency

Eduardo Gonçalves[1], Emanuel Marco Moniz[1], Saul Neves de Jesus[2]

[1]Department of Psychiatry and Mental Health of Hospital Center of Algarve, Faro, Portugal
[2]Department of Psychology of Faculty of Social and Human Sciences of University of Algarve, Faro, Portugal
Email: eduar.goncalves@gmail.com

Abstract

Economic insufficiency causes stress and negative affects. Poverty is self-perpetuated, also due to a particular pattern of economic behaviors induced by negative affects and stress. Often, loneliness occurs together with economic insufficiency. For this study, it has been selected a sample of convenience. A positive correlation between anxiety/depression and negative affects is presented. Dispositional optimism and social support, factors which contribute to health, serve as buffers, in negative correlation, of the negative impact of negative affects, due to financial restraint, on health. Financial management is negatively correlated with the lack of cardiovascular health, and cardiovascular dysfunction correlates positively with loneliness, in this study. Positive affects correlate positively with resilience skills, which correlate negatively with depression. Within this context, psychobiological therapeutic interventions and psychotherapy, which also target psychological dysfunction related to economic behavior of persons in a situation of poverty, would be beneficial.

Keywords

Poverty, Stress, Affects, Depression, Heart Rate Variability, Social Support, Resilience, Economic Behavior

1. Introduction (Theoretical Framework)

1.1. Stress and Negative Affects Caused by Economic Insufficiency (Poverty)

Poverty causes lack of opportunities, reduced accessibility to resources and is associated with a greater likelihood of life events with traumatic potential. By acting through stressors agents of socio-economic nature, such as unemployment and the difficulty of access to housing, it is much more likely that poverty precedes mental disorders, such as anxiety and depression, and it is an important risk factor for mental illness [1]. The relationship between poverty and mental illness is bidirectional, that is, poverty is a risk factor for certain mental illnesses, which, in turn, worsen the economic condition of the patient and their families. Some factors, such as education and employment, have a two-way relationship with poverty. The lack of employment results in financial difficulties, and poverty results in reduced opportunity to obtain gainful employment. Unemployed persons and those who fail to obtain employment have more depressive symptoms than individuals who can get a job [2]. Limited resources, resulting in reduced opportunity for education, which prevent access to most skilled jobs, increase individual vulnerability and insecurity contributing to a persistently low social capital. The prevalence of common mental disorders is higher among individuals with low levels of education. Chronic poverty is often associated with low levels of family and community support, alcoholism, insecurity and violent crime, family abuse and family desertion, particularly by men [1]. In a review of 115 studies, 79% showed a negative association between indicators of poverty and mental health [3]. Several studies have shown: high levels of cortisol in subjects with lower financial incomes and less education [4] [5]; lower economic status measured by occupational status [6] [7]. Measures, consisting generically in increased personal financial income, determine: reduction in hospitalization for mental health problems [8]; lower consumption of anxiolytics [9]; increased mental health [10]-[12]. Poverty causes negative affects and stress, and these effects alter the economic behavior of persons concerning time preference (*i.e.*, the degree of preference for present consumption over future consumption) and assumption of risky economic behavior, limiting economic decision-making, and thus favoring habitual behaviors, not oriented for objectives, perpetuating poverty itself [13]. Decision making requires individuals, in difficult circumstances of business transaction, *i.e.*, with less budget (and resulting lower capacity to acquire larger amount of desirable goods), to recruit scarce cognitive resources, which subsequently will be reflected in worse performances in tasks that require integrity of executive function, such as Stroop [14] [15]. Thus, cognitive deficit of executive function that characterizes economic insufficiency does not ensure the ability to defer rewards, implied in economic behavior related to time preference. There are three ways to break the cycle of economic insufficiency/poverty and improve well-being: the implementation of policy measures for direct poverty reduction; the management of the psychological consequences of economic insufficiency; the change in economic behavior arising from these [16]. Since the deteriorating effects of stress and negative affects in economic behavior can occur even in individuals who do not suffer from depression, therapeutic interventions of psychobiological nature and psychotherapy bring economic benefits even in non-clinical populations [17].

1.2. Stress, Positive and Negative Affects, Tripartite Model of Anxiety and Depression and Brain Electrophysiological Activity

Positive affectivity is a characteristic that describes how animals and humans experience positive emotions and interact with each other and their environments. Persons with increased positive affectivity are enthusiastic, energetic, confident, active and alert. Persons with low levels of positive affectivity are characterized by sadness, apathy, anxiety, stress and not rewarding social involvement. Happiness, high levels of well-being and self-esteem are often associated with increased levels of positive affectivity [18]. Positive affectivity provides a rupture of stress and supports ongoing efforts to replenish depleted resources from stress [19]. Positive affectivity and negative affectivity are not independent. Negative affectivity is a general dimension of subjective distress, due to stress and not satisfying social involvement, and encompasses a variety of aversive mood states, including anger, contempt, disgust, guilt, fear and nervousness. Low negative affectivity levels are characterized by a state of calm and serenity. Watson and Clark (1984) have defined negative affectivity as a dimension of dispositional mood that reflects individual differences relating to negative emotions and self-concept. These authors concluded that individuals who express high levels of negative affectivity envisage themselves and their involvement in generally negative terms [20]. Individuals with high negative affectivity levels have higher levels of stress, anxiety and dissatisfaction with life, and tend to focus on unpleasant aspects of themselves, the world, the future and others [21]. The tripartite model of anxiety and depression, developed by Clark and Watson (1991), proposes that anxiety and depressive disorders overlap considerably by a general, not specific, factor, negative affectivity, which reflects the level of aversive feelings present in an individual. The two remaining factors of this model are positive affectivity, which, when low, is relatively specific for depression, and physiological activation, which is relatively specific to anxiety [22]. Several authors consider anxiety and depression a single disorder's entity. Lovibond and Lovibond (1995), authors of anxiety, depression and stress scales (DASS), assume that psychological disorders are not categories, that is, the differences between depression, anxiety and stress, experienced by normal subjects and patients, are essentially level ones: depression is characterized mainly by the loss of self-esteem and motivation, and is associated with the perception of low probability of achieving life goals that are meaningful to the individual as a person; anxiety emphasizes the links between persistent state of anxiety and intense fear responses; stress suggests states of excitement and persistent tension, with low resistance to frustration and disappointment. According to this model, depression is defined by dysphoria, hopelessness, devaluation, self-depreciation, lack of interest, anhedonia and inertia, anxiety is defined by autonomic arousal, skeletal muscle effects, situational anxiety and subjective experience of anxious affect, and stress is defined by difficulty in relaxing, nervous excitation, easy agitation, irritability/excessive reactivity and impatience [23]. The components of the tripartite model of anxiety and depression have been linked to neurophysiological measures of anxiety and depression. Increased in left frontal electrophysiological activity is associated with an increased positive affectivity, i.e., the decrease of depressive states, while decreased left frontal electrophysiological activity is associated with decreased positive affectivity, i.e. the increase of depressive states. Anxiety disorders have repeatedly been associated with an increase in right prefrontal cortex and amygdala activity, abnormalities similar to those reported in depressed subjects [24]-[28]. Neuro-stimulation, in particular, high frequency (above 1 Hz) repetitive transcranial magnetic stimulation (rTMS) over the left dorso-lateral prefrontal cortex treats depressive states [29].

1.3. Loneliness

Loneliness is an unpleasant experience that occurs when personal network of social relationships is significantly deficient in quantity and/or quality. Predisposing factors that may increase personal risk for loneliness include individual differences in personality and behavior, such extreme shyness or lack of social skills. Within a society, social norms can also affect the tendency to feel lonely. The onset of loneliness is often initiated by a previous event, usually a change or loss in/of an emotional relationship, through death or divorce, or a disruption of social relationship created by the move to a new school, city or employment. The intensity of loneliness may increase if the individual evaluates his/her own situation as worse than that of their peers, or attributes the causes of their loneliness to personal inadequacies. Individuals with a solitary trait, compared to persons in a solitary state, are more likely to have poor social skills, attribute their loneliness to undesirable factors and have difficulty to overcoming their social deficits. Classically, it is distinguished emotional loneliness from social loneliness, wherein the first encompasses the lack of emotional ties inherent to intimate relationships, while bereavement, divorce or emptiness feelings within marriage are the likely background of this latter kind of loneliness. Loss of employment, exclusion from the peer group and not belonging to community organizations are the likely history of social loneliness. Several studies have shown that loneliness is more prevalent among lower financial income groups [30].

1.4. Dispositional Optimism

Well-being is the result of a cognitive and emotional subjective evaluation, and its level is determined by the individual's life satisfaction, satisfaction with leisure and professional practices, satisfaction with others and everyday experiences of positive emotions. Based on the behavioral theory of self-regulation, Scheier and Carver (1994) elaborated life orientation test (LOT), in order to measure dispositional optimism, as a personal construct [31]. Segerstrom and Nes (2006) found better psychological health indices associated with dispositional optimism [32]. Chang (1998) found that dispositional optimism is a significant moderator of the relationship between stress and psychological well-being [33]. Vickers and Vogeltanz (2000) found that the lack of optimism is a predictor of depression [34].

1.5. Social Support

Rodin and Salovey, cited by Pais-Ribeiro (1999), state that "social support relieves distress in crisis situation, can inhibit the development of diseases and, when one is ill, has a positive role in recovery from disease". A review of studies on the epidemiological evidence of the relationship between social support and health, held by Broadhead et al. (1983), cited by Pais-Ribeiro (1999), concluded that there is a strong correlation between the two variables [35].

1.6. Resilience

Taking into account a psycho-educational perspective on health promotion and well-being, Jardim and Pereira (2006) define resilience as the ability to operate knowledge, attitudes and skills in order to prevent, minimize or overcome the damaging effects of crises and adversity. A resilient person is someone, whom, having to face an adverse situation, is able to use their intra- and inter-personal resources in such a way as to develop the skills he/she needs to be successful in personal, social and professional life [36]. Wagnild (2010) had shown that resilience protects against negative emotions and, thus, has the potential to reduce their pathophysiological effects [37]. Resilience state scale (Wagnild, 1993) integrates four factors: perseverance; meaning of life; serenity; self-reliance and existential aloneness. Perseverance refers to the enthusiastic persistence in finding solutions to problems, overcoming adversity, and the will to continue to rebuild one live, trusting on oneself with a self-regulatory attitude. Meaning of life refers to the awareness that one have something meaningful to live, to the notion that life has a meaning (a reason) in which the individual focuses, avoiding being obsessed with disputes that one can't solve, involving determination and satisfaction with the achievement of defined objectives. Serenity depends on a balanced and focused perspective on the purpose of life itself, with the ability to accept the variety of experiences (even adverse), with calm and/or enthusiasm and to exercise self-esteem. Self-reliance and existential aloneness concern the sense of oneness, the awareness that each person's life path is unique and that certain steps are not faced in a group but in solitude, getting the person to be on his/her own and being able to depend essentially on himself/herself, referring to the belief in himself/herself, in his/her abilities and interest in life, recognizing limitations and being able to depend on him/herself [38]. Martins and Jesus (2007) discuss the transactional model of resilience proposed by Kumpfer (1999). Four main areas of influence and six basic predictors of resilience are identified: the stressors (or challenges); the environmental context; the individual-environment transaction process; the internal resilience factors; the resilience process; the results of reintegration. Kumpfer (1999) argues that resilient individuals, even in involvements of high social risk, are able to deal with situations in order to find support (their families, schools, communities and peer groups) for enabling them to face appropriate opportunities for positive and healthy development. Kumpfer (1999) adds that the subject can use different strategies to adapt or modify their involvement, mainly, the use of selective perceptions, cognitive recomposition, alteration of the involvement or active coping. The transactional model of resilience demonstrates that the stressors and challenges, not counterbalanced by protective environmental and social processes or bio-psycho-spiritual resilience factors, can lead to changes or disruption in homeostasis, with individual disorganization, which can be recovered and result in the reintegration of homeostasis, if environmental and social processes of support are present: the resilient reintegration occurs when the individual has acquired a heightened state of resilience; homeostatic reintegration occurs when the individual maintains the same resilience state he/she had before the exposure to stressors or challenges; not adaptive reintegration occurs when exposure to stressors or challenges results in continued low individual state of reintegration; dysfunctional reintegration occurs when exposure to stressors or challenges results in a greater reduction in positive reintegration [39] [40].

1.7. Monitoring of Cardiac Activity by Electrocardiography with Heart Rate Variability Function (HRV), Autonomic Influence on Heart Rate and Physiological and Pathophysiological Correlates of HRV Components

Heart rate and cardiac rhythm depend on their control by autonomic nervous system [41]. The sympathetic and parasympathetic/vagal activities target the sinus node and are characterized by electrochemical discharges in synchrony with each cardiac cycle which may also be modulated by central oscillators (vasomotor and respiratory centers) and peripheral (blood pressure oscillation and respiratory movements) [42]. In resting conditions, vagal tone prevails [43]. The parasympathetic system influences heart rate by releasing acetylcholine, and its muscarinic receptors respond with increased conductance of cell membrane to potassium ion [44]-[46]. The efferent vagal activity is the main contributor to the high frequency component (HF) of heart rate variability (HRV) [47] [48]. The increase of HF is induced by breath's control, cold stimulation of the face and rotational stimuli [49]. The sympathetic influence on heart rate is mediated by the release of adrenaline and noradrenaline, and the activation of beta-adrenergic receptors results in phosphorylation of membrane proteins mediated by adenosine 3',5'-cyclic monophosphate (cAMP) (molecular transductor of the signal within a cell, cellular second messenger). Low frequency component of heart rate variability (LF) is considered a marker of sympathetic modulation [50] [51]. Increased LF is induced by a variety of situations: orthostatic position, stress, moderate exercise in healthy subjects, moderate hypotension and coronary artery occlusion [50]. The LF/HF ratio reflects the sympathetic-vagal balance (or sympathetic modulation) of cardiac function. Autonomic failure (dysautonomia), as high levels of sympathetic activity, determines decreased HRV. Decreased HRV is caused by various heart disorders and other than heart diseases (diabetes). In accordance with the Task Force of the European Society of Cardiology and the North American Society of Pacing Electrophysiology, normal standard values of the most important HRV parameters are, in normalized units (nu): LF power equals 54 (average), with a standard deviation of 4; HF power equals 29 (average), with a standard deviation of 3; ratio LF/HF equals 1.5 - 2.0 (average) [52].

2. Empirical Study

2.1. Methods

It has been performed a recruitment of citizens with low financial incomes, without assigned diagnoses, particularly concerning neurological and/or psychiatric disorders, which integrates a convenience sample. The participants provided previous written, free and informed, consent. This is a transversal, quantitative, correlational, not experimental, study. The questionnaires and psychometric scales used are validated for Portuguese population. It has been performed a spectral analysis, with fast Fourier transform, of heart rate, during five minutes per participant, and evaluated the components/parameters of their heart rate variability (HRV), in accordance with standard procedures, as established by the Task Force of the European Society of Cardiology and the North American Society of Pacing Electrophysiology, in order to study the impact of stress, related with/caused by economic insufficiency (poverty), on cardiovascular function/health [52].

2.2. Participants

The sample consists of 33 elements. 48% of the participants are female. Data have been collected between 17 and 23 October of 2013. The age has a mean value of 53.8 years, with a dispersion of values of 11%. 97% of the participants live in the city of Olhão, Portugal. 24% of the participants are single, 49% are married, 3% are separated, 12% are divorced and 12% are widowed. On academic/literary abilities (scholarship), 40% of the participants have the primary 4th grade, 6% have the primary 5th grade, 21% have the primary 6th grade, 15% have the primary 9th grade, 3% have the primary 11th grade and 15% have the primary 12th grade. 40% of the participants are unemployed, 12% are retired, 6% are pensioners (the remaining participants do not answer). The net/liquid monthly income has a mean value of 337 euros, with a dispersion of values of 69%. The distribution of values of net/liquid monthly income is verified mainly between 200 and 500 euros. In the sample, the monthly expenses have a mean value of 376 euros, with a dispersion of values of 47%. The distribution of values of monthly expenses is verified mainly between 200 and 600 euros. The difference between incomes and expenses has a monthly mean value of −28.20 euros, with a dispersion of values of 746%. The distribution of the difference values between monthly incomes and expenses occurs mainly between −200 and −100 euros and between 0 and 100 euros. 94% of the participants believe that their financial situation has worsened over the past two years. 97% of participants believe that their financial situation will worsen in the coming years. 24% of the participants consider that past financial difficulties were mild, 36% moderate and 40% severe. 27% of the participants have not been involved in providing care and financial help to family and 73% respond affirmatively to the same question. 52% of participants say they do not suffer from chronic diseases. The remaining participants suffer from: cancer; diabetes; ischemic heart disease; arrhythmia; hypercholesterolemia; hypertension; myasthenia gravis.

2.3. Material

2.3.1. Questionnaire on Preoccupation
The questionnaire on preoccupation (QP) is an ordinal Likert scale with five possible answers ("1" to "5") between "I disagree very much" and "I agree very much". It consists of 16 items, which are organized in one dimension, and, for the items marked with an "R", the scale is recoded in the reverse order, because its formulation is held in a negative form: item R1—If I do not have time to do everything, I do not worry about it; item

2—My preoccupations dominate me; item R3 item—I tend not to worry about things; item 4—Many situations bother me; item 5—I know I should not concern myself with things, but I cannot prevent it; item 6—When I'm under pressure, I worry very much; item 7—I'm always worried; item R8—I believe it is easy to ignore troublesome thoughts; item 9—Once I've finished a task, I start worrying about everything else I have to do; item R10 item—I never worry about anything; item R11—When there's nothing I can do about a concern, I do not turn to look into it; item 12—I have always been a worried person; item 13—I notice that I have been worrying about things; item 14—When I start to worry, I can no longer stop to do so; item 15—I worry all the time; item 16—I worry about my projects until they are completed.

2.3.2. Questionnaire on Health Status

The questionnaire on health status (QHS) is an ordinal Likert scale with six possible answers (from "0" to "5") between "never" and "always." It consists of 12 items, which are organized in one dimension and, for items marked with an "R", the scale is recoded in reverse order, because its formulation is held in a negative form: item 1—Were you able to concentrate on what you were doing?; item R2—Have you lost sleep due to concerns?; item 3—Did you feel yourself to be useful in important things?; item 4—Were you able to make decisions about things?; item R5—Did you feel constantly under stress?; item R6—Did you feel that you were unable to overcome your difficulties?; item 7—Were you able to enjoy your daily activities?; item 8—Were you able to face your problems?; item R9—Have you been unhappy and depressed?; item R10—Have you lost self-confidence?; item R11—Have you thought on yourself as a worthless person?; item 12—Did you feel reasonably happy, all things considered?.

2.3.3. Questionnaire on Financial Management

The questionnaire on financial management (QFM) is an ordinal Likert scale with five possible answers ("1" to "5") between "I disagree very much" and "I agree very much". It consists of 8 items, which are organized in one dimension, and, for the items marked with an "R", the scale is recoded in reverse order, because its formulation is held in a negative form: item R1—I'm uncomfortable with the amount of debt that I have; item R2—I am concerned with the payment of my loans; item R3—I am concerned with the payment of my credit cards; item 4—I think I have a good financial condition; item R5—I think a lot about the debts that I have; item R6—I had discussions with other people (family, friends and significant others) about my spending level; item 7—Five years from now, I will not have debts with my credit cards; item 8—Within one year, I will not have debts with my credit cards.

2.3.4. Questionnaire on Financial Situation

The questionnaire on financial situation (QFS) is an ordinal Likert scale with five possible answers ("1" to "5") between "nothing" and "much". It consists of 6 items, which are organized in one dimension, and, for all items marked with an "R", the scale is recoded in reverse order, because its formulation is held in a negative form: item R1—How insecure do you feel?; item R2—How at risk do you feel?; item R3—How threatened do you feel?; item R4—How much do you worry about it?; item R5—How much do you think about it?; item R6—What is the probability to declare bankruptcy/failure to manage your debt?.

2.3.5. Questionnaire on Financial Restraints

The questionnaire on financial restraints (QFR) is an ordinal Likert scale with four possible answers ("1" to "4") between "never" and "often". It consists of 10 items, which are organized in one dimension: item 1—Did you cut in spending on social activities and entertainment?; item 2—Did you postpone major purchases for the home/ family?; item 3—Did you postpone the purchase of clothing?; item 4—Did you change the travel habits to save money?; item 5—Did you change the way to buy food or the eating habits to save money?; item 6—Did you decrease contributions to charity?; item 7—Did you reduce the use of utilities for home?; item 8—Did you sell some goods?; item 9—Did you postpone medical care to save money?; item 10—Did you have additional jobs to help pay the costs?.

2.3.6. Positive and Negative Affects Scale

Positive and negative affects scale (PANAS) is an ordinal Likert scale with five possible answers ("1" to "5") between "none or very little" and "extremely". It consists of 20 items, which are organized in two dimensions (one for positive affects, other for negative affects) [53] [54].

2.3.7. 21-Item Depression, Anxiety and Stress Scales

Depression, anxiety and stress scales (DASS) constitute an ordinal Likert scale with four response alternatives (from "0"a "3") between "not applied to me" and "applied to me, most of the time". The short version of DASS consists of 21 items, which are organized in three dimensions. Seven variables measure appropriately a single dimension, depression. The cutoff point for depression scale is greater than 7, that is the elements with a higher score than 7 exhibit depression. Seven variables measure appropriately a single dimension, anxiety. The cutoff point for anxiety scale is greater than 9, that is the elements with a higher feature score than 9 exhibit. Seven variables measure appropriately a single dimension, stress. The cutoff point for the stress range is greater than 14, that is the elements with a higher score than 14 show stress [55] [56].

2.3.8. Satisfaction with Social Support Scale

Satisfaction with social support scale (SSSS) is an ordinal Likert scale with five possible answers ("1" to "5") between "I totally agree" and "I totally disagree". It consists of 15 items, which are organized into four dimensions, and, for items marked with an "R", the scale is recoded in reverse because its formulation is held in the negative. This rating scale integrates the dimensions: satisfaction with friends; intimacy; satisfaction with family; social activities) [35] [57].

2.3.9. Revised Life Orientation Test

Revised life orientation test (LOT-R) is an ordinal Likert scale with five possible answers ("1" to "5") between "I totally disagree" and "I totally agree". It consists of 5 items, which are organized in one dimension, and for the items marked with an "R" range is recoded in reverse order, because its formulation is held in the negative [31] [58].

2.3.10. Resilience State Scale

Resilience state scale (RSS) is an ordinal Likert scale with seven possible answers ("1" to "7") between "I totally disagree" and "I totally agree". It consists of 23 items, which are organized in a single dimension. Their values were determined by calculating the sum of the items that constitute them. The minimum value is 23 and the maximum value is 161 [38] [59].

2.3.11. Loneliness Scale

Loneliness scale (LS) is an ordinal Likert scale with four response alternatives ("1" through "4") between "never" and "often". It consists of 18 items, which are organized in a single dimension and, for items marked with an "R", the scale is recoded in reverse because its formulation is held in the negative [60] [61].

3. Results

The QP has a mean value greater than the midpoint of the measurement scale, which is 48, and most of the values are found between 40 and 70. The QHS also has a mean value greater than the intermediate point of the measurement scale, which is 30, and the values are distributed between 20 and 55. The QFM has a mean value lower than the midpoint of the measurement scale, which is 24, and most of the values are located between 15 and 30. The same is true for QFS, with a mean value below the midpoint of the measurement scale, which is 18, and most of the values are located between 5 and 15. The QFR has a mean value above the midpoint of the measurement scale, which is 25, and most of the values are located between 30 and 40. PANAS for positive affects has a mean value of 30 (precisely at the midpoint of the measurement scale), and most of the values are located between 25 and 40. PANAS for negative affects has a mean value lower than the midpoint of the measurement scale, which is 30, and most of the values are located between 10 and 35. DASS for depression has a mean value below the midpoint of the measurement scale, and most of the values are located between 0 and 12. DASS for anxiety has a mean value lower than the midpoint of the measurement scale, which is 10.5, and most of the values are located between 0 and 9. DASS for stress has a mean value lower than the midpoint of the measurement scale, and most of the values are located between 0 and 12. LS has a mean value lower than the midpoint of the measurement scale, and most of the values are located between 30 and 55. SSSS has a mean value slightly higher than the midpoint of the measurement scale, and most of the values are located between 40 and 60. LOT-R for dispositional optimism has a mean value above the midpoint of the measurement scale, and most of the values are located between 15 and 25. RSS has a mean value of 129.2, well above the midpoint of the measurement scale, which is 92, and most of the values are located between 115 and 145. The internal consistency of the psychometric instruments used in this study are analyzed with Cronbach's alpha coefficient, and the obtained levels are good and very good (0.740 for QP; 0.805 for QHS; 0.796 for QFM; 0.904 for QFS; 0.862 for QFR; 0.703 for PANAS for positive affects; 0.890 for PANAS for negative affects; 0.836 for DASS for depression; 0.868 for DASS for anxiety; 0.896 for DASS for stress; 0.894 for SSSS; 0.816 for LOT-R for dispositional optimism; 0.695 for RSS; 0.873 for LS). Total power parameter of HRV has a mean value of 1344.6 with a dispersion of values of 202%, and the distribution of their values occurs mainly between 0 and 2000. Low frequency (LF) power parameter of HRV has a mean value of 64.95 with a dispersion of the values of 36%, and the distribution of their values occurs mainly between 70 and 90. High frequency (HF) power of HRV has a mean value of 21.88, with a distribution of values mostly between 5 and 25. Total mean heart rate (HR) value is 88.12 with a dispersion of values of 37%, and the distribution of the values occurs mainly between 70 to 100. LF/HF ratio has a mean value of 4.34, with a distribution of values mostly between 0 and 5. All variables whose relations are studied are quantitative and therefore can be analyzed using Pearson's correlation coefficient r. There are negative correlations between: RSS and DASS for depression, $r = -0.359$, $p = 0.040$; QFM and LS, $r = -0.404$, $p = 0.022$; QFS and PANAS for negative affects, $r = -0.382$, $p = 0.028$; QFS and LS, $r = -0.458$, $p = 0.008$; PANAS for negative affects and SSSS, $r = -0.550$, $p = 0.001$; PANAS for negative affects and LOT-R for dispositional optimism, $r = -0.465$, $p = 0.008$; DASS for depression and SSSS, $r = -0.447$, $p = 0.009$; DASS for depression and LOT-R for dispositional optimism, $r = -0.485$, $p = 0.006$; DASS for anxiety and SSSS, $r = -0.377$, $p = 0.030$; DASS for anxiety and LOT-R for dispositional optimism, $r = -0.483$, $p = 0.006$; DASS for stress and SSSS, $r = -0.388$, $p = 0.026$; DASS for stress and LOT-R for dispositional optimism, $r = -0.506$, $p = 0.004$; QFM and LF/HF, $r = -0.407$, $p = 0.019$. There are positive correlations between: DASS for stress and PANAS for negative affects, $r = 0.785$, $p < 0.001$; DASS for depression and PANAS for negative affects, $r = 0.711$, $p < 0.001$; DASS for anxiety and PANAS for negative affects, $r = 0.678$, $p < 0.001$; DASS for depression and LS, $r = 0.411$, $p = 0.019$; RSS and PANAS for positive affects, $r = 0.494$, $p = 0.003$; QFR and PANAS for negative affects, $r = 0.507$, $p = 0.003$; QFR and LS, $r = 0.480$, $p = 0.005$; QHS and SSSS $r = 0.382$, $p = 0.028$; QHS and LOT-R for dispositional optimism, $r = 0.427$, $p = 0.016$; LS and LF/HF ratio, $r = 0.399$, $p = 0.024$; QFM and HF power, $r = 0.450$, $p = 0.009$.

4. Discussion and Conclusions

In this study, the net/liquid monthly income has a mean value of 337 euros, and net/liquid monthly expenses have a mean value of 376 euros. Financial restraints (QFR) correlate positively with negative affects (PANAS). Measures consisting generically in increasing personal financial income determine: a reduction in hospitalization for mental health problems [8]; lower consumption of anxiolytics [9]; increased mental health [10]-[12]. Poverty causes negative affects and stress [13]. The majority of the participants don't hold any employment relationship. The lack of employment results in financial difficulties, and poverty results in reduced opportunity to obtain gainful employment. Unemployed persons and those who fail to obtain employment have more depressive symptoms than individuals who can get a job [2]. None of the participants has higher educational background (40% of the participants have the primary 4th grade, 6% have the primary 5th grade, 21% have the primary 6th grade, 15% have the primary 9th grade, 3% have the primary 11th grade and 15% have the primary 12th grade). Limited resources, resulting in reduced opportunity for education which prevents access to most skilled jobs, increase individual vulnerability and insecurity, contributing to a persistently low social capital. The prevalence of common mental disorders is higher among individuals with low levels of education [1]. In this work, negative affects (PANAS) correlate positively with depression, anxiety and stress (DASS). Watson and Clark (1984) concluded that individuals who express high levels of negative affectivity envisage themselves and their involvement in generally negative terms [20]. Individuals with high negative affectivity levels have higher levels of stress, anxiety and dissatisfaction with life, and tend to focus on unpleasant aspects of themselves, the world, the future and others [21]. The tripartite model of anxiety and depression, developed by Clark and Watson (1991), proposes that anxiety and depressive disorders overlap considerably by a general, not specific, factor, negative affectivity, which reflects the level of aversive feelings present in an individual. The two remaining factors of this model are positive affectivity, which, when low, is relatively specific for depression, and physiological activation, which is relatively specific to anxiety [22]. Lovibond and Lovibond (1995), authors of anxiety, depression and stress scales (DASS), assume that psychological disorders are not categories, that is, the differences between depression, anxiety and stress, experienced by normal subjects and patients, are essentially level ones: depression is characterized mainly by the loss of self-esteem and motivation, and is associated with the perception of low probability of achieving life goals that are meaningful to the individual as a person; anxiety emphasizes the links between persistent state of anxiety and intense fear responses; stress suggests states of excitement and persistent tension, with low resistance to frustration and disappointment [23]. The majority of the participants haven't marital life. In this work, loneliness correlates positively with economic insufficiency. The onset of loneliness is often initiated by a previous event, usually a change or loss in/of an emotional relationship, through death or divorce, or a disruption of social relationship created by the move to a new school, city or employment. Classically, it is distinguished emotional loneliness from social loneliness, wherein the first encompasses the lack of emotional ties inherent to intimate relationships, while bereavement, divorce or emptiness feelings within marriage are the likely background of this latter kind of loneliness. Loss of employment, exclusion from the peer group and not belonging to community organizations are the likely history of social loneliness. Several studies have shown that loneliness is more prevalent among lower financial income groups [30]. Dispositional optimism (LOT-R) and social support (SSSS), factors that positively support health (QHS), protect, in negative correlation, against the negative impact of negative affects (PANAS) associated with financial restraints (QFR), on health of the population which integrates this study. Chang (1998) found that dispositional optimism is a significant moderator of the relationship between stress and psychological well-being [33]. Vickers and Vogeltanz (2000) found that the lack of optimism is a predictor of depression [34]. Rodin and Salovey (1989), cited by Pais-Ribeiro (1999), state that "social support relieves distress in crisis situation, can inhibit the development of diseases and, when one is ill, has a positive role in recovery from disease" [35]. Financial management (QFM) is negatively correlated with the lack of cardiovascular health, and cardiovascular dysfunction correlates positively with loneliness (LS), in this study. Increased low frequency parameter of heart rate variability (HRV) LF is induced by a variety of situations, including stress [50]. Positive affects (PANAS) correlate positively with resilience skills (RSS), which correlate negatively with depression (DASS). Wagnild (2010) had shown that the resilience protects against negative emotions and, thus, has the potential to reduce their pathophysiological effects [37]. Positive affectivity provides a rupture of stress and supports ongoing efforts to replenish depleted resources from stress [19]. In summary, psychobiological therapeutic interventions and psychotherapy, which also target psychological dysfunction related with economic behavior of persons in a situation of poverty, would be beneficial.

References

[1] Patel, V. and Kleinman, A. (2003) Poverty and Common Mental Disorders in Developing Countries. *Bulletin of the World Health Organization*, **81**, 609-615.

[2] Simon, G.E., Revicki, D., Heiligenstein, J., Grothaus, L., VonKorff, M., Katon, W.J. and Hylan, T.R. (2000) Recovery from Depression, Work Productivity, and Health Care Costs among Primary Care Patients. *General Hospital Psychiatry*, **22**, 153-162. http://dx.doi.org/10.1016/S0163-8343(00)00072-4

[3] Lund, C., Breen, A., Flisher, A.J., Kakuma, R., Corrigall, J., Joska, J.A., Swartz, L. and Patel, V. (2010) Poverty and Common Mental Disorders in Low and Middle Income Countries: A Systematic Review. *Social Science & Medicine*, **71**, 517-528. http://dx.doi.org/10.1016/j.socscimed.2010.04.027

[4] Cohen, S., Schwartz, J.E., Epel, E., Kirschbaum, C., Sidney, S. and Seeman, T. (2006) Socioeconomic Status, Race, and Diurnal Cortisol Decline in the Coronary Artery Risk Development in Young Adults (CARDIA) Study. *Psychosomatic Medicine*, **68**, 41-50. http://dx.doi.org/10.1097/01.psy.0000195967.51768.ea

[5] Cohen, S., Doyle, W.J. and Baum, A. (2006) Socioeconomic Status Is Associated with Stress Hormones. *Psychosomatic Medicine*, **68**, 414-420. http://dx.doi.org/10.1097/01.psy.0000221236.37158.b9

[6] Li, L., Power, C., Kelly, S., Kirschbaum, C. and Hertzman, C. (2007) Life-Time Socio-Economic Position and Cortisol Patterns in Mid-Life. *Psychoneuroendocrinology*, **32**, 824-833. http://dx.doi.org/10.1016/j.psyneuen.2007.05.014

[7] Saridjan, N.S., Huizink, A.C., Koetsier, J.A., Jaddoe, V.W., Mackenbach, J.P., Hofman, A., Kirschbaum, C., Verhulst, F.C. and Tiemeier, H. (2010) Do Social Disadvantage and Early Family Adversity Affect the Diurnal Cortisol Rhythm

in Infants? The Generation R Study. *Hormones and Behavior*, **57**, 247-254.
http://dx.doi.org/10.1016/j.yhbeh.2009.12.001

[8]   Costello, E.J., Compton, S.N., Keeler, G. and Angold, A. (2003) Relationships between Poverty and Psychopathology: A Natural Experiment. *JAMA*, **290**, 2023-2029. http://dx.doi.org/10.1001/jama.290.15.2023

[9]   Cesarini, D., Lindqvist, E., Östling, R. and Wallace, B. (2013) Estimating the Causal Impact of Wealth on Health: Evidence from the Swedish Lottery Players. New York University Working Paper, New York.
http://webmeets.com/files/papers/res/2014/1050/Health%20RES.pdf

[10]   Case, A. (2004) Does Money Protect Health Status? Evidence from South African Pensions. In: Wise, D.A., Ed., *Perspectives on the Economics of Aging*, University of Chicago Press, Chicago, 287-312.
http://www.nber.org/chapters/c10346.pdf
http://dx.doi.org/10.7208/chicago/9780226903286.003.0008

[11]   Gardner, J. and Oswald, A.J. (2007) Money and Mental Wellbeing: A Longitudinal Study of Medium-Sized Lottery Wins. *Journal of Health Economics*, **26**, 49-60. http://dx.doi.org/10.1016/j.jhealeco.2006.08.004

[12]   Apouey, B. and Clark, A.E. (2014) Winning Big but Feeling No Better? The Effect of Lottery Prizes on Physical and Mental Health. *Health Economics*, **24**, 516-538. http://dx.doi.org/10.1002/hec.3035

[13]   Schwabe, L. and Wolf, O.T. (2009) Stress Prompts Habit Behavior in Humans. *Journal of Neuroscience*, **29**, 7191-7198. http://dx.doi.org/10.1523/JNEUROSCI.0979-09.2009

[14]   Spears, D. (2011) Economic Decision-Making in Poverty Depletes Behavioral Control. *The BE Journal of Economic Analysis & Policy*, **11**, 1935-1682. http://dx.doi.org/10.2202/1935-1682.2973

[15]   Muraven, M. and Baumeister, R.F. (2000) Self-Regulation and Depletion of Limited Resources: Does Self-Control Resemble a Muscle? *Psychological Bulletin*, **126**, 247-259. http://dx.doi.org/10.1037/0033-2909.126.2.247

[16]   Haushofer, J. and Fehr, E. (2014) On the Psychology of Poverty. *Science*, **344**, 862-867.
http://dx.doi.org/10.1126/science.1232491

[17]   Seligman, M.E., Steen, T.A., Park, N. and Peterson, C. (2005) Positive Psychology Progress: Empirical Validation of Interventions. *American Psychologist*, **60**, 410-421. http://dx.doi.org/10.1037/0003-066X.60.5.410

[18]   Naragon, K. and Watson, D. (2009) Positive Affectivity. In: Lopez, S., Ed., *The Encyclopedia of Positive Psychology*, Wiley-Blackwell, Hoboken, 707-711.

[19]   Southwick, S.M., Vythilingarn, M. and Charney, D.S. (2005) The Psychobiology of Depression and Resilience to Stress: Implications for Prevention and Treatment. *Annual Review of Clinical Psychology*, **1**, 255-291.
http://dx.doi.org/10.1146/annurev.clinpsy.1.102803.143948

[20]   Watson, D. and Clark, L.A. (1984) Negative Affectivity: The Disposition to Experience Negative Aversive Emotional States. *Psychological Bulletin*, **96**, 465-490. http://dx.doi.org/10.1037/0033-2909.96.3.465

[21]   Watson, D., Clark, L.A. and Carey, G. (1988) Positive and Negative Affectivity and Their Relation to Anxiety and Depressive Disorders. *Journal of Abnormal Psychology*, **97**, 346-353. http://dx.doi.org/10.1037/0021-843X.97.3.346

[22]   Clark, L.A. and Watson, D. (1991) Tripartite Model of Anxiety and Depression: Psychometric Evidence and Taxonomic Implications. *Journal of Abnormal Psychology*, **100**, 316-336.
http://dx.doi.org/10.1037/0021-843X.100.3.316

[23]   Lovibond P.F. and Lovibond, S.H. (1995) The Structure of Negative Emotional States: Comparison of the Depression Anxiety Stress Scales (DASS) with the Beck Depression and Anxiety Inventories. *Behaviour Research and Therapy*, **33**, 335-342. http://dx.doi.org/10.1016/0005-7967(94)00075-U

[24]   Jacobs, G.D. and Snyder, D. (1996) Frontal Brain Asymmetry Predicts Affective Style in Men. *Behavioral Neuroscience*, **110**, 3-6. http://dx.doi.org/10.1037/0735-7044.110.1.3

[25]   Tomarken, A.J. and Davidson, R.J. (1994) Frontal Brain Activation in Repressors and Nonrepressors. *Journal of Abnormal Psychology*, **103**, 339-349. http://dx.doi.org/10.1037/0021-843X.103.2.339

[26]   Allen, J.J., Iacono, W.G., Depue, R.A. and Arbisi, P. (1993) Regional Electroencephalographic Asymmetries in Bipolar Seasonal Affective Disorder before and after Exposure to Bright Light. *Biological Psychiatry*, **33**, 642-646.
http://dx.doi.org/10.1016/0006-3223(93)90104-L

[27]   Henriques, J.B. and Davidson, R.J. (1990) Regional Brain Electrical Asymmetries Discriminate between Previously Depressed and Healthy Control Subjects. *Journal of Abnormal Psychology*, **41**, 22-31.
http://dx.doi.org/10.1037/0021-843X.99.1.22

[28]   Henriques, J.B. and Davison, R.J. (1991) Left Frontal Hypoactivation in Depression. *Journal of Abnormal Psychology*, **100**, 535-545. http://dx.doi.org/10.1037/0021-843X.100.4.535

[29]   George, M.S. and Post, R.M. (2011) Daily Left Prefrontal Repetitive Transcranial Magnetic Stimulation for Acute Treatment of Medication-Resistant Depression. *Perspectives*, **168**, 356-364.

http://dx.doi.org/10.1176/appi.ajp.2010.10060864

[30] Perlman, D. and Peplau, L. (1998) Loneliness. In: Friedman, H.S., Ed., *Encyclopedia of Mental Health*, Vol. 2, Academic Press, San Diego, 571-581.

[31] Scheier, M.F., Carver, C.S. and Bridges, M.W. (1994) Distinguishing Optimism from Neuroticism (and Trait Anxiety, Self-Mastery, and Self-Esteem): A Re-Evaluation of the Life Orientation Test. *Journal of Personality and Social Psychology*, **67**, 1063-1078. http://dx.doi.org/10.1037/0022-3514.67.6.1063

[32] Segerstrom, S. and Nes, L. (2006) When Goals Conflict but People Prosper: The Case of Dispositional Optimism. *Journal of Research in Personality*, **40**, 675-693. http://dx.doi.org/10.1016/j.jrp.2005.08.001

[33] Chang, E. (1998) Does Dispositional Optimism Moderate the Relation between Perceived Stress and Psychological Well-Being? A Preliminary Investigation. *Personality and Individual Differences*, **25**, 233-240. http://dx.doi.org/10.1016/S0191-8869(98)00028-2

[34] Vickers, K. and Vogeltanz, N. (2000) Dispositional Optimism as a Predictor of Depressive Symptoms over Time. *Personalityand Individual Differences*, **28**, 259-272. http://dx.doi.org/10.1016/S0191-8869(99)00095-1

[35] Pais-Ribeiro, J. (1999) Escala de Satisfação com o Suporte Social (ESSS). *Análise Psicológica*, **3**, 547-558. http://hdl.handle.net/10216/5544

[36] Jardim, J. and Pereira, A. (2006) Competências pessoais e sociais: Guia prático para a mudança positiva. Edições ASA, Porto.

[37] Wagnild, G.M. (2010) Discovering Your Resilience Core. http://resiliencescale.net/papers.html

[38] Wagnild, G.M. and Young, H.M. (1993) Development and Psychometric Evaluation of the Resilience Scale. *Journal of Nursing Measurement*, **1**, 165-178.

[39] Martins, M. and Jesus, S. (2007) Factores de resiliência e bem-estar: Compreender e actuar para resistir. In: Siqueira, M.M.M., Jesus, S.N. and Oliveira, V.B., Orgs., *Psicologia da Saúde, Teoria e Pesquisa*, Universidade Metodista de São Paulo & Universidade do Algarve, São Bernardo do Campo, 85-113.

[40] Kumpfer, K.L. (1999) Factors and Processes Contributing to Resilience: The Resilience Framework. In: Glantz, M.D. and Johnson, J.L., Eds., *Resilience and Development: Positive Life Adaptations*, Kluwer, New York, 179-224.

[41] Jalife, J. and Michaels, D.C. (1994) Neural Control of Sinoatrial Pacemaker Activity. In: Levy, M.N. and Schwartz, P.J., Eds., *Vagal Control of the Heart: Experimental Basis and Clinical Implications*, Futura, Armonk, 173-205.

[42] Malliani, A., Pagani, M., Lombardi, F. and Cerutti, S. (1991) Cardiovascular Neural Regulation Explored in the Frequency Domain. *Circulation*, **84**, 1482-1492. http://dx.doi.org/10.1161/01.CIR.84.2.482

[43] Levy, M.N. (1971) Sympathetic-Parasympathetic Interactions in the Heart. *Circulation Research*, **29**, 437-445. http://dx.doi.org/10.1161/01.RES.29.5.437

[44] Noma, A. and Trautwein, W. (1978) Relaxation of the ACh-Induced Potassium Current in the Rabbit Sinoatrial Node Cell. *Pflügers Archiv*, **377**, 193-200. http://dx.doi.org/10.1007/BF00584272

[45] Osterrieder, W., Noma, A. and Trautwein, W. (1980) On the Kinetics of the Potassium Channel Activated by Acetylcholine in the S-A Node of the Rabbit Heart. *Pflügers Archiv*, **386**, 101-109. http://dx.doi.org/10.1007/BF00584196

[46] Sakmann, B., Noma, A. and Trautwein, W. (1983) Acetylcholine Activation of Single Muscarinic K^+ Channels in Isolated Pacemaker Cells of the Mammalian Heart. *Nature*, **303**, 250-253. http://dx.doi.org/10.1038/303250a0

[47] Akselrod, S., Gordon, D., Ubel, F.A., Shannon, D.C., Berger, A.C. and Cohen, R.J. (1981) Power Spectrum Analysis of Heart Rate Fluctuation: A Quantitative Probe of Beat to Beat Cardiovascular Control. *Science*, **213**, 220-222. http://dx.doi.org/10.1126/science.6166045

[48] Pomeranz, B., Macaulay, R.J.B., Caudill, M.A., Kutz, I., Adam, D., Gordon, D., *et al.* (1985) Assessment of Autonomic Function in Humans by Heart Rate Spectral Analysis. *American Journal of Physiology-Heart and Circulatory Physiology*, **248**, H151-H153. http://ajpheart.physiology.org/content/ajpheart/248/1/H151.full.pdf

[49] Kamath, M.V. and Fallen, E.L. (1992) Power Spectral Analysis of Heart Rate Variability: A Noninvasive Signature of Cardiac Autonomic Function. *Critical Reviews in Biomedical Engineering*, **21**, 245-311.

[50] Rimoldi, O., Pierini, S., Ferrari, A., Cerutti, S., Pagani, M., Malliani, A. (1990) Analysis of Short-Term Oscillations of R-R and Arterial Pressure in Conscious Dogs. *American Journal of Physiology-Heart and Circulatory Physiology*, **258**, H967-H976.

[51] Montano, N., Ruscone, T.G., Porta, A., Lombardi, F., Pagani, M. and Malliani, A. (1994) Power Spectrum Analysis of Heart Rate Variability to Assess the Changes in Sympathovagal Balance during Graded Orthostatic Tilt. *Circulation*, **90**, 1826-1831. http://dx.doi.org/10.1161/01.CIR.90.4.1826

[52] Malik, M., Bigger, J.T., Camm, A.J., Kleiger, R.E., Malliani, A., Moss, A.J. and Schwartz, P.J. (1996) Heart Rate Va-

riability Standards of Measurement, Physiological Interpretation, and Clinical Use. *European Heart Journal*, **17**, 354-381. http://dx.doi.org/10.1093/oxfordjournals.eurheartj.a014868

[53] Watson, D., Clark, L.A. and Tellegen, A. (1988) Development and Validation of Brief Measures of Positive Affect and Negative Affect: The PANAS Scales. *Journal of Personality and Social Psychology*, **54**, 1063-1070. http://dx.doi.org/10.1037/0022-3514.54.6.1063

[54] Galinha, I.C. and Pais-Ribeiro, J.L. (2005) Contribuição para o estudo da versão portuguesa da Positive and Negative Affect Schedule (PANAS): I—Abordagem teórica ao conceito de afecto. *Análise Psicológica*, **2**, 209-218. http://www.scielo.oces.mctes.pt/pdf/aps/v23n2/v23n2a11.pdf

[55] Lovibond, S.H. and Lovibond, P.F. (1995) Manual for the Depression Anxiety Stress Scales. 2nd Edition, Psychology Foundation of Australia, Sidney.

[56] Pais-Ribeiro, J., Honrado, A. and Leal, I. (2004) Contribuição para o estudo da Adaptação Portuguesa das Escalas de Ansiedade, Depressão e Stress (EADS) de 21 itens de Lovibond e Lovibond. *Psicologia, Saúde & Doenças*, **5**, 229-239. http://hdl.handle.net/10400.12/1058

[57] Sarason, I.G., Levine, H.M., Basham, R.B. and Sarason, B.R. (1983) Assessing Social Support: The Social Support Questionnaire. *Journal of Personality and Social Psychology*, **44**, 127-139. http://dx.doi.org/10.1037/0022-3514.44.1.127

[58] Pais-Ribeiro, J., Pedro, L. and Marques, S. (2012) Dispositional Optimism Is Unidimensional or Bidimensional? The Portuguese Revised Life Orientation Test. *The Spanish Journal of Psychology*, **15**, 1259-1271. http://dx.doi.org/10.5209/rev_SJOP.2012.v15.n3.39412

[59] de Carvalho Ng, C.A.F. and Pereira, I.D. (2012) Adaptação da "The Resilience Scale" para a população adulta portuguesa. *Psicologia USP*, **23**, 417-433. http://www.revistas.usp.br/psicousp/article/viewFile/42178/45851 http://dx.doi.org/10.1590/S0103-65642012005000008

[60] Russell, D., Peplau, L.A. and Ferguson, M.L. (1978) Developing a Measure of Loneliness. *Journal of Personality Assessment*, **42**, 290-294. http://dx.doi.org/10.1207/s15327752jpa4203_11

[61] Neto, F. (1989) Avaliação da solidão. *Psicologia Clínica*, **2**, 65-79.

Vulnerability and Resilience to Stress and Immune and Neuroendocrine Function in Portuguese Subjects with Psychic Anomaly (Anxiety and Depression)

Eduardo Goncalves[1], Saul Neves de Jesus[2]

[1]Department of Psychiatry and Mental Health of Hospital Center of Algarve, Faro, Portugal
[2]Department of Psychology of Faculty of Social and Human Sciences of University of Algarve, Faro, Portugal
Email: eduar.goncalves@gmail.com

Abstract

The present study aimed to investigate the impact of chronic psychosocial stress and resilience, including at a biological level (immune and neuroendocrine function) in Portuguese citizens with psychic anomaly/mental disorder. The sample aggregated 69 participants. It has been used the following psychometric instruments: 21-item depression, anxiety and stress scales (DASS-21), in the Portuguese validated version; measuring state resilience (MSR), in the Portuguese validated version; the Portuguese scale of 23 questions on vulnerability to stress. Serum levels of cortisol, dehydroepiandrosterone sulfate, antibodies anti-viral capsid antigen of Epstein-Barr virus, triglycerides, high density lipoprotein-cholesterol and body mass index have been measured. It has been concluded that factors of vulnerability to stress and chronic stress, of social nature (lack of social support, adverse living conditions), correlate positively with depression, anxiety and stress, and, through alostatic load, are involved in a greater propensity for immune and neuroendocrine dysfunction in this population.

Keywords

Vulnerability to Stress, Stress, Coping, Resilience, Alostatic Load, Anxiety, Depression, Cortisol, Dehydroepiandrosterone, Epstein-Barr Virus, Triglycerides, High Density Lipoprotein-Cholesterol, Body Mass Index

1. Introduction (Theoretical Framework)

1.1. Social Support, Stress, Appraisal, Coping, Evoked Emotions, Tripartite Model of Anxiety and Depression

The structural model of Smith and Lazarus (1993) [1] on stress appraisal stands six components of appraisal. Two components of primary appraisal include the motivational relevance, which consists of an assessment of the importance of the situation for the person, and the motivational congruence, that is, the assessment of the extent to which the situation is consistent or not with their current objectives (that is, if it is desirable or undesirable). Four secondary appraisal components include: self-accountability, *i.e.*, the an evaluation of the degree in which the individual himself is responsible for the situation; hetero-accountability, *i.e.*, an evaluation of the degree in which something or somebody is responsible; potential of problem-focused coping, *i.e.*, the perceived competence to act on the situation to maintain or increase its convenience; potential of emotion-focused coping, *i.e.*, the perceived competence for psychological adjustment and to deal with the situation if it is found that has become undesirable. Crossing the outcomes of the two types of appraisal will result in a mapping of these components in terms of the different emotions experienced (as proposed by Smith (1991) [2] and Smith and Lazarus (1993) [1]), and of the major outcomes of appraisals as described by Lazarus and colleagues, in the context of the theory of stress and coping: irrelevance, benefit, challenge, damage, threat [3]. A condition is evaluated as irrelevant to personal well-being if motivational relevance is low. High motivational relevance in combination with motivational congruence (situation appraised as important and desirable) defines the circumstances as beneficial and can evoke feelings of happiness [1] [2]. Beneficial appraisals of self-accountability evoke feelings of pride. Beneficial appraisals of hetero-accountability evoke feelings of gratitude. High motivational relevance appraisals and low motivational congruence (important and undesirable situation) define the circumstances as stressful. Self-accountability appraisals combined with primary appraisals of stress evoke guilt, shame (self-directed negative emotions). Hetero-accountability appraisals combined with primary appraisals of stress evoke anger. Appraisals of high potential of problem-focused coping combined with primary appraisals of stress define circumstances as an opportunity, indicate that the person has potential abilities to change the circumstances in order to make them more syntonic to their wishes and evoke feelings of challenge, determination, that motivate the individual to get involved in the situation and work to make it more desirable [1] [2]. Appraisals of low potential of problem-focused coping combined with primary appraisals of stress define circumstances as damage, indicate that the person is in a precarious situation, for which little can be done to improve and evoke feelings of sadness and resignation, that motivate the person to seek help and possibly to resign on harmful situation, allowing his/her involvement in another one [1] [4]. Appraisals of high potential of emotion-focused coping,. *i.e*, assessments of competencies to adapt to circumstances which do not function as desired, allow the person to keep calm, facing conditions evaluated as stressful. Appraisals of low potential of emotion-focused coping, *i.e*, evaluations of incompetence to adapt to circumstances which do not function as desired, define the situation as threat and evoke feelings of fear, anxiety, motivating the person to be vigilant and to take care in an attempt to avoid undesirable results [1]. Stress results from combined high motivational relevance and motivational incongruence, that is, it occurs when a person evaluates their circumstances as important, but undesirable, *i.e.*, stress can be identified as a subjectively important discrepancy between what one wants (motivational state) and what one have in a given situation (situational state), and then it follows that coping consists of individual efforts to reduce the magnitude of this discrepancy. Acting on the circumstances for change in order to put them more in line with wishes corresponds to problem-focused coping [3]. Acting on desires or beliefs so that conditions become more desirable, without change, which can be achieved by strategies as reprioritization objectives [4], evaluate the circumstances in accordance with a more positive perspective, reinterpret the relevance of circumstances with respect to objectives, corresponds to emotion-focused coping, as described by Lazarus and Folkman (1984) [3], and, more appropriately, to accommodative coping, as described by Walker and colleagues (1997) [5].

Subjects with low levels of positive affectivity are characterized by sadness, apathy, anxiety, stress and not rewarding social involvement. The negative affectivity and positive affectivity are not independent. The positive affectivity provides a rupture of stress and supports ongoing efforts to replenish depleted resources from stress [6] [7]. The tripartite model of anxiety and depression, developed by Clark and Watson (1991) [8], proposes that anxiety and depressive disorders overlap considerably by a general, not specific, factor, negative affectivity, which reflects the level of aversive feelings present in an individual. The two remaining factors of this model are positive affectivity, which, when low, is relatively specific for depression, and physiological activation, which is relatively specific to anxiety. Lovibond and Lovibond (1995) [9], authors of anxiety, depression and stress scales (DASS), assume that psychological disorders are not categories, that is, the differences between depression, anxiety and stress, experienced by normal subjects and patients, are essentially level ones: depression is characterized mainly by the loss of self-esteem and motivation, and is associated with the perception of low probability of achieving life goals that are meaningful to the individual as a person; anxiety emphasizes the links between persistent state of anxiety and intense fear responses; stress suggests states of excitement and persistent tension, with low resistance to frustration and disappointment.

1.2. Vulnerability and Resilience to Stress, Anxiety and Depression, and Alostatic Load

Resilience is a multidimensional phenomenon, defined by Reich, Zautra and Hall (2010) [10] as the result of successful adaptation to adversity. Although the resilient response can be almost universal, it is unlikely that this capacity is equally distributed in population, such as environmental, social, factors that strengthen or weaken the individual resilience to stress [10]. Within an ecological perspective, Holling, Schindler, Walker and Roughgarden (1995) [11] argue that resilience is defined assistem's ability to absorb disturbance prior to the occurrence of fundamental changes in system's state [11]. Intense stress and pain decrease individual ability to distinguish between the presence of positive emotion and the absence of negative emotion, reducing thereby the sustainability of coping strategies concerning positive emotional involvement. According to Reich *et al.* (2010) [10], psychic and organic homeostasis is sustained, not by emotional neutrality but, by an intentional emotional engagement process. In line with this view, resilience extends beyond the individual ability for recovering from disease's state, and, within this sense, resilience is considered as the amount of stress that a person can withstand without a fundamental change in his/her ability to pursue objectives that give meaning to life. The higher individual ability to stay in a satisfactory life course is, the greater his/her resilience is. However, as resilient recovery relates with passive aspects of resilience, resilience's sustainability meets its proactive, positive, side, that is, for relevant results in the preservation of important commitments and involvements in living tasks (work, leisure and social relationships). Consciousness and choice characterize the development of human values and sustainable objectives [10]. Exceptions to rapid and full recovery, and that challenge homeostatic fundamentals, examples of which, facing stress chronicity, are dysregulation of the hypothalamic-pituitary-adrenal axis, hypercortisolemia or hypocortisolemia, metabolic syndrome, anxiety and depression, present in some people within the concept of alostatic load [12] [13]. Deprivation of means of full understanding of a highly threatening experience that characterizes younger age groups, determines that they are kept not recovered, for years, from emotional after-effects, so early abuse and trauma may later invade the consciousness, interfering in homeostasis, through the determination of a chronic elevation of central operation of psychophysiological processes [14] [15]. Resiliency resources are not positive qualities found in the other end of a single risk continuum but, rather an inseparable factor of global well-being, which gives unique physical and mental benefits, not taken into account through relative risk assessments [16]. The necessary distinction between factors stems from joining several motivational processes, the need for protection and protection against damage, on one hand, and the need to extend individual reach relating to positive objectives, on the other hand [17], being evident the distinct neuronal structures responsible for the regulation of positive emotional responses and for the negative emotional responses [18]. Also, the underlying cognitions of personal control demonstrate the existence of two factors [19], one for agency, optimism and hope, another for helplessness, pessimism and despair. Within research's framework of public health, there have been studied processes taken as buffer's function providers in relation to stress and vulnerability to stress, such as social support [20] and individual control [21] [22]. Rates of risk factors are listed as following (biological, individual, inter-personal/family, community/organizational). Biological ones include: diastolic blood pressure greater than 90 mmHg; systolic blood pressure greater than 140 mmHg; total cholesterol greater than 240 mg/dl; glucose at rest greater than 124 mg/dl; body mass index (BMI) greater than 25; genetic factors associated with anxiety; elevated C-reactive protein and/or other increases in inflammatory processes. Individual ones include: history of mental disease; depression/helplessness; traumatic brain injury. Inter-personal/familiar ones are: history of childhood trauma/adult abuse; chronic social stress. Community/organizational ones include: presence of environmental accidents; high rates of violent crime; stressful working environment. The corresponding indices of resiliency resources include heart rate variability (HRV), regular physical exercise, genetic factors associated with resilience to stress, immune responsiveness and regulation (biological), positive emotional resources, hope/optimism/agency, cognitive functioning, learning/memory, high executive functioning (individual), safe kinship relationships, close social ties (inter-personal/family), green spaces, involvement in activities in a natural environment (for example, community gardening), voluntarism, satisfactory professional life (community/organizational). Active coping strategies, such as planning and problems solving have been associated with a higher degree of well-being and ability to cope with stress, trauma and disease [6]. Denial and behavioral divestment before stressful situations are associated with higher levels of distress [7]. Those subjects with post-traumatic stress disorder avoid coping with trauma-related memories, which contributes to the maintenance of conditioned fear. According to Fredrickson (2001) [23], positive emotions provide a buffer function in relation to the adverse consequences of stress, by decreasing autonomic activation, determined by negative emotions, and increased processes of thought's flexibility (cognitive flexibility) and problem solving. Ability for cognitive revaluation/reappraisal allows reformulation of adverse experiences, through the adduction of positive meaning and mood [23]. Affiliative behaviors, in animals and humans, mitigate the effects of stress, physical injury and infection [24]. High levels of anti-Epstein Barr virus antibodies (EBV-ab) are indicative of decreased cell-mediated immunity that has been related to psychosocial stress. A low function of cell-mediated immunity increases an individual's risk for B-cell lymphoproliferative disorder. Individuals with negative tests for anti-EBV antibodies have increased risk for severe disease associated with EBV, when infected at advanced ages [25]. Repeated or prolonged stress can determine dysregulation or suppression of immune function. Chronic stress suppresses immune-protective parameters such as production of antibodies [26]. The presence of objectives in life, as well as a set of beliefs about what is ethically correct and incorrect, has been associated with resilience. Beliefs and religious or spiritual practices provide, to many people, a structural frame that facilitates recovery and meeting of meaning, upon the occurrence of traumatic or associated with high load stress experiences [27]. Initial adverse living experiences increase the risk of depression and post-traumatic stress disorder in adulthood, through prolonged production of hormones, neurotransmitters and alterations of the central nervous system, which thereafter will affect the resistance to stress [28]. A key factor identified in trained children to overcome adversity is a close relationship with an adult caregiver [29]. Stress at an early age is associated with chronic elevation of corticotrophin releasing hormone levels during adulthood [28]. Changes in the function of the hypothalamic-pituitary-adrenal axis differ according to the specific nature of psychiatric disorder: major depressive disorder is associated with elevated levels of corticotrophin releasing hormone in cerebrospinal fluids and plasma cortisol; post-traumatic stress disorder is associated with elevated levels of corticotrophin releasing hormone and low levels of cortisol [30]. Dehydroepiandrosterone (DHEA), simultaneously secreted with cortisol, in response to stress, may increase stress resistance, protecting against neuronal injury induced by corticosteroids, particularly in the hippocampus resulting from the prolonged activity of the hypothalamic-pituitary-adrenal axis [31]. Higher serum levels of DHEA in patients with post-traumatic stress disorder are associated with lower disease severity and higher recovery of symptomatology. Higher values of DHEA sulphate/cortisol ratios during stress can be protective in healthy individuals [32]. Within the context of the dysfunction of the hypothalamic-pituitary-adrenal axis, several mechanisms have been proposed concerning the evolution towards low cortisol states. A model suggests that, under the influence of chronic stress, initial adaptive response of hypercortisolism, over time, becomes a self-protecting state of hypocortisolism, in order to preserve the endocrine-metabolic system and the brain. Other potential mechanisms of states of hypocortisolism centrally induced include the down-regulation of pituitary receptors of corticotrophin releasing factor, in response to elevations of corticotrophin releasing hormone and to negative feedback, induced by hypercortisolism at central nervous system, over sustained release of stimulating hormones. Relative states of hypocortisolism, or resistance to cortisol, may also occur despite the presence of normal, or even elevated, levels of cortisol [33] [34]. Obesity, an actual public health problem worldwide, in conjunction with metabolic syndrome and the clinical picture of type II diabetes mellitus, integrates the concept of alostatic load [13], which groups several anomalies, including insulin resistance, dyslipidemia and markers of cardiovascular disease. The increased triglycerides (TGL)/high density lipoprotein-cholesterol (HDL) ratio identifies individuals with overweight, insulin resistance, atherogenic particles of low density lipoprotein-cholesterol (LDL), constituting a predictive marker for the presence of atherosclerotic coronary lesions and cardiovascular accident. In addition, low serum HDL levels, in combination with increased serum concentrations of TGL, has predictive value for the development of type II diabetes mellitus [35] [37]. Alostatic load determines long-term effects on cardiovascular system (determining atherosclerosis and cardiovascular disease), brain (with decreased neurogenesis and increased dendritic remodeling in the hippocampus, causing loss of the ability to adapt to environmental requirements), adipose tissue and muscle (determining the development of obesity and metabolic syndrome) and immune system (increasing the risk of infection and autoimmune disease) [38]. The mediterranean diet is beneficial in this context, because it is poor in saturated fat (lipid) and rich in monounsaturated fats (consumption of fish and olive oil) and fiber (vegetable consumption). Recent meta-analysis on the effects of the mediterranean diet on metabolic syndrome has highlighted its association with lower values of blood pressure, glucose and triglycerides [39]. Locus coeruleus-norepinephrine system interferes with the functioning of the sympathetic nervous system and the responses of the hypothalamic-pituitary-adrenal axis to stress. Locus coeruleus sustains a general alarm function, in response to potential threats, triggering the release of norepinephrine in amygdala, nucleus accumbens, prefrontal cortex and hippocampus, and its activation also inhibits neurovegetative function, including sleep and eating behavior. A chronically hyperactived locus coeruleus-norepinephrine system predisposes the organism to high levels of anxiety, by inhibition of prefrontal cortex, thus interfering with the regulation of more complex cognitive and emotional processes, and determining cardiovascular clinical problems [40] [41]. Beta-adrenergic receptors blocking in amygdala prevents the development of aversive memories, in animals and humans [42]. Thus, resilience is associated to the reduction of the response of locus coeruleus-norepinephrine system. Serotonin/5-hdroxi-tryptamine (5-HT) has neuro-modulatory effects on other neurotransmitter systems involved in the regulation of mood and anxiety. Stress experiences at an early age can lead to decreased stress tolerance in adult life, through increasing levels of releasing corticotrophin hormone and cortisol, which, in turn, decreases the activity of serotoninergic 5-HT-1A receptors [43]. Dopaminergic neurons are activated by rewarding stimuli and inhibited by aversive stimuli, wherein stress activates dopamine releasing in neurons in medial prefrontal cortex and inhibits its release in nucleus accumbens, a key component of rewarding circuitry. Excessive dopamine release at meso-cortical level after stressful events may be associated with increased vulnerability to stress. Signaling of dopamine facilitates fear extinction, but its role in resilience is not yet totally clarified [44]. Neuronal circuit of fear regulation involves mainly amygdala, hippocampus and ventro-medial prefrontal cortex. Amygdala mediates fear conditioning [45]. Hippocampus mediates contextual and temporal aspects of conditioned fear [46]. Over time, it may occur reactivation and reconsolidation through strengthening, or weakening, by extinction of memories. Amygdala and ventro-medial prefrontal cortex are involved in successful extinction, a process which involves the formation of new memories [47]. The pathophysiology of post-traumatic stress disorder may involve an abnormal fear learning and underlying dysfunction of neural circuitry of fear [48]. Post-traumatic stress disorder patients tend to generalize, from specific conditioned stimuli, to other stimuli in their environment that also become associated with its original trauma, and are therefore fear inductors. Resilience may involve the ability to avoid this generalization of fear. Recently, it was found that, in healthy individuals, the lateral prefrontal cortex, activated by cognitive regulation of emotions can act, through connections of ventro-medial prefrontal cortex with amygdala, in order to decrease fear responses [47]. Phillips, Drevets, Rauch and Lane (2003) [49] described a neuronal model of emotional regulation which comprises a ventral system (integrating amygdala, insula, ventral striatum, ventral anterior cingulate cortex and ventral prefrontal cortex), responsible for the identification of emotional stimuli and production of suitable emotional response, and a dorsal system (including hippocampus, dorsal anterior cingulate cortex and dorsal prefrontal cortex), responsible for the regulation of emotional responses [49]. It has been shown that disturbances of mood and anxiety correlated more consistently with defects in the amygdala, hippocampus, subgenual anterior cingulate cortex and prefrontal cortex [50]. Cognitive reevaluation (reappraisal) is a mechanism by which resilient individuals can reduce or control emotional responses to stressful situations. Recent studies of functional brain imaging, with participants instructed to reappraise the significance of negative images, demonstrate the involvement of medial and lateral prefrontal cortex in the regulation of emotional responses, through top-down control of amygdala activation during cognitive reappraisal [51]. Greater use of cognitive reappraisal in everyday life has also been linked to increased activation of the prefrontal cortex and less activation of the amygdala, in face of negative stimuli [52], suggesting the existence of a possible neuronal mechanism by which cognitive reappraisal increases the resistance to stress. In short, resilience can be related to a greater ability for emotional regulation, while psychopathology may be associated with abnormalities in emotional regulation systems [53]. The rewarding system includes dopaminergic neurons in midbrain, especially in ventral tegmental area, which project in nucleus accumbens and other limbic regions. Recently, it has been highlighted a dysfunction of neural circuitry of rewarding, in patients with major depression [54] and post-traumatic stress disorder [55], as well as in young adults with history of abuse in childhood [56]. A large body of epidemiological research suggests that individuals with lack of social support are at greater risk for problems of mental and physical health, and low social support is related to higher levels of depression, anxiety and dissatisfaction with life. The existence of social support is also associated with low mortality from all causes, but particularly due to cardiovascular disease. The interface between social support and processes related with stress is crucial in understanding these epidemiological associations [57]. Research suggests that oxytocin, neuropeptide involved in pro-social behavior and neuroendocrine responses to stress in animals, may mediate some of the protective effects and reducing anxiety that characterize affiliative behaviors [58]. In humans, the combination of social support with oxytocin is more effective in reducing anxiety and reactivity of the hypothalamic-pituitary-adrenal axis in response to psychosocial stress. Oxytocin can also facilitate individual ability of inference of the mental states of others [59]. The ability to empathize may be related to social competence, a characteristic of resilient individuals. The mirror neuron system, working in conjunction with limbic areas, may play a role in understanding the emotions and intentions of others [60].

2. Empirical Study

2.1. Participants

In the present study, a convenience sampling has been selected, with subjects residents in Olhão, Portugal, referred by general practitioners, to a first psychiatric appointment at the outpatient consultation of psychiatry of hospital of Faro, Portugal, with attributed generic diagnostic hypothesis of anxiety and mood disorders (depression), according to the tenth edition of the international classification of diseases of world health organization [61], with chronic evolution, not subjected to previous interventions of psychopharmacology and psychotherapy. The research protocol has been accepted by the ethics committee of this hospital, and has been in compliance with Helsinki declaration (concerning medical research). Participants provided their written informed consent. The sample is initially composed by 75 elements, 77% female. The age presents a mean value of 45.3 years (standard deviation: 14.3). Six elements did not answered the measurement scales used, whereby the sample has been reduced to 69 elements.

2.2. Material and Methods

The scales have been validated for their use by Portuguese population. It is presented a brief description of the psychometric scales used in this work.

2.2.1. 23 Questions on Vulnerability to Stress

The Portuguese scale of 23 questions on vulnerability to stress (23QVS) [62] is an ordinal Likert scale with five possible answers ("0" to "4") between "absolutely agree" and "absolutely disagree" for items 1, 3, 4, 6, 7, 8 and 20 and, conversely, between "absolutely disagree" and "absolutely agree", for the remaining items. It consists of 23 items, which are organized into seven factors: perfectionism and intolerance to frustration; inhibition and functional dependence; lack of social support; adverse living conditions; dramatization of existence; subjugation; deprivation of affection and rejection. The cutoff point for this scale is greater than 43 (that is, scores higher than 43 mean the existence of vulnerability to stress).

2.2.2. 21 Items Depression, Anxiety and Stress Scales

21-items depression, anxiety and stress scales (DASS) [9] [63] is an ordinal Likert scale with four response alternatives (from "0" to "3") between "not applied to me at all" and "applied to me most of the time". It consists of 21 items, which are organized in three dimensions. Seven variables measure appropriately a single dimension, depression, and the cutoff point for depression scale is greater than 7. Seven variables measure appropriately a single dimension, anxiety, and the cutoff point for anxiety scale is greater than 9. Seven variables measure appropriately a single dimension, stress, and the cutoff point for stress scale is greater than 14. Lovibond and Lovibond (1995) [9] define depression, anxiety and stress as follows: depression includes dysphoria, hopelessness, devaluation, self-depreciation, lack of interest, anhedonia and inertia; anxiety integrates autonomic arousal, skeletal muscle effects, situational anxiety and subjective experience of anxious affect; stress integrates difficulty to relaxing, nervous excitation, easy agitation, irritability/excessive reactivity and impatience.

2.3. Measuring State Resilience

The scale for measuring state resilience(MSR) [64] [65] is an ordinal Likert scale with five possible answers ("1" to "5") between "I totally disagree 'and' I totally agree" and consists of 14 items. The cutoff point is greater than the median, 57.

The departure point of this research focused on the biological impact, particularly at the level of immune and neuroendocrine functions, of vulnerability to stress and chronic stress in patients with psychopathological symptomatology (anxiety and depression). The clinical diagnosis has been confirmed according to the results provided by DASS. In line with technical methodology used at laboratorial medicine unit of hospital of Faro, Portugal, there have been collected morning (08:00 AM) blood samples in peripheral venous blood, for: dosing cortisol (chemical luminescence method); titrating levels of antibodies against viral capsid antigen of Epstein-Barr virus (EBV-ab) (EIA method); determining triglycerides (TGL)/high density lipoprotein-cholesterol (HDL) ratio (enzyme method GPO PAP) (biochemical indicators of vulnerability/risk); titrating levels of dehydroe-piandrosteronesulfate (DHEA-S) (chemical luminescence method) (biochemical indicator of protection/resilience factor). It has been calculated body mass index (BMI). For ethical and deontological reasons, it was not considered a subjects-control group (for not requesting diagnostic tests to healthy subjects). This study is descriptive, transversal and quantitative, correlational, not experimental. It has been used Pearson correlation coefficient r.

2.4. Results

The internal consistency values of all used scales are high, attesting the reliability of the results. Cronbach's alpha coefficient is: 0.864, for 23QVS; 0.945, for DASS-depression; 0.886, for DASS-anxiety; 0.899, for DASS-stress; 0.838, for MSR. Concerning the existence of disorders in participants, taking as references the cutoff points indicated by the used scales, in 62% of the subjects there is vulnerability to stress, 54% exhibit depression, 65% manifest anxiety, 58% have stress and 43% of the participants have resilience. Cortisol levels have an average value of 14.8, with a dispersion of values of 44% (normal range values: 5 - 25 micrograms per deciliter), 89% of the elements present normal cortisol levels, 5% have hypocortisolemia and 6% have hypercortisolemia (with 5 missing values). DHEA-S levels have an average value of 146.7, with a dispersion of values of 82% (normal range values: 35 - 430 micrograms per deciliter), 8% of the elements have values of DHEA-S lower than normal and 3% have higher than normal values (with 5 missing values). EBV-ab levels have an average value of 67.8, with a dispersion of values of 54% (the cutoff point is equal to or greater than 10 Units per milliliter), and 92% of the elements have values greater than EBV-ab normal values (with 5 missing values). The TGL/HDL ratios have an average value of 2.88, with a dispersion of values of 104% (the cutoff point is greater than 3.5), 23% of the elements have values of TGL/HDL ratios higher than normal (with 4 missing values). The BMI have an average value of 26.1, with a dispersion of values of 20% (the cutoff point is greater than 25), 46% of the elements present BMI greater than normal, *i.e.*, overweight (with 2 missing values). In terms of medical comorbidity, 31% of the participants have endocrine and metabolic disease (predominantly, hypercholesterolemia, diabetes) and hypertension, 40% have oncological diseases (predominantly, breast cancer, uterine cancer, prostatic cancer), and auto-immune disease (lupus) (29% of respondents have no comorbidity). When analysis is performed in terms of absolute values, for each variable obtained with the application of 23QVS and biological/physiological measures, it is verified the occurrence of a statistically significant negative correlation between full scale values (vulnerability to stress) and values of EBV-ab, $r = -0.274$; $p = 0.029$. Apart from this, there are levels of statistical significance in the correlations between factor 3 of 23QVS (lack of social support) and cortisol values, $r = -0.248$, $p = 0.048$, between factor 3 of 23QVS (lack of social support) and EBV-ab, $r = -0.264$; $p = 0.035$ and between the factor 4 of 23QVS (adverse living conditions) and EBV-ab, $r = -0.277$; $p = 0.027$, remaining negative. The negative correlation between the DASS dimensions and MSR are related in a statistically significant way ($r = -0.437$, $p < 0.01$, for the negative correlation between MRS and DASS-depression; $r = -0.374$, $p < 0.01$, for the negative correlation between MRS and DASS-anxiety; $r = -0.318$, $p < 0.01$, for the negative correlation between MSR and DASS-stress).The 23QVS (vulnerability to stress) and all its dimensions are positively correlated with all dimensions of DASS (depression, anxiety and stress). There have been more strong correlations (above 0.5) between: 23QVS and depression, $r = 0.714$, $p < 0.001$; 23QVS and anxiety, $r = 0.691$, $p < 0.001$; 23QVS and stress, $r = 0.663$, $p < 0.001$; Factor 1 of 23 QVS (perfectionism and intolerance to frustration) and anxiety, $r = 0.558$, $p < 0.001$; Factor 1 of 23QVS (perfectionism and intolerance to frustration) and stress, r = 0.599, p < 0.001; Factor 2 of 23QVS (inhibition and functional dependence) and depression, r = 0.656, p < 0.001; Factor 2 of 23 QVS (inhibition and functional dependence) and anxiety, r = 0.579, p < 0.001; Factor 2 of 23 QVS (inhibition and functional dependence) and stress, r = 0.554, p < 0.001; Factor 6 of 23QVS (subjugation) and depression, r = 0.535, p < 0.001; Factor 6 of 23QVS (subjugation) and anxiety, r = 0.547, p < 0.001; Factor 7 of 23QVS (deprivation of affection and rejection) and depression, r = 0.635, p < 0.001; Factor 7 of 23QVS (deprivation of affection and rejection) and anxiety. r = 0.647, p < 0.001; Factor 7 of 23QVS (deprivation of affection and rejection) and stress, r = 0.578, p < 0.001.

2.5. Discussion and Conclusions

In this empirical study, vulnerability to stress correlates positively with depression, anxiety and stress. Also, depression, anxiety and stress correlate negatively with resilience. It has been shown that disturbances of mood and anxiety correlated more consistently with defects in the amygdala, hippocampus, subgenual anterior cingulate cortex and prefrontal cortex [50]. Cognitive reevaluation (reappraisal) is a mechanism by which resilient individuals can reduce or control emotional responses to stressful situations. Recent studies of functional brain imaging, with participants instructed to reappraise the significance of negative images, demonstrate the involvement of medial and lateral prefrontal cortex in the regulation of emotional responses, through top-down control of amygdala activation during cognitive reappraisal [51]. Greater use of cognitive reappraisal in everyday life has also been linked to increased activation of the prefrontal cortex and less activation of the amygdala, in face of negative stimuli [52], suggesting the existence of a possible neuronal mechanism by which cognitive reappraisal increases the resistance to stress. In short, resilience can be related to a greater ability for emotional regulation, while psychopathology may be associated with abnormalities in emotional regulation systems [53].

The lack of social support correlates negatively with serum levels of cortisol. The factor, of vulnerability to stress, lack of social support integrates two dimensions/items (3. When I have problems that bother me I can count on one or more friends to serve me as confidants; 6. When I have a problem to solve I usually have someone for helping me). A large body of epidemiological research suggests that individuals with lack of social support are at greater risk for mental and physical health problems. The low social support is related to higher levels of depression, anxiety and dissatisfaction with life. The existence of social support is also associated with low mortality from all causes, but particularly due to cardiovascular disease. The interface between social support and processes related stress is crucial in understanding these epidemiological associations [57]. Within the context of the dysfunction of the hypothalamic-pituitary-adrenal axis, several mechanisms have been proposed concerning the evolution towards low cortisol states. A model suggests that, under the influence of chronic stress, initial adaptive response of hypercortisolism, over time, becomes a self-protecting state of hypocortisolism, in order to preserve the endocrine-metabolic system and the brain. Other potential mechanisms of states of hypocortisolism centrally induced include the down-regulation of pituitary receptors of corticotrophin releasing factor, in response to elevations of corticotrophin releasing hormone and to negative feedback, induced by hypercortisolism at central nervous system, over sustained release of stimulating hormones. Relative states of hypocortisolism, or resistance to cortisol, may also occur despite the presence of normal, or even elevated, levels of cortisol [33] [34]. Exceptions to rapid and full recovery, and that challenge homeostatic fundamentals, examples of which, facing stress chronicity, are dysregulation of the hypothalamic-pituitary-adrenal axis, hypercortisolemia or hypocortisolemia, metabolic syndrome, anxiety and depression , present in some people within the concept of alostatic load [12] [13].

The lack of social support and adverse living conditions correlate negatively with serum levels of anti-Epstein-virus antibodies. The factor, of vulnerability to stress, adverse living conditions, integrates two dimensions/items (4. Often I have enough money to meet my personal needs; 21. The amount of money I have isn't enough to use it in my essential expenses). Repeated or prolonged stress can determine dysregulation or suppression of immune function. Chronic stress suppresses immune-protective parameters such as the production of antibodies [26].

In this study, 23% of participants present triglyceride (TGL)/high density lipoprotein-cholesterol (HDL) ratio levels higher than normal; 46% of participants present body mass index (BMI) greater than normal, and, in terms of medical comorbidity, 31% of the participants have endocrine-metabolic disorder (mainly, hypercholesterolemia, diabetes) and hypertension; 40% have oncological disease (predominantly, breast cancer, uterine cancer, neoplasia prostate), and auto-immune disease (lupus). Alostatic load determines long-term effects on cardiovascular system (determining atherosclerosis and cardiovascular disease), brain (with decreased neurogenesis and increased dendritic remodeling in the hippocampus, causing loss of the ability to adapt to environmental requirements), adipose tissue and muscle (determining the development of obesity and metabolic syndrome) and immune system (increasing the risk of infection and autoimmune disease) [38].

Chronic stress, associated with increased alostatic load, in persons with psychic anomaly/mental disorder may depress immune function (with decreased production of antibodies) and neuroendocrine function (with decreased formation and release of cortisol). This trend is observed in this study, placing subjects with psychic anomaly/mental disorder at risk for infectious, oncologic, autoimmune and endocrine diseases.

References

[1] Smith, C.A. and Lazarus, R.S. (1993) Appraisal Components, Core Relational Themes and the Emotions. *Cognition and Emotion*, **7**, 233-269. http://dx.doi.org/10.1080/02699939308409189

[2] Smith, C.A. (1991) The Self, Appraisal, and Coping. In: Snyder, C.R. and Forsyth, O.R., Eds., *Handbook of Social and Clinical Psychology: The Health Perspective*, Pergamon Press, New York, 116-137.

[3] Lazarus, R.S. and Folkman, S. (1984) Stress, Appraisal, and Coping. Springer, New York.

[4] Rasmussen, H.N., Wrosch, C., Scheier, M.F. and Carver, C.S. (2006) Self-Regulation Processes and Health: The Importance of Optimism and Goal Adjustment. *Journal of Personality*, **74**, 1721-1747. http://dx.doi.org/10.1111/j.1467-6494.2006.00426.x

[5] Walker, L.S., Smith, C.A., Garber, J. and Van Slyke, D.A. (1997) Development and Validation of the Pain Response Inventory for Children. *Psychological Assessment*, **9**, 392-405. http://dx.doi.org/10.1037/1040-3590.9.4.392

[6] Southwick, S.M., Vythilingam, M. and Charney, D.S. (2005) The Psychobiology of Depression and Resilience to Stress: Implications for Prevention and Treatment. *Annual Review of Clinical Psychology*, **1**, 255-291. http://dx.doi.org/10.1146/annurev.clinpsy.1.102803.143948

[7] Carver, C.S. (1997) You Want to Measure Coping but Your Protocol's Too Long: Consider the Brief COPE. *International Journal of Behavioral Medicine*, **4**, 92-100. http://dx.doi.org/10.1207/s15327558ijbm0401_6

[8] Clark, L.A. and Watson, D. (1991) Tripartite Model of Anxiety and Depression: Psychometric Evidence and Taxonomic Implications. *Journal of Abnormal Psychology*, **100**, 316-336. http://dx.doi.org/10.1037/0021-843X.100.3.316

[9] Lovibond, S.H. and Lovibond, P.F. (1995) Manual for the Depression Anxiety Stress Scales. 2nd Edition, Psychology Foundation of Australia, Sidney.

[10] Reich, J.W., Zautra, A. and Hall, J.S. (2010) Handbook of Adult Resilience. The Guilford Press, New York.

[11] Holling, C.S., Schindler, D.W., Walker, B.W. and Roughgarden, J. (1995) Biodiversity in the Functioning of Ecosystems: An Ecological Synthesis. In: Perrings, C., Maler, L.G., Folke, C., Holling, C.S. and Jansson, B.O., Eds., *Biodiversity and Loss: Economic and Ecological Issues*, Cambridge University Press, Cambridge, 44-83. http://dx.doi.org/10.1017/cbo9781139174329.005

[12] McEwen, B.S. (1998) Stress Adaptation and Disease: Allostasis and Allostatic Load. *Annals of the New York Academy of Sciences*, **840**, 33-44. http://dx.doi.org/10.1111/j.1749-6632.1998.tb09546.x

[13] McEwen, B.S. and Wingfield, J.C. (2003) The Concept of Allostasis in Biology and Biomedicine. *Hormones and Behavior*, **43**, 2-15. http://dx.doi.org/10.1016/S0018-506X(02)00024-7

[14] Luecken, L.J. and Appelhans, B.M. (2006) Early Parental Loss and Cortisol Stress Responses in Young Adulthood: The Moderating Role of Family Environment. *Development and Psychopathology*, **18**, 295-308. http://dx.doi.org/10.1017/S0954579406060160

[15] Luecken, L.J., Appelhans, B.M., Kraft, A. and Brown, A. (2006) Never Far from Home: A Cognitive-Affective Model of the Impact of Early-Life Family Relationships on Physiological Stress Responses in Adulthood. *Journal of Social and Personal Relationships*, **23**, 189-203. http://dx.doi.org/10.1177/0265407506062466

[16] Steptoe, A., Wardle, J. and Marmot, M. (2005) Positive Affect and Health-Related Neuroendocrine, Cardiovascular, and Inflammatory Processes. *Proceedings of the National Academy of Sciences of the United States of America*, **102**, 6508-6512. http://dx.doi.org/10.1073/pnas.0409174102

[17] Bernston, G.C., Caccioppo, J.T. and Gardner, W.L. (1999) The Affect System Has Parallel and Integrative Processing Components: Form Follows Function. *Journal of Personality and Social Psychology*, **76**, 839-855. http://dx.doi.org/10.1037/0022-3514.76.5.839

[18] Canli, T., Zhao, Z., Desmond, J.E., Kang, E., Gross, J. and Gabrieli, J.D. (2001) An fMRI Study of Personality Influences on Brain Reactivity to Emotional Stimuli. *Behavioral Neuroscience*, **115**, 33-42. http://dx.doi.org/10.1037/0735-7044.115.1.33

[19] Reich, J.W. and Zautra, A.J. (1991) Experimental and Measurement Approaches to Internal Control in Older Adults. *Journal of Social Issues*, **47**, 143-188. http://dx.doi.org/10.1111/j.1540-4560.1991.tb01839.x

[20] Berkman, L.F. and Glass, T.A. (2000) Social Integration, Social Networks, Social Support, and Health. In: Berkman, L.F. and Kawachi, I., Eds., *Social Epidemiology*, Oxford University Press, New York, 137-173.

[21] Pearlin, L.I. and Schooler, C. (1978) The Structure of Coping. *Journal of Health and Social Behavior*, **19**, 2-21. http://dx.doi.org/10.2307/2136319

[22] Reich, J.W. and Zautra, A.J. (1990) Dispositional Control Beliefs and the Consequences of a Control-Enhancing Intervention. *Journal of Gerontology*, **45**, 46-51. http://dx.doi.org/10.1093/geronj/45.2.P46

[23] Fredrickson, B.L. (2001) The Role of Positive Emotions in Positive Psychology. The Broaden-and-Build Theory of Positive Emotions. *American Psychologist*, **56**, 218-226. http://dx.doi.org/10.1037/0003-066X.56.3.218

[24] DeVries, A.C., Glasper, E.R. and Detillion, C.E. (2003) Social Modulation of Stress Responses. *Physiology and Behavior*, **79**, 399-407. http://dx.doi.org/10.1016/S0031-9384(03)00152-5

[25] Mihai, A., McDade, T., Williams, S. and Lindau, S. (2008) Blood Spot Measurement of Epstein Barr Virus Antibody Titers in Wave I of the National Social Life, Health & Aging Project (NSHAP). NORC and the University of Chicago. http://biomarkers.bsd.uchicago.edu/pdfs/TR-EBV.pdf

[26] Dhabhar, F.S. (2011) Effects of Stress on Immune Function: Implications for Immunoprotection and Immunopathology. In: Contrada, R.J. and Baum, A., Eds., *The Handbook of Stress Science: Biology, Psychology and Health*, Springer Publishing Company, New York, 55.

[27] Pargament, K.I., Smith, B.W., Koenig, H.G. and Perez, L. (1998) Patterns of Positive and Negative Religious Coping with Major Life Stressors. *Journal for the Scientific Study of Religion*, **37**, 710-724. http://dx.doi.org/10.2307/1388152

[28] Heim, C. and Nemeroff, C.B. (2001) The Role of Childhood Trauma in the Neurobiology of Mood and Anxiety Disorders: Preclinical and Clinical Studies. *Biological Psychiatry*, **49**, 1023-1039. http://dx.doi.org/10.1016/S0006-3223(01)01157-X

[29] Masten, A.S., Best, K.M. and Garmezy, N. (1990) Resilience and Development: Contributions from the Study of Children Who Overcome Adversity. *Development and Psychopathology*, **2**, 425-444. http://dx.doi.org/10.1017/S0954579400005812

[30] De Kloet, E.R., Joëls, M. and Holsboer, F. (2005) Stress and the Brain: From Adaptation to Disease. *Nature Reviews Neuroscience*, **6**, 463-475. http://dx.doi.org/10.1038/nrn1683

[31] Morfin, R. and Starka, L. (2001) Neurosteroid 7-Hydroxylation Products in the Brain. *International Review of Neurobiology*, **46**, 79-95. http://dx.doi.org/10.1016/S0074-7742(01)46059-4

[32] Yehuda, R., Brand, S.R., Golier, J.A. and Yang, R.K. (2006) Clinical Correlates of DHEA Associated with Post-Traumatic Stress Disorder. *Acta Psychiatrica Scandinavica*, **114**, 187-193. http://dx.doi.org/10.1111/j.1600-0447.2006.00801.x

[33] Edwards, L. and Guilliams, T.G. (2010) Chronic Stress and the HPA Axis: Clinical Assessment and Therapeutic Considerations. *The Standard*, **9**, 1-12. http://www.pointinstitute.org/wpcontent/uploads/2012/10/standard_v_9.2_hpa_axis.pdf

[34] Fries, E., Hesse, J., Hellhammer, J. and Hellhammer, D.H. (2005) A New View on Hypocortisolism. *Psychoneuroendocrinology*, **30**, 1010-1016. http://dx.doi.org/10.1016/j.psyneuen.2005.04.006

[35] Reynolds, K. and He, J. (2005) Epidemiology of the Metabolic Syndrome. *The American Journal of the Medical Sciences*, **330**, 273-279. http://dx.doi.org/10.1097/00000441-200512000-00004

[36] Reaven, G.M. (2005) Insulin Resistance, the Insulin Resistance Syndrome, and Cardiovascular Disease. *Panminerva Medica*, **47**, 201-210.

[37] Laws, A., King, A.C., Haskell, W.L. and Reaven, G.M. (1991) Relation of Fasting Plasma Insulin Concentration to High Density Lipoprotein Cholesterol and Triglyceride Concentrations in Men. *Arteriosclerosis, Thrombosis, and Vascular Biology*, **11**, 1636-1642. http://dx.doi.org/10.1161/01.ATV.11.6.1636

[38] Korte, S.M., Koolhaas, J.M., Wingfield, J.C. and McEwen, B.S. (2005) The Darwinian Concept of Stress: Benefits of Allostasis and Costs of Allostatic Load and the Trade-Offs in Health and Disease. *Neuroscience & Biobehavioral Reviews*, **29**, 3-38. http://dx.doi.org/10.1016/j.neubiorev.2004.08.009

[39] Kastorini, C.M., Milionis, H.J., Esposito, K., Giugliano, D., Goudevenos, J.A. and Panagiotakos, D.B. (2011) The Effect of Mediterranean Diet on Metabolic Syndrome and Its Components: A Meta-Analysis of 50 Studies and 534, 906 Individuals. *Journal of the American College of Cardiology*, **57**, 1299-1313. http://dx.doi.org/10.1016/j.jacc.2010.09.073

[40] Charney, D.S. (2003) Neuroanatomical Circuits Modulating Fear and Anxiety Behaviors. *Acta Psychiatrica Scandinavica*, **108**, 38-50. http://dx.doi.org/10.1034/j.1600-0447.108.s417.3.x

[41] Charney, D.S. (2004) Psychobiological Mechanisms of Resilience and Vulnerability: Implications for Successful Adaptation to Extreme Stress. *American Journal of Psychiatry*, **2**, 369-391. http://dx.doi.org/10.1176/foc.2.3.368

[42] McGaugh, J.L. (2004) The Amygdala Modulates the Consolidation of Memories of Emotionally Arousing Experiences. *Annual Review of Neuroscience*, **27**, 1-28. http://dx.doi.org/10.1146/annurev.neuro.27.070203.144157

[43] Lanzenberger, R.R., Mitterhauser, M., Spindelegger, C., Wadsak, W., Klein, N., Mien, L.-K., *et al.* (2007) Reduced Serotonin-1A Receptor Binding in Social Anxiety Disorder. *Biological Psychiatry*, **61**, 1081-1089. http://dx.doi.org/10.1016/j.biopsych.2006.05.022

[44] Cabib, S., Ventura, R. and Puglisi-Allegra, S. (2002) Opposite Imbalances between Mesocortical and Mesoaccumbens Dopamine Responses to Stress by the Same Genotype Depending on Living Conditions. *Behavioural Brain Research*, **129**, 179-185. http://dx.doi.org/10.1016/S0166-4328(01)00339-4

[45] Delgado, M.R., Olsson, A. and Phelps, E.A. (2006) Extending Animal Models of Fear Conditioning to Humans. *Biological Psychology*, **73**, 39-48. http://dx.doi.org/10.1016/j.biopsycho.2006.01.006

[46] Bast, T. (2007) Toward an Integrative Perspective on Hippocampal Function: From the Rapid Encoding of Experience to Adaptive Behavior. *Reviews in the Neurosciences*, **18**, 253-281. http://dx.doi.org/10.1515/REVNEURO.2007.18.3-4.253

[47] Delgado, M.R., Nearing, K.L., LeDoux, J.E. and Phelps, E.A. (2008) Neural Circuitry Underlying the Regulation of Conditioned Fear and Its Relation to Extinction. *Neuron*, **59**, 829-838. http://dx.doi.org/10.1016/j.neuron.2008.06.029

[48] Yehuda, R. and LeDoux, J. (2007) Response Variation Following Trauma: A Translational Neuroscience Approach to Understanding PTSD. *Neuron*, **56**, 19-32. http://dx.doi.org/10.1016/j.neuron.2007.09.006

[49] Phillips, M.L., Drevets, W.C., Rauch, S.L. and Lane, R. (2003) Neurobiology of Emotion Perception I: The Neural Basis of Normal Emotion Perception. *Biological Psychiatry*, **54**, 504-514. http://dx.doi.org/10.1016/S0006-3223(03)00168-9

[50] Ressler, K.J. and Mayberg, H.S. (2007) Targeting Abnormal Neural Circuits in Mood and Anxiety Disorders: From the Laboratory to the Clinic. *Nature Neuroscience*, **10**, 1116-1124. http://dx.doi.org/10.1038/nn1944

[51] Goldin, P.R., McRae, K., Ramel, W. and Gross, J.J. (2008) The Neural Bases of Emotion Regulation: Reappraisal and Suppression of Negative Emotion. *Biological Psychiatry*, **63**, 577-586. http://dx.doi.org/10.1016/j.biopsych.2007.05.031

[52] Drabant, E.M., McRae, K., Manuck, S.B., Hariri, A.R. and Gross, J.J. (2009) Individual Differences in Typical Reappraisal Use Predict Amygdala and Prefrontal Responses. *Biological Psychiatry*, **65**, 367-373. http://dx.doi.org/10.1016/j.biopsych.2008.09.007

[53] Johnstone, T., van Reekum, C.M., Urry, H.L., Kalin, N.H. and Davidson, R.J. (2007) Failure to Regulate: Counterproductive Recruitment of Top-Down Prefrontal-Subcortical Circuitry in Major Depression. *Journal of Neuroscience*, **27**, 8877-8884. http://dx.doi.org/10.1523/JNEUROSCI.2063-07.2007

[54] Forbes, E.E., Hariri, A.R., Martin, S.L., Silk, J.S., Moyles, D.L., Fisher, P.M., *et al.* (2009) Altered Striatal Activation Predicting Real-World Positive Affect in Adolescent Major Depressive Disorder. *American Journal of Psychiatry*, **166**, 64-73. http://dx.doi.org/10.1176/appi.ajp.2008.07081336

[55] Sailer, U., Robinson, S., Fischmeister, F.P.S., König, D., Oppenauer, C., Lueger-Schuster, B., *et al.* (2008) Altered Reward Processing in the Nucleus Accumbens and Mesial Prefrontal Cortex of Patients with Posttraumatic Stress Disorder. *Neuropsychologia*, **46**, 2836-2844. http://dx.doi.org/10.1016/j.neuropsychologia.2008.05.022

[56] Dillon, D.G., Holmes, A.J., Birk, J.L., Brooks, N., Lyons-Ruth, K. and Pizzagalli, D.A. (2009) Childhood Adversity Is Associated with Left Basal Ganglia Dysfunction during Reward Anticipation in Adulthood. *Biological Psychiatry*, **66**, 206-213. http://dx.doi.org/10.1016/j.biopsych.2009.02.019

[57] Uchino, B.N. and Birmingham, W. (2011) Stress and Support Processes. In: Contrada, R.J. and Braum, A., Eds., *The Handbook of Stress Science: Biology, Psychology, and Health*, Springer Publishing Company, New York, 111-121.

[58] Kosfeld, M., Heinrichs, M., Zak, P.J., Fischbacher, U. and Fehr, E. (2005) Oxytocin Increases Trust in Humans. *Nature*, **435**, 673-676. http://dx.doi.org/10.1038/nature03701

[59] Domes, G., Heinrichs, M., Michel, A., Berger, C. and Herpertz, S.C. (2007) Oxytocin Improves "Mind-Reading" in Humans. *Biological Psychiatry*, **61**, 731-733. http://dx.doi.org/10.1016/j.biopsych.2006.07.015

[60] Schulre-Rurher, M., Markowirsch, H.I., Fink, G.R. and Piefke, M. (2007) Mirror Neuron and Theory of Mind Mechanisms Involved in Face-to-Face Interactions: A Functional Magnetic Resonance Imaging Approach to Empathy. *Journal of Cognitive Neuroscience*, **19**, 1354-1372. http://dx.doi.org/10.1162/jocn.2007.19.8.1354

[61] Medicode (2015) International Classification of Diseases. 10th Edition (ICD-10), World Health Organization (WHO), Geneva.

[62] Vaz-Serra, A. (2000) Construção de uma escla para avaliar a vulnerabilidade ao stress: A 23QVS. *Psiquiatria Clínica*,

21, 278-308.

[63] Pais-Ribeiro, J., Honrado, A. and Leal, I. (2004) Contribuição para o estudo da Adaptação Portuguesa das Escalas de Ansiedade, Depressão e Stress (EADS) de 21 itens de Lovibond e Lovibond. *Psicologia, Saúde & Doenças*, **5**, 229-239. http://hdl.handle.net/10400.12/1058

[64] Hiew, C.C. (1999) Development of a State Resilience Scale. *Annual Meeting of the International Council of Psychologists*, Salem, 15-19 August 1999.

[65] Martins, M.H.V. (2005) Contribuições para a análise de crianças e jovens em situação de risco—Resiliência e desenvolvimento. Tese de doutoramento, Faculdade de Ciências Humanas e Sociais, Universidade do Algarve, Faro.

Permissions

List of Contributors

Benedict Francis and Subash Kumar Pillai
Department of Psychiatry, University Malaya Medical Center, Kuala Lumpur, Malaysia
The Mind Faculty, Solaris Mont Kiara, Kuala Lumpur, Malaysia

Stephen Thevananthan Jambunathan
Department of Psychiatry, University Malaya Medical Center, Kuala Lumpur, Malaysia
The Mind Faculty, Solaris Mont Kiara, Kuala Lumpur, Malaysia

Bengt Svensson, Ulrika Bejerholm, Mona Eklund, Amanda Lundvik Gyllensten, Christel Leufstadius and Lars Hansson
Department of Health Sciences, Lund University, Lund, Sweden

David Brunt
School of Health Sciences and Social Work, Linnean University, Växjö, Sweden

Urban Markström
Department of Social Work, Umeå University, Umeå, Sweden

Mikael Sandlund
Department of Clinical Sciences/Psychiatry, Umeå University, Umeå, Sweden

Margareta Östman
Faculty of Health and Society, Malmö University, Malmö, Sweden

Yasuko Takanashi, Shuntaro Itagaki, Hiromichi Ishikawa and Shin-Ichi Niwa
Fukushima General Health and Welfare Center, Fukushima, Japan

Hirobumi Mashiko
Department of Neuropsychiatry, Fukushima Medical University School of Medicine, Fukushima, Japan
Fukushima General Health and Welfare Center, Fukushima, Japan

Hirohide Yokokawa
Department of Public Health, Fukushima Medical University School of Medicine, Fukushima, Japan
Department of General Medicine, Juntendo University School of Medicine, Tokyo, Japan

Yoko Kawasaki
Musasino Child Development Clinic, Tokyo, Japan

Norihiro Miyashita
Department of Neuropsychiatry, Fukushima Medical University School of Medicine, Fukushima, Japan
Hanawakousei Hospital, Fukushima, Japan

Yasuaki Hayashi
Landic Nihonbashi Clinic, Tokyo, Japan

Asako Kudo
Hoshigaoka Hospital, Fukushima, Japan

Kentaro Oga
Surugadai Nihon University Hospital, Tokyo, Japan

Rieko Matsuura
Shiba Clinic, Tokyo, Japan

Kay M. Jones and Leon Piterman
Office of the Pro Vice-Chancellor, Peninsula Campus, Monash University, Frankston, Australia

Rajeevan Rasasingham
University of Toronto, Toronto, Canada
Harvard University, Cambridge, MA, USA

Setsuko Taneichi, Fumiharu Togo and Tsukasa Sasaki
Laboratory of Health Education, Graduate School of Education, Tokyo, Japan

Ahmed Mohamed Abdel Shafi
Barts and The London School of Medicine and Dentistry, London, UK

Reem Mohamed Abdel Shafi
Fremantle Hospital, Fremantle, Australia

Takashi Ikeno and Hiroto Ito
Department of Social Psychiatry, National Institute of Mental Health, National Center of Neurology and Psychiatry, Tokyo, Japan
Faculty of Medicine, Graduate School of Medical Science, University of Yamanashi, Yamanashi, Japan

Kiyotaka Kugiyama
Faculty of Medicine, Graduate School of Medical Science, University of Yamanashi, Yamanashi, Japan

Yngvar Reichelt
Department of Mathematics, University of Oslo, Oslo, Norway

Karl L. Reichelt
Lab 1, No 1337, Sandvika, Norway and Kleve 4541 m, University of Oslo, Oslo, Norway

Emel Serap Monkul, Mark Bangs, Mary Anne Dellva, Jonna Ahl and Celine Goldberger
Eli Lilly and Company, Indianapolis, IN, USA

Keita Asato, Masashi Takahashi and Yasushi Takita
Eli Lilly Japan K.K. Office, Kobe, Japan

Henning Værøy
Department for Research and Development, Division of Mental Health Services, Akershus University Hospital, Lørenskog, Norway

Lee S. Berk
Allied Health Studies, School of Allied Health Professions, Loma Linda University, Loma Linda, USA
Department of Pathology and Human Anatomy, School of Medicine, Loma Linda University, Loma Linda, USA
Center for Spirituality, Theology and Health, Duke University, Durham, USA

Harold G. Koenig
Center for Spirituality, Theology and Health, Duke University, Durham, USA
Department of Psychiatry and Behavioral Sciences, Duke University Medical Center, Durham, USA
Department of Medicine, Duke University Medical Center, Durham, USA
Department of Medicine, King Abdulaziz University, Jeddah, Saudi Arabia

Noha Daher
Allied Health Studies, School of Allied Health Professions, Loma Linda University, Loma Linda, USA
Epidemiology, Biostatistics, and Population Medicine, School of Public Health, Loma Linda University, Loma Linda, USA

Michelle J. Pearce
Center for Spirituality, Theology and Health, Duke University, Durham, USA
Department of Psychiatry and Behavioral Sciences, Duke University Medical Center, Durham, USA
School of Medicine, University of Maryland, Baltimore, USA

Clive J. Robins
Department of Psychiatry and Behavioral Sciences, Duke University Medical Center, Durham, USA
Department of Psychology and Neuroscience, Duke University Medical Center, Durham, USA

Bruce Nelson and Sally F. Shaw
Department of Research, Glendale Adventist Medical Center, Glendale, USA

Michael B. King
Division of Psychiatry, Faculty of Brain Sciences, University College, London, UK

Harvey Jay Cohen
Center for Spirituality, Theology and Health, Duke University, Durham, USA
Department of Medicine, Duke University Medical Center, Durham, USA

Denise L. Bellinger
Department of Pathology and Human Anatomy, School of Medicine, Loma Linda University, Loma Linda, USA

Masayo Uji
Department of Bioethics, Kumamoto University Graduate School of Medical Sciences, Kumamoto, Japan

Hossein Jenaabadi
Faculty of Educational Sciences and Psychology, University of Sistan and Baluchestan, Zahedan, Iran

Bahareh Azizi Nejad
Department of Educational Science, Payame Noor University, Tehran, Iran

Ghazal Fatehrad
Department of Management and Economic, Science and Research Branch, Islamic Azad University, Tehran, Iran

Yueren Zhao and Nakao Iwata
Fujita Health University, Toyoake, Japan

Yuko Yasuhara, Tetsuya Tanioka, Sakiko Sakamaki, Masahito Tomotake and Rozzano C. Locsin
Tokushima University, Tokushima, Japan

Beth King
Florida Atlantic University, Boca Raton, USA

Milton Kramer
Psychiatry Department, College of Medicine, University of Cincinnati, Cincinnati, Ohio, USA

Kay M. Jones and Leon Piterman
Office of the Pro Vice-Chancellor, Peninsula Campus, Monash University, Frankston, Australia

Wilfried Dimpfel
Justus-Liebig-University c/o NeuroCode AG, Wetzlar, Germany

Winfried Wedekind
NeuroCode AG, Wetzlar, Germany

Angelika Dienel
Dr. Willmar Schwabe GmbH & Co. KG, Karlsruhe, Germany

Michihiro Takahashi
Takahashi Psychiatric Clinic, Ashiya, Japan
Medical Science, Lilly Research Laboratories Japan, Eli Lilly Japan K.K., Kobe, Japan

Shinji Fujikoshi
Statistical Science, Lilly Research Laboratories Japan, Eli Lilly Japan K.K., Kobe, Japan

Jumpei Funai
Science Communications, Lilly Research Laboratories Japan, Eli Lilly Japan K.K., Kobe, Japan

Levent Alev
Medical Science, Lilly Research Laboratories Japan, Eli Lilly Japan K.K., Kobe, Japan

Masaomi Iyo
Department of Psychiatry, Graduate School of Medicine, Chiba University, Chiba, Japan

Arsia Taghva, Mohammad Reza Hatami and Vahid Donyavi
Department of Psychiatry, AJA University of Medical Sciences, Tehran, Iran

Masoud Azizi
Department of English Language, Amirkabir University, Tehran, Iran

Abdelgadir H. Osman
Department of Psychiatry, Faculty of Medicine University of Khartoum, Khartoum, Sudan

Taissier Y. Hagar and Abdelaziz A. Osman
Formerly Registrar in Sudan Medical Council, Currently Specialists in Saudi Arabia

Hussein Suliaman
Khartoum Neuropsychiatric Centre, Khartoum, Sudan

Senyo Gudugbe and Jonathan Lamptey
Department of Surgery, Korle Bu Teaching Hospital, Accra, Ghana

Mathew Y. Kyei and Isaac Asiedu
Urology Unit, Department of Surgery, School of Medicine and Dentistry, College of Health Sciences, University of Ghana, Accra, Ghana

Kenneth Baidoo
Otolaryngology Unit, Department of Surgery, School of Medicine and Dentistry, College of Health Sciences, University of Ghana, Accra, Ghana

Anatoly Boleslavovich Smulevich, Natalia Alekseevna Ilyina and Victoria Valentinovna Chitlova
National Centre of Mental Health of the Russian Academy of Medical Sciences, Moscow, Russia

W. John Martin
Institute of Progressive Medicine, South Pasadena, CA, USA

Eduardo Gonçalves
Department of Psychiatry and Mental Health of Hospital Center of Algarve, Faro, Portugal

Saul Neves de Jesus
Department of Psychology of Faculty of Social and Human Sciences of University of Algarve, Faro, Portugal

Leslie Lim, Justine Goh and Shi-Hui Poon
Department of Psychiatry, Singapore General Hospital, Republic of Singapore

Yiong-Huak Chan
National University Health System, National University of Singapore, Republic of Singapore

Amit Chauhan
Department of Orthopedics, Park Hospital, Gurgaon, Haryana, India

Shravani Chauhan
Department of Psychiatry, VIMHANS, New Delhi, India

Eduardo Gonçalves and Emanuel Marco Moniz
Department of Psychiatry and Mental Health of Hospital Center of Algarve, Faro, Portugal

Saul Neves de Jesus
Department of Psychology of Faculty of Social and Human Sciences of University of Algarve, Faro, Portugal

Eduardo Goncalves
Department of Psychiatry and Mental Health of Hospital Center of Algarve, Faro, Portugal

Saul Neves de Jesus
Department of Psychology of Faculty of Social and Human Sciences of University of Algarve, Faro, Portugal